Diagnosis and classification are considered essential but [difficult by] mental health practitioners and trainees. Here is a book that will dispel this notion and bring alive the excitement and nuances of diagnosis of mental health conditions. Led by world-renowned editors and a global cast of authors, this publication is a must-read for all in the caring profession.

—Shekhar Saxena, MD, Professor of the Practice of Global Mental Health, Harvard T. H. Chan School of Public Health, Boston, MA, United States

This book is a gift of invaluable knowledge to the global community of mental health professionals, crafted by scientists from the international elite. The clinician is equipped with in-depth explanations of psychopathology pivotal for *ICD-11* diagnostics and treatment planning. A key companion to WHO's *Clinical Descriptions and Diagnostic Requirements (CDDR)* covering changes of diagnostic definitions from *ICD-10* to *ICD-11*, epidemiology, maintaining factors for psychopathology, and prospects for new diagnoses. Momentous and handy!

—Klaus Pedersen, MSc, Specialist Psychologist in General Psychiatry, Psychopathology & Psychotherapy, Aarhus University Hospital Psychiatry, Aarhus, Denmark

This volume is a comprehensive compendium for classification and diagnosis of behavioral and mental disorders. The editors have assembled an outstanding cadre of chapter authors from around the world who are recognized for their expertise and scientific contributions to the field of behavioral and mental disorders. The insightful chapters detail the update of the *ICD* supported by an exceptionally strong evidence base developed through innovative methodology and confirmatory field studies. This important contribution fulfills the need for a psychological understanding based on robust empirical and clinical information for the global professional community serving mental health needs.

—Michael C. Roberts, PhD, ABPP, Professor Emeritus, Clinical Child Psychology Program, University of Kansas, Lawrence, KS, United States

A timely new perspective from leaders in the field. This book masterfully bridges the gap between diagnosis and treatment to support a more holistic, psychologically informed approach. Essential applied reading!

—Corinna Hackmann, PhD, DClinPsy, Norfolk and Suffolk Foundation Trust, University of East Anglia, Norwich, England

A Psychological Approach to Diagnosis

A Psychological Approach to Diagnosis

Using the ICD-11 as a Framework

Editors

Geoffrey M. Reed
Pierre L.-J. Ritchie
Andreas Maercker

Associate Editor

Tahilia J. Rebello

Foreword by Michael B. First

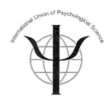

 AMERICAN PSYCHOLOGICAL ASSOCIATION

Published by
American Psychological Association
750 First Street, NE
Washington, DC 20002
https://www.apa.org

International Union of Psychological Science
PH-G 6300 Place Northcrest
Montreal (Quebec), H3S 2W3
Canada

Order Department
https://www.apa.org/pubs/books
order@apa.org

Typeset in Meridien and Ortodoxa by Circle Graphics, Inc., Reisterstown, MD

Printer: Sheridan Books, Chelsea, MI
Cover Designer: Beth Schlenoff Design, Bethesda, MD

Library of Congress Cataloging-in-Publication Data

Names: Reed, Geoffrey M., editor.
Title: A psychological approach to diagnosis : using the ICD-11 as a
  framework / edited by Geoffrey M. Reed, Pierre L.-J. Ritchie, and
  Andreas Maercker; associate editor: Tahilia J. Rebello.
Description: Washington, DC : American Psychological Association, [2024] |
  Includes bibliographical references and index.
Identifiers: LCCN 2023034721 (print) | LCCN 2023034722 (ebook) |
  ISBN 9781433832680 (paperback) | ISBN 9781433837241 (ebook)
Subjects: LCSH: Mental illness--Diagnosis. | Diagnosis--Psychological
  aspects. | BISAC: PSYCHOLOGY / Clinical Psychology | PSYCHOLOGY /
  Psychotherapy / General
Classification: LCC RC469 .P7668 2024 (print) | LCC RC469 (ebook) |
  DDC 616.89/075--dc23/eng/20231013
LC record available at https://lccn.loc.gov/2023034721
LC ebook record available at https://lccn.loc.gov/2023034722

https://doi.org/10.1037/0000392-000

Printed in the United States of America

10 9 8 7 6 5 4 3 2 1

The editors and authors of this volume represent only a small portion of the hundreds of experts and thousands of clinicians around the world on whose contributions this book is based and to whom it is dedicated. In particular, we acknowledge Suzanne Bennett Johnson, Shekhar Saxena, and Ann D. Watts, without whose strategic vision; political acumen; and sustained commitment, collaboration, and support this book and the work behind it would not have been possible.

CONTENTS

CONTRIBUTORS

Iván Arango-de Montis, MD, Instituto Nacional de Psiquiatría Ramón de la Fuente Muñiz, Mexico City, Mexico

Elham Atallah, MD, Ibn Al-Nafaees Hospital, Manama, Kingdom of Bahrain

José Luis Ayuso-Mateos, PhD, MD, Universidad Autónoma de Madrid, CIBERSAM, Madrid, Spain

Gillian Baird, MD, Guy's and St Thomas' NHS Foundation Trust and King's Health Partners, London, England

Joël Billieux, PhD, University of Lausanne and Centre for Excessive Gambling, Lausanne University Hospitals, Lausanne, Switzerland

Chris R. Brewin, PhD, University College London, London, England

Rachel Bryant-Waugh, PhD, South London and Maudsley NHS Foundation Trust, London, England

Gualberto Buela-Casal, PhD, Universidad de Granada, Granada, Spain

Almudena Carneiro-Barrera, PhD, Universidad Loyola Andalucía, Seville, Spain

Amy Y. M. Chow, PhD, The University of Hong Kong, Hong Kong SAR, PR China

Lee Anna Clark, PhD, University of Notre Dame, Notre Dame, IN, United States

Marylène Cloitre, PhD, National Center for PTSD Dissemination and Training Division and Stanford University, Palo Alto, CA, United States

Jason P. Connor, PhD, The University of Queensland, Brisbane, Australia

Francisco R. de la Peña, MD, Instituto Nacional de Psiquiatría Ramón de la Fuente Muñiz, Mexico City, Mexico

Paul M. G. Emmelkamp, PhD, University of Amsterdam, Amsterdam, The Netherlands

Spencer C. Evans, PhD, University of Miami, Coral Gables, FL, United States

Alireza Farnam, MD, Tabriz University of Medical Sciences, Tabriz, Iran

Naomi A. Fineberg, MBBS, University of Hertfordshire, Hatfield, Hertfordshire, England; Hertfordshire Partnership University NHS Trust, Welwyn Garden City, England

Michael B. First, MD, Columbia University Vagelos College of Physicians and Surgeons, New York, NY, United States

Paul French, PhD, Pennine Care NHS Foundation Trust, Manchester Metropolitan University, Manchester, England

Ana Fresán, PhD, Instituto Nacional de Psiquiatría Ramón de la Fuente Muñiz, Mexico City, Mexico

Claudia García-Moreno, MD, MSc, World Health Organization, Geneva, Switzerland

Janna Glozman, PhD, Moscow State University, Moscow, Russian Federation

Kirstin Greaves-Lord, PhD, University of Groningen and Lentis Psychiatric Institute, Groningen, The Netherlands

Oye Gureje, MD, DSc, University of Ibadan, Ibadan, Nigeria

Richard E. Heyman, PhD, New York University, New York, NY, United States

Steven H. Jones, PhD, Lancaster University, Lancaster, England

Brigitte Khoury, PhD, American University of Beirut Medical Center, Beirut, Lebanon

Daniel L. King, PhD, Flinders University, Adelaide, Australia

Cary S. Kogan, PhD, University of Ottawa, Ottawa, Ontario, Canada

Theophilus Lazarus, PhD, Neuropsychology Practice, Durban, South Africa and Emory University, Atlanta, GA, United States

Tatia M. C. Lee, PhD, The University of Hong Kong, Hong Kong SAR, PR China

Roberto Lewis-Fernández, MD, Columbia University Vagelos College of Physicians and Surgeons, New York, NY, United States

Tania Lincoln, PhD, Universität Hamburg, Hamburg, Germany

John E. Lochman, PhD, University of Alabama, Tuscaloosa, AL, United States

Christine Lochner, PhD, Stellenbosch University, Cape Town, South Africa

Andreas Maercker, PhD, MD, University of Zurich, Zurich, Switzerland

Walter Matthys, MD, PhD, Utrecht University, Utrecht, The Netherlands

Thomas D. Meyer, PhD, University of Texas Health Science Center, Houston, TX, United States

Katie Moraes de Almondes, PhD, Federal University of Rio Grande do Norte, Natal, Rio Grande do Norte, Brazil

Alexander Moreira-Almeida, MD, PhD, Universidade Federal de Juiz de Fora, Juiz de Fora, Minas Gerais, Brazil

Andrew Moskowitz, PhD, George Washington University, Washington, DC, United States

Ellert Nijenhuis, PhD, Psychiatrische Klinik, Littenheid, Switzerland

Akin Ojagbemi, MD, PhD, University of Ibadan, Ibadan, Nigeria

Sharon J. Parish, MD, Weill Cornell Medical College, New York, NY, United States

Miguel Pérez-García, PhD, Universidad de Granada, Granada, Spain

Tania Perich, PhD, Western Sydney University, Sydney, Australia

Kathleen M. Pike, PhD, Columbia University Vagelos College of Physicians and Surgeons, New York, NY, United States

Antonio E. Puente, PhD, University of North Carolina Wilmington, Wilmington, NC, United States

Tahilia J. Rebello, PhD, Columbia University Vagelos College of Physicians and Surgeons, New York, NY, United States

Geoffrey M. Reed, PhD, Columbia University Vagelos College of Physicians and Surgeons, New York, NY, United States

Pierre L.-J. Ritchie, PhD, University of Ottawa, Ottawa, Ontario, Canada (emeritus) and International Union of Psychological Science (past secretary general)

Rebeca Robles, PhD, Instituto Nacional de Psiquiatría Ramón de la Fuente Muñiz, Mexico City, Mexico

Graccielle Rodrigues da Cunha, MD, Universidade Federale de São Paulo, São Paulo, Brazil

Ashok Roy, MBBS, Coventry and Warwickshire Partnership NHS Trust, Birmingham, England

Hans-Jürgen Rumpf, PhD, University of Lübeck, Lübeck, Germany

John B. Saunders, MD, The University of Queensland, Brisbane, Australia

David Skuse, MD, University College London, London, England

Amy M. Smith Slep, PhD, New York University, New York, NY, United States

Dan J. Stein, MD, PhD, University of Cape Town, Cape Town, South Africa

Paulomi M. Sudhir, PhD, National Institute of Mental Health and Neurosciences, Bengaluru, Karnataka, India

Michaela A. Swales, PhD, Bangor University, Bangor, Wales

Robyn Sysko, PhD, Icahn School of Medicine at Mount Sinai, New York, NY, United States

Chee-Wing Wong, PsychD, The University of Hong Kong, Hong Kong SAR, PR China

FOREWORD

It is widely acknowledged that the publication of third edition of the *Diagnostic and Statistical Manual of Mental Disorders* (*DSM-III*) by the American Psychiatric Association (1980) marked a paradigm shift in the classification of mental disorders. A principal element of this shift was the adoption of a descriptive approach to diagnostic criteria, in which disorders were defined strictly in terms of their symptomatic presentations. Diagnostic criteria focused on what could be visibly observed or reported by the patient and studiously avoided incorporating theories about causality into the definitions. (It has been pointed out that this approach is not truly "atheoretical" given that the approach itself constitutes a theory.) Around the same time, there was also a move toward objective descriptive definitions of mental disorders related to the World Health Organization's *International Classification of Diseases* (*ICD*), but these were much more fully realized in the *DSM-III*.

Despite important differences between the *ICD* and the *DSM* (First et al., 2021), this descriptive approach continues to characterize the latest version of the diagnostic manuals for both systems: the *Clinical Descriptions and Diagnostic Requirements for ICD-11 Mental, Behavioural and Neurodevelopmental Disorders* (*CDDR*; World Health Organization, 2024) and the text revision of the fifth edition of the *DSM* (*DSM-5-TR*; American Psychiatric Association, 2022). In the *ICD-11 CDDR*, for each disorder the section on essential (required) features defines the disorder descriptively in terms of how it presents symptomatically. Moreover, across all of the additional sections that provide information about each disorder in the *CDDR*—additional clinical features, boundary with normality (threshold), course features, developmental features, culture-related features, sex and/or gender-related features, and boundaries with other disorders and conditions—a conscious effort has been made to confine the diagnostic material to information relevant to the process of making the diagnosis and not to include information about either hypothesized etiological factors or about treatment selection.

However, although making an accurate diagnosis is a necessary and essential component in the management of mental disorders, it is only the first step. What is generally of greatest importance to clinicians is the selection and implementation of the treatment most likely to reduce the patient's suffering and consequently to improve their psychosocial functioning and quality of life. Similarly, the essential diagnostic features are not in themselves an adequate basis for case conceptualization. In fact, the World Health Organization International Advisory Group for *ICD-11* mental, behavioral, and neurodevelopmental disorders

> took the position that diagnostic classification is only *a part* of patient assessment and that the classification system should not attempt to function as a guide to patient care or a comprehensive textbook of psychiatry. The focus of the *ICD* is on the classification of *disorders* and not the assessment and treatment of *people*. . . . Additional information beyond the diagnostic categories and descriptions is clearly needed to improve the quality of care and the impact of services for mental and behavioural disorders. (International Advisory Group for the Revision of *ICD-10* Mental and Behavioural Disorders, 2011, p. 91, italics in original)

This book helps bridge the gap between diagnosis and treatment by focusing on the psychological mechanisms associated with the *ICD-11* mental and behavioral disorders. As noted in Chapter 1, "a psychological approach to diagnosis is one that focuses on psychological mechanisms and principles as an aspect of diagnostic practice and case formulation, regardless of professional discipline. It considers the psychological factors—including cognitions, emotions, and behaviors—involved in the development and maintenance of each major grouping of mental disorders and their linkage with treatment considerations." For example, the essential features in *ICD-11 CDDR* for obsessive-compulsive and related disorders (OCRD) focus on their symptomatic presentations (i.e., presence of persistent obsessions and/or compulsions in obsessive-compulsive disorder; persistent preoccupation with one or more perceived defects or flaws in appearance in body dysmorphic disorder; persistent preoccupation about emitting a foul or offensive odor in olfactory reference disorder; persistent preoccupation or fear about the possibility of having one or more serious, progressive or life-threatening illnesses in hypochondriasis; and accumulation of possessions that results in living spaces becoming cluttered to the point that their use or safety is compromised in hoarding disorder).

In contrast, in Chapter 9 of this book, a section titled "A Psychological Approach to OCRDs," goes beyond superficial symptomatic manifestations and focuses on the underlying psychological mechanisms. The chapter notes that cognitive behavioral models emphasize the role of faulty appraisals and dysfunctional beliefs in the development and maintenance of OCRD. In particular, misappraisals of the significance of intrusive thoughts—as informative, important, dangerous, or predictive of harm—lead to increased anxiety and distress and to the performance of behaviors aimed at reducing these emotions or the perceived likelihood of catastrophic consequences occurring and thus preserving the symptoms through negative reinforcement. Similarly, Chapter 16, "Disorders Due to Addictive Behaviors and Impulse Control Disorders," describes the urgency-premeditation-perseverance-sensation seeking (UPPS) impulsivity model as a particularly useful framework for understanding these disorders.

The chapters of this book are intended to provide clinicians with tools that go beyond phenomenology and help to conceptualize the underlying psychological mechanisms for different groups of disorders. This information is directly relevant to the provision of effective psychological treatment. The editors of the book emphasize in Chapter 1 that the articulation of psychological mechanisms is not intended to suggest that these represent the necessary and sufficient causes of the disorders described. At the same time, they are based on scientific evidence about how disorders and specific symptoms develop, how they relate to one another, and how they are maintained over time. They make an important contribution to case conceptualization and signal important avenues for psychological intervention. This will be of use to both students and clinicians, given that many of the clinical interventions known to be effective for mental disorders are based on psychological treatment methods, alone or in combination with pharmacological treatment.

The highest priority in the construction of the *CDDR* was to maximize clinical utility. As such, the *CDDR* avoids arbitrary cutoffs and overly precise requirements related to symptom counts and duration unless these have been empirically established or there is another compelling reason to include them. This approach is intended to conform to the way clinicians actually make diagnoses, with the flexible exercise of clinical judgment, and to increase clinical utility by allowing for individual and cultural variations in presentation. This places a greater emphasis on understanding the nature of the clinical expression of the essential features, as opposed to imposing precise rules, and is also compatible with a deeper understanding of the mechanisms underlying the presenting symptoms.

This book is an invaluable supplement to the *ICD-11 CDDR* that can be highly recommended to both clinicians and trainees involved in the treatment of individuals with mental disorders, regardless of discipline. Its focus on taking a psychological approach to *ICD-11* diagnosis will help the clinician in selecting the psychological treatments most likely to be effective for a particular patient as well as enhance the likelihood of developing a successful therapeutic alliance.

—Michael B. First
Department of Psychiatry, Columbia University
Vagelos College of Physicians and Surgeons

REFERENCES

American Psychiatric Association. (1980). *Diagnostic and statistical manual of mental disorders* (3rd ed.).

American Psychiatric Association. (2022). *Diagnostic and statistical manual of mental disorders* (5th ed., text rev.).

First, M. B., Gaebel, W., Maj, M., Stein, D. J., Kogan, C. S., Saunders, J. B., Poznyak, V. B., Gureje, O., Lewis-Fernández, R., Maercker, A., Brewin, C. R., Cloitre, M., Claudino, A., Pike, K. M., Baird, G., Skuse, D., Krueger, R. B., Briken, P., Burke, J. D., . . . Reed, G. M. (2021). An organization and category-level comparison of diagnostic requirements for mental disorders in *ICD-11* and *DSM-5*. *World Psychiatry, 20*(1), 34–51. https://doi.org/10.1002/wps.20825

International Advisory Group for the Revision of *ICD-10* Mental and Behavioural Disorders. (2011). A conceptual framework for the revision of the *ICD-10* classification of mental and behavioural disorders. *World Psychiatry, 10*(2), 86–92. https://doi.org/10.1002/j.2051-5545.2011.tb00022.x

World Health Organization. (2024). *Clinical descriptions and diagnostic requirements for ICD-11 mental, behavioural and neurodevelopmental disorders.* https://www.who.int/publications/i/item/9789240077263

A Psychological Approach to Diagnosis

1

A Psychological Approach to Diagnosis

Andreas Maercker, Tahilia J. Rebello, Pierre L.-J. Ritchie, and Geoffrey M. Reed

This book is intended as an essential resource for mental health practitioners and educators around the world who will implement the World Health Organization's (WHO's) *Clinical Descriptions and Diagnostic Requirements for ICD-11 Mental, Behavioural and Neurodevelopmental Disorders* (*CDDR*; WHO, 2024) in their clinical practice, teaching, and training. This book is not intended to replace the *CDDR* and does not duplicate their text. Rather, it is intended as an important tool to be used together with the *CDDR* to facilitate understanding as well as accurate and skillful implementation of the *International Classification of Diseases–11th Revision (ICD-11)* classification of mental, behavioral and neurodevelopmental disorders in health care and other clinical settings.

A Psychological Approach to Diagnosis: Using the ICD-11 as a Framework offers a structured approach to implementing the *CDDR* in clinical practice that is vital not only for practitioners and trainees in psychology but also for mental health professionals in psychiatry, nursing, social work, and other disciplines who aim to deliver high-quality, empirically informed mental health care. A psychological approach to diagnosis is one that focuses on psychological mechanisms and principles as an aspect of diagnostic practice and case formulation, regardless of professional discipline. It considers the psychological factors—including cognitions, emotions, and behaviors—involved in the development and maintenance of each major grouping of mental disorders and their linkage with treatment considerations.

https://doi.org/10.1037/0000392-001
A Psychological Approach to Diagnosis: Using the ICD-11 as a Framework, G. M. Reed, P. L.-J. Ritchie, and A. Maercker (Editors)

The etiologies of mental, behavioral, and neurodevelopmental disorders are complex and, in most cases, not clearly understood. There are some exceptions, such as specific genetic syndromes that are linked to certain neurodevelopmental disorders (see Chapter 3). The classification of neurocognitive disorders includes specific forms of dementia that are attributable to identified underlying disease processes (Chapter 18), and the use of psychoactive substances has been shown to cause a variety of substance-induced mental disorders (Chapter 15). Even in these cases, where the etiology is considered established, there is a broad spectrum of symptom expression and co-occurring disorders that vary unpredictably across individuals.

For the majority of disorders, there is not a one-to-one relationship between a particular etiology and a particular syndrome. A variety of genetic, epigenetic, familial, neurochemical and neurophysiological, emotional, psychological, social, and environmental factors have been identified as risk and protective factors in the development, symptomatic expression, and course of mental, behavioral, and neurodevelopmental disorders. Even in posttraumatic stress disorder (PTSD), which is generally believed to have a clear etiology because it develops in response to an event or situation of an extremely threatening or horrific nature, other factors are clearly relevant. Many people who experience these events do not develop a mental disorder, whereas others do not develop PTSD but rather other disorders such as anxiety disorders, depressive disorders, or disorders due to substance use (see Chapter 10).

One reason it is important to emphasize the issues related to etiology is that neither the editors nor any of the authors of this book intend to communicate that the psychological mechanisms described for a particular disorder or set of disorders represent the necessary and sufficient cause of the disorder. Rather, evidence described in the chapters suggests that these psychological mechanisms can be relevant to how disorders and specific symptoms develop, how they relate to one another, and how they are maintained over time. They represent an important basis for case conceptualization and signal important avenues for psychological intervention. Although a detailed discussion of disorder-specific psychological interventions is beyond the scope of this book, a large body of evidence indicates that the most effective interventions for a wide range of disorders are psychological ones (Nathan & Gorman, 2015). For other disorders, psychological interventions are often combined with pharmacological interventions, and such combination treatment has generally been found to be more effective than either alone (Leichsenring et al., 2022).

This book is written to be useful to practitioners, residents, interns, teachers, and students in psychology and to be responsive to the unique context of psychological practice. Moreover, an understanding of psychological mechanisms and principles as they relate to the diagnosis of mental disorders also has a place in the unique body of knowledge and training of a range of mental health disciplines and health disciplines. Accordingly, although many of the chapter authors are renowned psychologists from across the world, experts from psychiatry and other disciplines are also important contributors to this book.

STRUCTURE AND CONTENT OF THIS BOOK

This first chapter provides the conceptual framework for the psychological approach to diagnosis, which serves as a unifying perspective across the book. The second chapter focuses on *ICD-11*'s global approach, embodied in its development and testing, its characteristics, and its implementation. The largest block of chapters, comprising Chapter 3, on disorders of intellectual development and developmental learning disorder, through Chapter 18, on neurocognitive disorders, cover the major groupings of *ICD-11* mental, behavioral, and neurodevelopmental disorders. Each of these chapters further elaborates the ways in which an awareness of psychological mechanisms and principles contributes to diagnosis and case conceptualization in each respective disorder area.

In most cases, the content of these chapters corresponds to the major disorder groupings in the *ICD-11*, such as schizophrenia and other primary psychotic disorders (Chapter 5), anxiety and fear-related disorders (Chapter 8), and personality disorders and related traits (Chapter 17). The order of the chapters in this book correspond to the order of the groupings in the *ICD-11*. This order is intended to approximate a developmental perspective on psychopathology based on the stages of life in which their onset is most typical, although the *ICD-11* does not adhere perfectly to this principle. An exception to the correspondence between chapters of this book and the groupings of the *ICD-11* is neurodevelopmental disorders, which is the longest section in the *CDDR*. Specific components of neurodevelopmental disorders are highly important to psychological practice, so these have been divided across Chapter 3, which covers disorders of intellectual development and developmental learning disorder; Chapter 4 on autism spectrum disorder; and Chapter 14, which covers attention deficit hyperactivity disorder (ADHD; a neurodevelopmental disorder) alongside the *ICD-11* grouping of disruptive behavior and dissocial disorder due to their overlapping presentations and high rate of co-occurrence. Similarly, the *ICD-11* overarching grouping of mood disorders is covered by Chapter 6, on depressive disorders, and Chapter 7, on bipolar and related disorders. This book's treatment of the *ICD-11* grouping of disorders due to substance use and addictive behaviors, which contains more categories than any other grouping of mental disorders, is also divided across Chapter 15, on disorders due to substance use, and Chapter 16, on disorders due to addictive behaviors. Although disorders due to substance use and those due to addictive behaviors have overlapping symptoms, psychological mechanisms, and assessment strategies, there are also important differences. Chapter 16 also includes a discussion of compulsive sexual behavior disorder, which shares the characteristic of behavioral dysregulation but is not classified as an addiction but rather as an impulse control disorder.

Three additional chapters cover areas that, although not classified as mental disorders, are directly relevant to the psychological practice and with which it is important that psychologists and other mental health professionals be conversant. The first of these is sexual dysfunctions and sexual pain disorders (Chapter 19) and the second is sleep–wake disorders (Chapter 20). The classification of both these areas in *ICD-10* (WHO, 1992a, 1992b) relied on their now obsolete division into organic and nonorganic disorders. The term *organic* implied that a disorder had some basis in the brain or some "real" medical causation, whereas *nonorganic* denoted that it was "functional" or purely psychological (i.e., the possibility of medical etiology had been ruled out). We wish to emphasize that this is not at all how the term *psychological* is used in this book.

The current state of the evidence clearly demonstrates that most sexual dysfunctions and sleep–wake disorders—like most mental disorders—involve both physiological and psychological/behavioral components that are further influenced by a variety of environmental and other contextual factors (American Academy of Sleep Medicine, 2014; Reed et al., 2016). A major innovation in the *ICD-11* was the introduction of two new chapters—on conditions related to sexual health and sleep–wake disorders, respectively—that bring together categories comprising these two sets of disorders that were previously distributed across several chapters in the *ICD-10*. These innovations more accurately reflect current scientific knowledge about these two groups of disorders, eliminate the "mind–body" split on which their previous classification was based, and provide clinicians with an integrated and accurate guide that serves to enhance understanding and improve diagnostic accuracy (Reed et al., 2019).

The final chapter of the book (Chapter 21) focuses on relationship problems and maltreatment. This chapter starts from WHO's 1946 definition of health as "a state of complete physical, mental and social well-being and not merely the absence of disease or infirmity" (as cited in WHO, 2020, p. 1). The chapter observes that social well-being depends on the health of the relationships individuals form, most notably those with parents (or other primary caregivers), intimate partners, children, and other family members, that strongly affect individuals' mental and physical health and well-being. Sometimes the behaviors that occur within these relationships are disturbed enough to constitute maltreatment or abuse. This may create specific legal and ethical obligations for psychologists and other mental health professionals to protect vulnerable parties.

Each of these chapters contains a set of common elements. They begin by describing the overarching logic for the classificatory arrangement of the disorders discussed in the chapter. The arrangement of mental disorders categories within the *ICD-11* was partly based on studies conducted for this revision on how clinicians think about mental disorders and their relationship to one another (Reed et al., 2013; Roberts et al., 2012). Each chapter also provides a discussion of the elements of a psychological approach to that set of disorders, including psychological models for conceptualizing their symptoms and recommendations for psychological assessment. The chapters also discuss presentations and symptom patterns for the disorders covered, specifiers and subtypes, boundaries with normality, differential diagnoses, co-occurring disorders, developmental course, cultural and contextual considerations, and gender-related features. This material parallels and supplements the *CDDR* for the same set of disorders.

Together, these chapters cover the majority of conditions with which people are likely to present in the clinical practice of psychologists and other mental health professionals. However, their coverage of the *ICD-11* mental, behavioral, or neurodevelopmental disorders is not completely comprehensive. Practice in certain areas, such as elimination disorders, paraphilic disorders, and factitious disorders, is not covered in this book and will require more specialized resources.

Another major change in the *ICD-11* that has important implications for psychological practice is that transgender identity is no longer considered to be a mental disorder (Reed et al., 2016, 2019). The *ICD-10* chapter on mental and behavioral disorders included a grouping called gender identity disorders. Two of the categories in this grouping have been renamed and reconceptualized in the *ICD-11* and have been moved from the mental disorders chapter to the new chapter on conditions related to sexual health. The new categories are gender incongruence of adolescence and adulthood and gender incongruence of childhood; other categories from the *ICD-10* grouping of gender identity disorders have been eliminated. The *ICD-11* explicitly states that gender variant behavior and preferences alone are not sufficient for a diagnosis of gender incongruence (WHO, 2023). Gender incongruence was not proposed for elimination in the *ICD-11* because in many countries a qualifying diagnosis is required to access health services. The new conceptualization of gender incongruence and its removal from the *ICD-11* chapter on mental disorders were supported by a large study of transgender people in Mexico City (Robles et al., 2016), as well as replications in five other countries (Robles et al., 2022).

Psychologists and other mental health professionals should adopt a clinical stance consistent with WHO's policy that being transgender is not a mental disorder. They should recognize the particular vulnerability of this population to stigmatization and violence, as well as the difficult history and negative experiences many transgender individuals have had with the health system (Robles et al., 2016; WHO, 2015). All mental health professionals should be prepared to assess and provide equitable and nonstigmatizing services responsive to the mental health needs of transgender individuals. At the same time, the diagnosis of gender incongruence per se is a rapidly evolving and controversial area, and the interested clinician is referred to more specialized resources (Coleman et al., 2022) for further information.

In all areas, it is expected that psychologists and other mental health professionals "provide services, teach, and conduct research with populations and in areas only within the boundaries of their competence, based on their education, training, supervised experience, consultation, study, or professional experience" (American Psychological Association, 2017). This book, along with the *CDDR*, provides a fundamental step toward competent diagnostic practice using the *ICD-11*.

DEFINING A PSYCHOLOGICAL APPROACH TO PSYCHOPATHOLOGY

The science of psychopathology is in large part the systematic description of mental disorders and their correlates and substrates, starting with the identification of emotions, thoughts, and behaviors that are characteristic of mental disorders and the disturbances in psychological processes that underlie them. When these experiences and behaviors reach an agreed-upon threshold of severity, dysfunction, or distress, they may be characterized as symptoms. In this regard, the diagnostic process proceeds from an understanding of psychopathology.

A psychological approach to psychopathology is grounded in an understanding of how people think, feel, and act as individuals as well as in the context of their intimate and other proximate relationships and their broader social and environmental context. While the psychological approach is person-centered, emotions, thoughts and actions are most often subjectively experienced through interactions with others and with the environment. This is a distinct and scientifically informed strategy anchored in inquiry regarding relevant cognitive, emotional, motivational, interpersonal, and other psychological processes.

The chapters of this book describe psychological models that are relevant for conceptualizing the expression of disorders in a particular individual. For example, Chapter 5, on schizophrenia and other primary psychotic disorders, reviews evidence of a very strong genetic component in schizophrenia but also indicates what appears to be inherited is a vulnerability to schizophrenia and related disorders rather than the disorder. The likelihood that this vulnerability will be expressed in a diagnosable disorder is increased by factors that have a psychological impact, such as exposure to childhood trauma, migration, and discrimination. Factors associated with symptom expression and maintenance also vary across symptoms. For example, negative symptoms may be linked to social withdrawal, and incoherent speech to interpersonal stress. The *ICD-11* therefore provides an inherently more psychological model of psychotic symptoms, which has replaced the *ICD-10* system of schizophrenia subtypes (e.g., paranoid, hebephrenic), which has been shown to lack validity, with ratings of specific symptom domains (e.g., positive symptoms, negative symptoms, cognitive symptoms) as they are currently experienced. These symptom domains provide a stronger basis for conceptualizing currently needed interventions and can be used to assess change and improvement over time, making them more compatible with a recovery-based approach.

The discussion of psychological mechanisms in obsessive-compulsive disorder (OCD) in Chapter 9 emphasizes cognitive factors including misappraisals of intrusive thoughts as informative, important, dangerous, or predictive of harm, leading to increased anxiety and distress. In turn, compulsions are aimed at reducing these emotions or reducing the likelihood of the feared catastrophic consequence, thus strengthening and maintaining the symptom through negative reinforcement. Dysfunctional beliefs such as an inflated sense of responsibility, perfectionism, or the belief that thoughts are equivalent to actions can increase the likelihood of misappraisals. Although there is no question that important neuroanatomical, neurochemical, and genetic features are etiologically important in OCD, an understanding of psychological processes in OCD is important in conceptualizing the development and maintenance of obsessions and compulsions as well as suggesting avenues for intervention. This model relates directly to the provision of specifiers in the *ICD-11* for the level of insight associated with OCD and related disorders. The use of cognitive intervention strategies would be appropriate for individuals with fair to good insight, allowing them to consider, at least some of the time, that their thoughts may not be true and possibly to accept an alternative explanation. For people with poor to absent insight, more purely behavioral strategies such as exposure and response prevention are more likely to be effective.

Chapter 16, on disorders due to addictive behaviors and compulsive sexual behavior disorder, applies the urgency–premeditation–perseverance–sensation-seeking (UPPS) impulsivity model to these disorders. The *urgency* component of the UPPS model encompasses emotion-related impulsivity and reduced inhibitory control; the (lack of) *premeditation* component is related to inability to delay rewards, poor decision-making, and poor problem-solving; the (lack of) *perseverance* component relates to difficulty remaining focused on tasks that are boring or cognitively demanding, increasing the likelihood of memory intrusions that promote subjective states of urge or craving; and the *sensation-seeking* component is a risk factor for the initiation of various problematic behaviors (e.g., drug use, delinquent acts, gambling, risky sexual behaviors), although other aspects of the model appear to be more important in their maintenance.

A psychological approach promotes a comprehensive understanding of disorder or dysfunction by considering the person's subjective experience, whether they are distressed by it, and whether they negatively impact the lives of others, especially those in their proximate interpersonal context. A psychological approach leads to more informed and deeper case conceptualization, regardless of the presumed etiology of disorder, strengthening intellectual coherence and supporting the clinical application of the *CDDR*. Moreover, many of the effective clinical interventions for mental disorders, either alone or in combination with other therapies (e.g., pharmacotherapy), are based on psychological treatment methods (Norcross et al., 2016). This book focuses on diagnosis, and thus a detailed discussion of interventions is beyond its scope. However, the preceding examples make clear that a psychological approach to diagnosis informs clinical interventions to improve the mental health and functioning of the person who is experiencing a mental disorder.

HOW DO THE *CDDR* SUPPORT A PSYCHOLOGICAL APPROACH?

The *CDDR* draw on research and clinical findings in psychology in their description of the disorders covered in this book. The *CDDR* guide clinicians in making a diagnosis through evidence-informed descriptions of the presentations and symptom patterns and other diagnostic material in a consistent manner across all diagnostic categories in the *ICD-11* chapter on mental, behavioral, and neurodevelopmental disorders (First et al., 2015). These elements, shown in Box 1.1, support clinicians in making a differential diagnosis and developing a case formulation based on a psychological approach. Multilingual field testing of the *CDDR* through Internet- and clinic-based studies involving

BOX 1.1 | **INFORMATION PROVIDED FOR THE MAIN DISORDER CATEGORIES IN THE *CLINICAL DESCRIPTIONS AND DIAGNOSTIC REQUIREMENTS FOR ICD-11 MENTAL, BEHAVIORAL AND NEURODEVELOPMENTAL DISORDERS***

Essential (required) features
Additional clinical features
Boundary with normality (threshold)
Course features
Developmental presentations
Culture-related features
Sex- and/or gender-related features
Boundaries with other disorders and conditions (differential diagnosis)

Note. ICD-11 = International Classification of Diseases–11th Revision.

thousands of mental health professionals from across the world also allowed for the validation and evidence-based improvements in clinical utility, global applicability, and reliability of the *CDDR* for assessment and diagnosis (Keeley et al., 2016; Reed et al., 2019). When used by well-trained clinicians, the *CDDR* provide considerable enhancements that increase the probability of accurate diagnoses. They provide practical means for collecting useful information and enable clinicians to make evidence-informed ratings of functioning and impairment through detailed descriptions and examples of functional impact for disorders, at varying severity levels, across a range of domains. The use of multidimensional assessments and profiles in diagnosis and management is a key feature of the psychological approach. The use of psychological tests and other forms of psychometric assessment is an integral part of this practice.

A Dimensional Approach to Psychopathology

One of the most profound changes in the *ICD-11* classification of mental, behavioral, and neurodevelopmental disorders is that structural innovations in the now fully digital classification have made it possible to create linkages among categories and integrate dimensional assessments in the context of the categorical classification system (Reed et al., 2019). As mentioned previously, this is the case for schizophrenia and other primary psychotic disorders, where severity and functional impact can be specified as none, mild, moderate, or severe for six classes of symptoms: positive and negative symptoms, depressed and manic mood, psychomotor symptoms, and cognition (see Chapter 5). The *CDDR* include detailed guidance for assigning these ratings to generate a detailed and individualized profile of symptoms and functional impact at a given point in time. Also consistent with a psychological approach, improvement in these symptom domains may be a critical outcome of treatment, which might be more directed at improving functioning and quality of life than on curing or eliminating the underlying disorder. This is in marked contrast to the process of assigning a label in *ICD-10* (e.g., paranoid schizophrenia, undifferentiated schizophrenia) that supposedly represented a type of schizophrenia with the implication that this pattern would be durable over time.

Similarly, in disorders of intellectual development, diagnosis and assessment is supported by inclusion in the *CDDR* of behavioral indicators by age group (early childhood, childhood and adolescence, adulthood) to capture a person's intellectual functioning as well as their adaptive behavior functioning in the domains of conceptual, social, and practical skills (see Chapter 3). Impairment or limitations in each area experienced by the individual being assessed can be rated as mild, moderate, severe, or profound, and these scores are integrated to form an overall rating of disorder severity. These ratings show specific areas in which people with disorders of intellectual development need support as well as what they are able to do on their own, consistent with a psychological approach.

To take another example, syndromal diagnoses of dementia (see Chapter 18) are rated for severity (mild, moderate, severe) and are linked to diagnosis of the underlying cause, if known (e.g., Alzheimer disease, cerebrovascular disease, chronic use of alcohol, Parkinson disease, HIV). In addition, specifiers for behavioral or psychological disturbances in dementia (psychotic symptoms, mood symptoms, anxiety symptoms, apathy, agitation or aggression, disinhibition, and wandering) can be appended to the diagnosis. As many of these specifiers can be used as necessary to describe specific needs for intervention for the individual being evaluated.

The area of personality disorders has also undergone a profound shift toward both a dimensional model and the integration of a psychological approach, as described in Chapter 17. In the *ICD-10*, there were general diagnostic requirements for personality disorder, followed by nine specific personality disorders (e.g., paranoid personality disorder, dissocial personality disorder, emotionally unstable personality disorder, borderline type), plus additional categories for "other" and "unspecified" personality disorders. The *ICD-11* has retained updated general diagnostic requirements for personality disorder. If these are met, the severity of the disorder is classified, based on (a) the degree and pervasiveness of disturbance in the person's relationships and their sense of self; (b) the intensity and breadth of the emotional, cognitive, and behavioral manifestations of personality dysfunction; (c) the extent to which these patterns and problems cause distress or psychosocial impairment; and (d) the level of risk of harm to self and others. This approach clearly locates personality disturbance along a continuum with normal functioning. The severity-based classification is important because severity is a major driver of the need for complex treatments compared with simpler treatments. It is also intended to be useful in nonspecialist settings and to assist in tracking changes in the severity of the disturbance over time.

The personality disturbance can be further characterized by five trait domain specifiers that are based on extensive psychological research (see Chapter 17) and continuous with personality traits in individuals who do not have personality disorders. The trait domains are negative affectivity, detachment, dissociality, disinhibition, and anankastia. Multiple specifiers may be applied, as necessary, to describe characteristics of the personality disturbance in an individual case. The trait domain specifiers are not diagnostic categories; rather, they represent a set of dimensions that correspond to the underlying structure of an individual's personality. The model provided by the *ICD-11* of how traits interact in the expression of personality is specifically psychological. To fully operationalize and reliably implement a more complex and individualized dimensional model compared with a categorical one, the development of reliable and valid psychological tests will be important and indeed is well underway (e.g., Bach et al., 2021; Clark et al., 2021; Oltmanns & Widiger, 2021).

A Developmental Approach

Consistent with the perspective of developmental psychology, the *ICD-11* has adopted a lifespan approach to the classification and description of mental disorders, reflected in the material provided in the *CDDR* and in this book. This approach emphasizes the continuity of expressions of psychological distress and mental health conditions among children, adolescents, and adults, including older adults. In the *ICD-11*, separate disorder groupings specific to childhood and adolescence were eliminated, and these disorders distributed to corresponding groupings. For example, separation anxiety disorder was moved to the anxiety and fear-related disorders grouping, and adult presentations are specifically described. For all main disorder categories, the *CDDR* provide information, where available, describing variations in the presentation of the disorder among children and adolescents as well as among older adults. Although the diagnosis of neurodevelopmental disorders requires that they have their onset during the developmental period (before the age of 18), adult presentations are also described. Important examples include disorders of intellectual development (see Chapter 3), autism spectrum disorder (see Chapter 4), and ADHD (see Chapter 14). Adult forms of disruptive behavior and dissocial disorders are also considered (see Chapter 14).

To expand on the example of ADHD, Schmidt and Petermann (2009) describe the ways in which ADHD manifests over the life course. From an early age, people who are later diagnosed with ADHD already show a higher motor activity level and increased negative emotionality. At preschool age, problems with attention and difficulty following instructions develop. If the disorder is recognized and treated at this early point, the symptoms can diminish, but otherwise they will typically intensify. At school age, there are notable ADHD symptoms; these may be accompanied by symptoms of other conditions such as dyslexia or dyscalculia. Intervention at this developmental stage can mitigate the effects of the disorder and yield positive outcomes at home, school, and in social lives. If ADHD persists or worsens in adolescence and adulthood, the core symptoms may expand to include disorganization, emotional reactivity, and a higher risk of co-occurring disorders such as disorders due to substance use, depressive disorders, and anxiety or fear-related disorders. The *CDDR* support the early detection and consistent monitoring of ADHD by describing its manifestations throughout the life course. The *CDDR* include sections on Course Features and Developmental Presentations that provide clinical guidance regarding typical onset and natural history of each disorder.

Another aspect of this developmental perspective relates to the longitudinal course of disorders. Many mental disorders are chronic, but most are also episodic such that phases of adaptation, maladaptation, and positive changes can alternate several times over a person's life. For example, a child might develop depressive episodes that remit during adolescence, then reappear in adulthood. The person may recover again and regain a stable sense of well-being that can last into old age, or they may continue to suffer recurrent depressive episodes for the remainder of their life. These trajectories and their determinants and outcomes have been studied for a variety of mental disorders (e.g., Hoffmann et al., 2021; Veldman et al., 2015). The *ICD-11* provides a variety of mechanisms for specifying the course of mental disorders in a particular case (e.g., schizophrenia, first episode, currently symptomatic; acute and transient psychotic disorder, multiple episodes, in partial remission; recurrent depressive disorder, current episode severe, without psychotic symptoms, with seasonal pattern; bipolar type I disorder, current episode manic, with psychotic symptoms). These specifiers provide a substantial amount of valuable information about a person's clinical trajectory, with important implications for treatment.

A PSYCHOLOGICAL APPROACH TO DIAGNOSTIC ASSESSMENT

A diagnostic evaluation is most commonly prompted when a person seeks care due to either (a) subjectively experienced distress, impairment, or related dysfunction that reduces their psychological, physical, or interpersonal well-being; or (b) initiation by someone else who is close to the person and is distressed, concerned, or otherwise affected by the person's behavior (e.g., a spouse or partner, a parent or child, a workplace manager). Diagnostic evaluations may also be requested based on a person's interaction with the legal system, which raises a complex set of issues related to practice in the forensic context that is largely beyond the scope of this book.

There are a range of methodologies for assessing psychopathological symptoms, disturbed psychological process, and related mental and interpersonal distress. Much information about symptoms experienced by the person as distressing can be obtained through self-report. This can be aided by appropriately normed and valid self-report measures. All chapters of this book that focus on specific groups of disorders contain information about measures that may be relevant in assessing those disorders, with priority given to instruments freely available in multiple languages.

In some cases, information necessary for making a diagnosis must be gathered more directly by the clinician through direct observation or clinician-administered psychological tests. For example, this is considered the optimal approach for diagnosing disorders of intellectual development and developmental learning disorder (as described in Chapter 3) as well as neurocognitive disorders (as described in Chapter 18). Structured clinical interviews are also being developed for *ICD-11* that are intended to be useful as a means of systematically gathering information about symptoms and differential diagnoses. Interviews with other informants (e.g., parents or other caretakers, teachers) are typically important for children or adolescents, as well as for adults with certain types of problems. For example, during some phases of certain disorders, the person may not be aware of the dysfunction associated with their symptoms (e.g., euphoric mood during a manic episode, hallucinations during an episode of schizophrenia, hoarding behavior).

Establishing a diagnosis is a fundamental step toward developing a treatment plan. A diagnosis is made based on an integrative evaluation of the collected findings from all available sources of information. Depending on the presenting problems, these may include a summary of symptoms, functional assessments, clinical interviews, and case history including personal, educational/vocational, family, medical, and social history, as well as results from psychological and other tests. It is critical for the clinician to be aware that the diagnostic process can be prone to errors, particularly those due to the clinician's biases or customary patterns of practice (Kildahl et al., 2023; Liu et al., 2022). Using multiple assessment methods and multiple sources of information reduces the risk of the clinician leaping prematurely from an initial clinical impression to a diagnosis without adequately assessing pertinent and potentially contradictory information.

A fundamental strategy for reducing the impact of bias is the systematic and objective consideration of differential diagnoses when the evaluation reveals elements that could be indicative of more than one diagnosis. All essential features included in the *CDDR* for the disorders being considered in the differential should be carefully evaluated. The person being evaluated may also be experiencing co-occurring disorders, and multiple diagnoses may be warranted. Clinicians should be aware of the potential for the symptoms of one disorder (e.g., a disorder due to substance use) to mask those of another (e.g., a depressive disorder). The *CDDR* provides extensive information on differential diagnoses for each disorder. Similarly, alternative explanations for the observed findings (e.g., a medical condition, the effects of a substance or medication, intense anxiety in the testing situation) must be considered.

The *CDDR* also provide information on distinguishing each disorder from normal variation or subclinical presentations. The mere presence of symptoms does not necessarily warrant a diagnosis. For example, significant symptoms of grief that impact functioning which are present in response to the recent loss of a spouse or partner would not be considered a disorder. However, when the nature, severity, and duration of these symptoms markedly exceeds social, cultural, or religious norms for the individual's culture and context and results in significant impairment in personal, family, social, educational, occupational, or other important areas of functioning, a diagnosis of prolonged grief disorder may be warranted.

A psychological approach considers people within their social and environmental context. When significant variations in affect, behavior, and thinking meet established requirements, a diagnosis can be made. Nonetheless, competent practitioners will exercise informed clinical judgment in determining whether a diagnosis is warranted. Clinical judgment is not an expression of individual beliefs or externally driven ideology. Rather, it is a thoughtful consideration of factors (e.g., culture, learned adaptive behaviors) that may explain behavioral variations. For example, expressions of unusual thoughts may make others uncomfortable but are not inherently an expression of a psychotic disorder. The absence of crying in response to an important loss when crying is culturally normative is most often not due to a lack of empathy or avoidance of grief. However, in both instances, the person or others in their environment may be concerned about atypical behaviors or the absence of socially mandated expressions. When the clinician concludes that a diagnosable disorder is not present, it may be important to assist the person in recognizing that there is nothing inherently problematic about their individual experience and expression, even if it varies from the norms of their community, culture, or family. Clinicians may also assist others in close relationships with the identified patient to understand, accept, or at least tolerate behavior they consider to be unusual.

The essential features of most *ICD-11* mental, behavioral, and neurodevelopmental disorders include significant impairment in personal, family, social, educational, occupational, or other important areas of functioning. Systematic assessment of these areas of functioning, in terms of how each is being affected by the presenting symptoms, provides a much more comprehensive understanding of the person. The functional impact of mental disorders is often cumulative and interacts with symptoms over time; earlier episodes can affect behaviors, choices, and opportunities that may confer greater vulnerability to later episodes. Moreover, the same disorder has different impacts on the psychosocial functioning of affected persons, producing different forms of subjective suffering and differing degrees of impairment. Sometimes people who are experiencing substantial emotional and psychological distress may avoid showing overt dysfunction such as relationship disruption or problems in occupational performance through significant additional effort. However, having to expend this degree of effort can be considered a type of functional impairment. For example, the *CDDR* describe how some individuals with autism spectrum disorder may function adequately in many contexts through exceptional effort, such that their deficits are not apparent to others. A diagnosis of autism spectrum disorder is still appropriate in such cases when other diagnostic requirements are met. Often, functional impairment emerges over time—for example, as developing children are faced with increasing social demands that eventually exceed their capacity to compensate.

Individual History

History-taking is also a part of diagnostic assessment because it helps the clinician to understand the impact of the individual's disorder in terms of its risk factors, precursors, onset, and course over the person's life as well as the experiences, vulnerabilities, strengths, and resources that may affect case conceptualization and treatment. History may be collected in an unstructured, semistructured (e.g., with coverage of specific prescribed areas), or fully structured (e.g., a standard history interview) manner. Although there are common generic features, the process of history-taking varies across the lifespan, requiring different methodologies, expertise, and experience.

As an illustration, key information collected during history-taking via a detailed clinical interview with adult persons may include the following:

- Sociodemographic: age, gender, education, occupation, religion, relationship status, and contact details; biographical and family information such as childhood characteristics, emotional relationship to the nuclear family, peer relationships, psychosexual development, nonnormative life events such as abuse, traumatic life events, or any legal issues

- Social–interpersonal: relationships in adulthood, previous occupational history, family composition, financial circumstances, and notable transitions such as children moving out of the home or retirement

- Mental disorders: any previous episodes of the presenting complaint as well as any other past or ongoing mental health problems; pertinent family history, such as the presence of mental disorders within the nuclear and extended family across the current and previous two generations

- Medical/biological: current and previous illnesses (e.g., cardiovascular, respiratory, endocrine, gynecological, renal) and systemic illnesses (e.g., autoimmune, infectious, cancers, intoxication); current and previous medications

The social–interpersonal and psychological components of history-taking provide important information for case conceptualization (discussed next), including factors related to the development and maintenance of the current mental disorder(s) as well as starting points for interventions. It is also important that the patient's current social environment is evaluated (e.g., to enable planning social support measures for isolated persons with severe mental disorders). In addition to its diagnostic importance, the medical/biological component facilitates integration of care and coordination among health professionals who are concurrently treating comorbid medical conditions.

Case Conceptualization

Case conceptualization, also known as case formulation or problem formulation, often represents an important product of a psychological approach to assessment. The case conceptualization consolidates different sources of diagnostic and contextual information about the individual based on a comprehensive bio-psycho-socio-cultural framework that supports a comprehensive understanding of the person. Elements of such a framework are shown in Box 1.2, which is intended to be illustrative and does not include all the factors that may merit detailed inquiry in an individual case.

BOX 1.2 | **EXAMPLE ELEMENTS OF A BIO-PSYCHO-SOCIO-CULTURAL FRAMEWORK AS A BASIS FOR CASE CONCEPTUALIZATION**

Biological elements

Are there indications of genetic, metabolic, neurological, autoimmune, and other influences on the disorder?

Is it known whether a first-degree relative had a severe mental disorder such as bipolar disorder, dementia, or schizophrenia?

Psychological elements

What are the important affective, cognitive, motivational, values, and other characteristics that enable coping and resilience?

Are there individual, family, or other experiences such as developmental problems, financial issues, personal autonomy or relatedness, or issues related to sexual orientation or gender identity?

Social elements

What is the person's social situation—their social, occupational, and other relationships?

What are other socioenvironmental factors? These might include poverty, unemployment, social conflict, or exposure to civil conflict or war.

Cultural elements

What is the role of religion or spirituality in the person's life? How might basic cultural factors such as individualistic versus collectivistic values be relevant to the person's experience and their expression of distress and symptoms?

Are there culturally determined gender role differences (e.g., norms or rules about contact with the other sex or childcare and work outside the home), or identity-forming affiliations with specific ethnic groups or subcultures (e.g., activities/programs to reinforce ethnic identity)?

The use of stand-alone mental disorder diagnoses has long been criticized for being overly medicalized, uninformative regarding etiology, and unhelpful for intervention (Macneil et al., 2012). The assignment of a diagnosis has also sometimes been contrasted with both case conceptualization and recovery-based approaches (British Psychological Society, 2011). In truth, they are not incompatible. As a part of their systematic review of service user, clinician, and caregiver perspectives on mental health diagnosis, Perkins and colleagues (2018) pointed out that the many clinicians who value diagnosis are supportive of recovery-based approaches. They concluded that the experience of diagnosis can be improved by integrating principles of psychological case conceptualization, including "collaboratively developing a holistic understanding of a person's difficulties that addresses etiology, and then using diagnosis as a tool to guide treatment and recovery" (p. 761).

Dawson and Moghaddam (2015) developed evaluation criteria to promote the coherence and quality of case conceptualization. These are (a) clarity and parsimony, where key concepts are used specifically and nonredundantly; (b) precision and testability, meaning that the components of the case conceptualization are potentially measurable and/or lead to testable hypotheses that are relevant to diagnosis, treatment, and outcomes; (c) comprehensiveness and relative generalizability—for example, the case conceptualization is applicable across a range of situations and clinical phenomena; (d) utility—that is, it facilitates shared meaning among clinicians as well as between clinician and patient; and (e) applied value, related to the effectiveness of interventions based on the conceptualization.

A solid case conceptualization facilitates the selection of treatments from the wide spectrum of evidence-informed psychological interventions that are available for mental disorders. Additional forms of intervention such as pharmacotherapy and social–environmental interventions (e.g., supported employment for individuals living with schizophrenia) may also be indicated. A case conceptualization should provide a coherent integration of multiple intervention methods based on the patient's individual combination of cognitive, developmental, personality, relational, social, and other factors in combination with the characteristics of one or more mental disorders. To ensure that the various methods are coordinated in a goal-oriented manner, each treatment should have a specified focus and objectives to orient the contributions of multiple clinicians. As Perkins and colleagues (2018) concluded, a case formulation approach "could enable the diagnostic process to be implemented in a way that is concordant with recovery principles. It particularly supports collaboration, person centered care, and service user agency and empowerment, reflecting recommendations about service user participation" (p. 761).

Consistent with a case conceptualization approach, an important component of the diagnostic process is effective communication of the results of the assessment to the person being evaluated. Thoughtfully prepared communication is a fundamental responsibility of clinicians. When appropriate, and with the patient's consent, feedback may also be given to others in close relationships with the person. It is important for the clinician to be aware of those aspects of the diagnostic formulation that have the potential to be experienced as confusing or even stigmatizing, as documented in *ICD-11* field studies conducted with service users (Askevis-Leherpeux et al., 2022; Hackmann et al., 2019).

As the preceding discussion suggests, the psychological approach is a collaborative one, emphasizing shared decision-making based on the principles of autonomy and self-determination (Joosten et al., 2008). These principles can be operationalized by several components: (a) agreement between the clinician and patient that assessment results and diagnoses will be communicated; (b) comprehensive information is provided about the disorder and treatment options, including evidence and alternatives; (c) patient preferences are determined, and the clinician's recommendations are made explicit; (d) understanding the options and asking about alternatives are encouraged; and (e) in the case of severe mental disorders, when applicable, full adherence to the legal framework for substitute decision-making during a temporary assumption of responsibility by the clinician or a designated other person, often a partner or family member.

Participatory decision-making generally has beneficial effects on compliance (e.g., fewer premature terminations of treatment, greater adherence to therapeutic protocols), treatment success, and patient satisfaction (Joosten et al., 2008; Thompson & McCabe, 2012). Of course, these principles must also be implemented in a way that is congruent with the patient's need for a diagnostic assessment conducted by a competent clinician–expert. In providing diagnostic information, conclusions, and recommendations, the clinician's challenge is to be authoritative without being controlling or authoritarian.

CONCLUSIONS

The development of the *ICD-11* chapter on mental, behavioral, and neurodevelopmental disorders as well as the *CDDR* included an unprecedented degree of leadership and participation by psychologists in the development of the classification and diagnostic guidance, as well as participation of thousands of psychologists across the world in field-testing the proposed guidelines before their finalization and publication. At the same time, it is critical to emphasize that the entire process was multidisciplinary in nature, incorporating the most current knowledge and best practices from psychiatry and other disciplines. When we refer to a psychological approach, we do not mean one that is exclusive or proprietary to the discipline of psychology. Rather, a psychological approach focuses on psychological mechanisms and principles as an aspect of diagnostic practice and case formulation, regardless of professional discipline.

Each disorder-specific chapter in this book highlights the ways in which the *CDDR* promote the application of the core principles of a psychological approach. Along with the *CDDR,* this book equips clinicians to understand the core aspects of the relevant clinical phenomena as well as to use their clinical judgment and their understanding of the person (e.g., developmental stage, social and cultural environment) to consider whether a given patient meets the diagnostic requirements for a given diagnosis. The *CDDR* are intentionally flexible to allow for clinical judgment and cultural variability; this flexibility has been shown to improve clinical utility without sacrificing reliability (Reed et al., 2018, 2019). The dimensional elements of the *ICD-11* and the *CDDR* allow for more granular tracking of a patient's clinical course, which can be valuable in assessing responsiveness to treatments (e.g., the person transitions from a severe to a moderate personality disorder after an intervention) and assessing clinical trajectories and prognoses. A range of specifiers are provided that allows for a more nuanced diagnosis and the incorporation of current and historical information.

In summary, the *CDDR* align strongly with core psychological principles, and their implementation is further guided by this book. Together, this book and the *CDDR* provide mental health professionals, primary care clinicians, educators, and trainees with essential tools for the competent practice of diagnosis using the *ICD-11* as a framework. As editors of this book, our intention is to facilitate the implementation of the *ICD-11* around the world, contributing to reducing the global disease burden of mental disorders by helping to bridge the gap between those who need psychologically competent services and those who receive them.

REFERENCES

American Academy of Sleep Medicine. (2014). *International classification of sleep disorders* (3rd ed.). American Academy of Sleep Medicine.

American Psychological Association. (2017). *Ethical principles of psychologists and code of conduct* (2002, amended effective June 1, 2010 and January 1, 2017). https://www.apa.org/ethics/code/

Askevis-Leherpeux, F., Hazo, J. B., Agoub, M., Baleige, A., Barikova, V., Benmessaoud, D., Brunet, F., Carta, M. G., Castelpietra, G., Crepaz-Keay, D., Daumerie, N., Demassiet, V., Fontaine, A., Grigutyte, N., Guernut, M., Kishore, J., Kiss, M., Koenig, M., Laporta, M., . . . Roelandt, J. L. (2022). Accessibility of psychiatric vocabulary: An international study about schizophrenia essential features. *Schizophrenia Research*, *243*(6), 463–464. https://doi.org/10.1016/j.schres.2022.03.001

Bach, B., Brown, T. A., Mulder, R. T., Newton-Howes, G., Simonsen, E., & Sellbom, M. (2021). Development and initial evaluation of the *ICD-11* personality disorder severity scale: PDS-*ICD-11*. *Personality and Mental Health*, *15*(3), 223–236. https://doi.org/10.1002/pmh.1510

British Psychological Society. (2011). *Good practice guidelines on the use of psychological formulation*. https://doi.org/10.53841/bpsrep.2011.rep100

Clark, L. A., Corona-Espinosa, A., Khoo, S., Kotelnikova, Y., Levin-Aspenson, H. F., Serapio-García, G., & Watson, D. (2021). Preliminary scales for *ICD-11* personality disorder: Self and interpersonal dysfunction plus five personality disorder trait domains. *Frontiers in Psychology*, *12*, Article 668724. https://doi.org/10.3389/fpsyg.2021.668724

Coleman, E., Radix, A. E., Bouman, W. P., Brown, G. R., de Vries, A. L. C., Deutsch, M. B., Ettner, R., Fraser, L., Goodman, M., Green, J., Hancock, A. B., Johnson, T. W., Karasic, D. H., Knudson, G. A., Leibowitz, S. F., Meyer-Bahlburg, H. F. L., Monstrey, S. J., Motmans, J., Nahata, L., . . . Arcelus, J. (2022). Standards of care for the health of transgender and gender diverse people, version 8. *International Journal of Transgender Health*, *23*(Suppl. 1), S1–S259. https://doi.org/10.1080/26895269.2022.2100644

Dawson, D., & Moghaddam, N. (2015). *Formulation in action: Applying psychological theory to clinical practice*. de Gruyter Open. https://doi.org/10.1515/9783110471014

First, M. B., Reed, G. M., Hyman, S. E., & Saxena, S. (2015). The development of the *ICD-11* clinical descriptions and diagnostic guidelines for mental and behavioural disorders. *World Psychiatry*, *14*(1), 82–90. https://doi.org/10.1002/wps.20189

Hackmann, C., Balhara, Y. P. S., Clayman, K., Nemec, P. B., Notley, C., Pike, K., Reed, G. M., Sharan, P., Rana, M. S., Silver, J., Swarbrick, M., Wilson, J., Zeilig, H., & Shakespeare, T. (2019). Perspectives on *ICD-11* to understand and improve mental health diagnosis using expertise by experience (INCLUDE study): An international qualitative study. *The Lancet Psychiatry*, *6*(9), 778–785. https://doi.org/10.1016/S2215-0366(19)30093-8

Hoffmann, M. S., McDaid, D., Salum, G. A., Silva-Ribeiro, W., Ziebold, C., King, D., Gadelha, A., Miguel, E. C., Mari, J. J., Rohde, L. A., Pan, P. M., Bressan, R. A., Mojtabai, R., & Evans-Lacko, S. (2021). The impact of child psychiatric conditions on future educational outcomes among a community cohort in Brazil. *Epidemiology and Psychiatric Sciences*, *30*, e69. https://doi.org/10.1017/S2045796021000561

Joosten, E. A., DeFuentes-Merillas, L., de Weert, G. H., Sensky, T., van der Staak, C. P. F., & de Jong, C. A. (2008). Systematic review of the effects of shared decision-making on patient satisfaction, treatment adherence and health status. *Psychotherapy and Psychosomatics, 77*(4), 219–226. https://doi.org/10.1159/000126073

Keeley, J. W., Reed, G. M., Roberts, M. C., Evans, S. C., Medina-Mora, M. E., Robles, R., Rebello, T., Sharan, P., Gureje, O., First, M. B., Andrews, H. F., Ayuso-Mateos, J. L., Gaebel, W., Zielasek, J., & Saxena, S. (2016). Developing a science of clinical utility in diagnostic classification systems field study strategies for *ICD-11* mental and behavioral disorders. *American Psychologist, 71*(1), 3–16. https://doi.org/10.1037/a0039972

Kildahl, A. N., Oddli, H. W., & Helverschou, S. B. (2023). Bias in assessment of co-occurring mental disorder in individuals with intellectual disabilities: Theoretical perspectives and implications for clinical practice. *Journal of Intellectual Disabilities*, 17446295231154119. https://doi.org/10.1177/17446295231154119

Leichsenring, F., Steinert, C., Rabung, S., & Ioannidis, J. P. A. (2022). The efficacy of psychotherapies and pharmacotherapies for mental disorders in adults: An umbrella review and meta-analytic evaluation of recent meta-analyses. *World Psychiatry, 21*(1), 133–145. https://doi.org/10.1002/wps.20941

Liu, F. F., Coifman, J., McRee, E., Stone, J., Law, A., Gaias, L., Reyes, R., Lai, C. K., Blair, I. V., Yu, C. L., Cook, H., & Lyon, A. R. (2022). A brief online implicit bias intervention for school mental health clinicians. *International Journal of Environmental Research and Public Health, 19*(2), 679. https://doi.org/10.3390/ijerph19020679

Macneil, C. A., Hasty, M. K., Conus, P., & Berk, M. (2012). Is diagnosis enough to guide interventions in mental health? Using case formulation in clinical practice. *BMC Medicine, 10*(1), 111. https://doi.org/10.1186/1741-7015-10-111

Nathan, P., & Gorman, J. M. (Eds.). (2015). *A guide to treatments that work* (4th ed.). Oxford University Press.

Norcross, J. C., VandenBos, G. R., Freedheim, D. K., & Krishnamurthy, R. E. (Eds.). (2016). *APA handbook of clinical psychology: Vol. 3. Applications and methods*. American Psychological Association. https://doi.org/10.1037/14861-000

Oltmanns, J. R., & Widiger, T. A. (2021). The self- and informant-personality inventories for *ICD-11*: Agreement, structure, and relations with health, social, and satisfaction variables in older adults. *Psychological Assessment, 33*(4), 300–310. https://doi.org/10.1037/pas0000982

Perkins, A., Ridler, J., Browes, D., Peryer, G., Notley, C., & Hackmann, C. (2018). Experiencing mental health diagnosis: A systematic review of service user, clinician, and carer perspectives across clinical settings. *The Lancet Psychiatry, 5*(9), 747–764. https://doi.org/10.1016/S2215-0366(18)30095-6

Reed, G. M., Drescher, J., Krueger, R. B., Atalla, E., Cochran, S. D., First, M. B., Cohen-Kettenis, P. T., Arango-de Montis, I., Parish, S. J., Cottler, S., Briken, P., & Saxena, S. (2016). Disorders related to sexuality and gender identity in the *ICD-11*: Revising the *ICD-10* classification based on current scientific evidence, best clinical practices, and human rights considerations. *World Psychiatry, 15*(3), 205–221. https://doi.org/10.1002/wps.20354

Reed, G. M., First, M. B., Kogan, C. S., Hyman, S. E., Gureje, O., Gaebel, W., Maj, M., Stein, D. J., Maercker, A., Tyrer, P., Claudino, A., Garralda, E., Salvador-Carulla, L., Ray, R., Saunders, J. B., Dua, T., Poznyak, V., Medina-Mora, M. E., Pike, K. M., . . . Saxena, S. (2019). Innovations and changes in the *ICD-11* classification of mental, behavioural and neurodevelopmental disorders. *World Psychiatry, 18*(1), 3–19. https://doi.org/10.1002/wps.20611

Reed, G. M., Roberts, M. C., Keeley, J., Hooppell, C., Matsumoto, C., Sharan, P., Robles, R., Carvalho, H., Wu, C., Gureje, O., Leal-Leturia, I., Flanagan, E. H., Correia, J. M., Maruta, T., Ayuso-Mateos, J. L., de Jesus Mari, J., Xiao, Z., Evans, S. C., Saxena, S.,

& Medina-Mora, M. E. (2013). Mental health professionals' natural taxonomies of mental disorders: Implications for the clinical utility of the *ICD-11* and the *DSM-5*. *Journal of Clinical Psychology, 69*(12), 1191–1212. https://doi.org/10.1002/jclp.22031

Reed, G. M., Sharan, P., Rebello, T. J., Keeley, J. W., Medina-Mora, M. E., Gureje, O., Ayuso-Mateos, J. L., Kanba, S., Khoury, B., Kogan, C. S., Krasnov, V. N., Maj, M., de Jesus Mari, J., Stein, D. J., Zhao, M., Akiyama, T., Andrews, H. F., Asevedo, E., Cheour, M., . . . Pike, K. M. (2018). The *ICD-11* developmental field study of reliability of diagnoses of high-burden mental disorders: Results among adult patients in mental health settings of 13 countries. *World Psychiatry, 17*(2), 174–186. https://doi.org/10.1002/wps.20524

Roberts, M. C., Reed, G. M., Medina-Mora, M. E., Keeley, J. W., Sharan, P., Johnson, D. K., de Jesus Mari, J., Ayuso-Mateos, J. L., Gureje, O., Xiao, Z., Maruta, T., Khoury, B., Robles, R., & Saxena, S. (2012). A global clinicians' map of mental disorders to improve *ICD-11*: Analysing meta-structure to enhance clinical utility. *International Review of Psychiatry, 24*(6), 578–590. https://doi.org/10.3109/09540261.2012.736368

Robles, R., Fresán, A., Vega-Ramírez, H., Cruz-Islas, J., Rodríguez-Pérez, V., Domínguez-Martínez, T., & Reed, G. M. (2016). Removing transgender identity from the classification of mental disorders: A Mexican field study for *ICD-11*. *The Lancet Psychiatry, 3*(9), 850–859. https://doi.org/10.1016/S2215-0366(16)30165-1

Robles, R., Keeley, J. W., Vega-Ramírez, H., Cruz-Islas, J., Rodríguez-Pérez, V., Sharan, P., Purnima, S., Rao, R., Rodrigues-Lobato, M. I., Soll, B., Askevis-Leherpeux, F., Roelandt, J. L., Campbell, M., Grobler, G., Stein, D. J., Khoury, B., Khoury, J. E., Fresán, A., Medina-Mora, M. E., & Reed, G. M. (2022). Validity of categories related to gender identity in *ICD-11* and *DSM-5* among transgender individuals who seek gender-affirming medical procedures. *International Journal of Clinical and Health Psychology, 22*(1), Article 100281. https://doi.org/10.1016/j.ijchp.2021.100281

Schmidt, S., & Petermann, F. (2009). Developmental psychopathology: Attention deficit hyperactivity disorder (ADHD). *BMC Psychiatry, 9*(1), 58. https://doi.org/10.1186/1471-244X-9-58

Thompson, L., & McCabe, R. (2012). The effect of clinician-patient alliance and communication on treatment adherence in mental health care: A systematic review. *BMC Psychiatry, 12*, Article 87. https://doi.org/10.1186/1471-244X-12-87

Veldman, K., Reijneveld, S. A., Ortiz, J. A., Verhulst, F. C., & Bültmann, U. (2015). Mental health trajectories from childhood to young adulthood affect the educational and employment status of young adults: Results from the TRAILS study. *Journal of Epidemiology and Community Health, 69*(6), 588–593. https://doi.org/10.1136/jech-2014-204421

World Health Organization. (1992a). *The ICD-10 classification of mental and behavioural disorders: Clinical descriptions and diagnostic guidelines.* https://www.who.int/publications/i/item/9241544228

World Health Organization. (1992b). *International statistical classification of diseases and related health problems* (10th rev.).

World Health Organization. (2015). *Sexual health, human rights and the law.* https://apps.who.int/iris/handle/10665/175556

World Health Organization. (2020). *Basic documents* (49th ed., amended effective May 31, 2019). https://apps.who.int/gb/bd/

World Health Organization. (2023). *ICD-11 for mortality and morbidity statistics* (Version: 01/2023). https://icd.who.int/browse11/l-m/en#/

World Health Organization. (2024). *Clinical descriptions and diagnostic requirements for ICD-11 mental, behavioural and neurodevelopmental disorders.* https://www.who.int/publications/i/item/9789240077263

2

A Global Approach to Diagnosis

Geoffrey M. Reed

The World Health Organization (WHO) is a specialized, autonomous agency of the United Nations and the world's foremost public health authority. Founded in 1948, the WHO provides leadership and technical assistance on matters related to health to its 194 member states (countries), including global efforts to expand health coverage, directing and coordinating the world's response to public health emergencies, and promoting the highest possible level of health for all people through science-based policies and programs. WHO's 1946 Constitution defines health as "a state of complete physical, mental and social well-being and not merely the absence of disease or infirmity" (as cited in WHO, 2020, p. 2). Therefore, from the time of its founding, mental health has been an integral part of the WHO's mission. Moreover, a right to universal mental health coverage is grounded in the WHO Constitution: "The enjoyment of the highest attainable standard of health is one of the fundamental rights of every human being without distinction of race, religion, political belief, economic or social condition" and "is fundamental to the attainment of peace and security and is dependent upon the fullest co-operation of individuals and States" (p. 2).

The 11th revision of the WHO's *International Classification of Diseases* (*ICD-11*) was approved by the World Health Assembly on May 25, 2019 (WHO, 2019). The World Health Assembly is the WHO's governing body, made up of the ministers/secretaries of health from all member states. The *ICD* is a core constitutional function of the WHO; two of the explicitly identified purposes for which WHO was established are "to establish and revise as necessary international

https://doi.org/10.1037/0000392-002
A Psychological Approach to Diagnosis: Using the ICD-11 as a Framework, G. M. Reed, P. L.-J. Ritchie, and A. Maercker (Editors)

nomenclatures of diseases, of causes of death and public health practices" and "to standardize diagnostic procedures as necessary" (WHO, 2020, p. 3). The *ICD-11* covers all areas of health and is designed to be used for the classification of both causes of death (mortality) and diseases, disorders, injuries, and other health conditions (morbidity). The WHO's 1946 Constitution (see WHO, 2020) also defines the obligations of its 194 member states, which include using the *ICD* as the framework for the reporting of health information to the WHO. Global reporting of health statistics based on the *ICD* provides a critical part of the basis for monitoring epidemics and other threats to public health, calculating the global burden of disease, identifying vulnerable and at-risk populations, and creating accountability for the achievement of public health objectives by member states. The *ICD-11* replaced the 10th revision (*ICD-10*) as the reporting standard for mortality and morbidity statistics on January 1, 2022 (WHO, 2022).

For most countries, diagnostic classification based on the *ICD* also provides a large part of the framework for defining the government's obligations to provide free or subsidized health care, social services, and disability benefits to its citizens (International Advisory Group for the Revision of *ICD-10* Mental and Behavioural Disorders, 2011). Typically, a particular diagnosis determines the range of treatments and services an individual is eligible to receive. Implemented as a part of heath care systems, the common language of the *ICD* facilitates access to appropriate health care services, provides a basis for developing and implementing clinical guidelines and standards of practice, and supports research into more effective prevention and treatment strategies.

The *ICD-11* is organized into 26 chapters, often based on the affected organ system (e.g., diseases of the immune system; diseases of the respiratory system) or on classes of etiology (e.g., neoplasms; certain infectious or parasitic diseases). Chapter 6 covers mental, behavioral, and neurodevelopmental disorders and is the primary focus of this book. The WHO Department of Mental Health and Substance Use led the development of the version of Chapter 6 used for global health statistics, called the *ICD-11* for Mortality and Morbidity Statistics (MMS; WHO, 2023). The department also developed the *ICD-11* diagnostic manual for use in clinical settings—the *Clinical Descriptions and Diagnostic Requirements for ICD-11 Mental, Behavioural and Neurodevelopmental Disorders* (*CDDR*; WHO, 2024*)*. This book is intended as a tool to deepen and expand the material in the *CDDR* and comprises chapters organized around the major *ICD-11* diagnostic groupings, such as depressive disorders (Chapter 6), disorders specifically associated with stress (Chapter 10), and disruptive behavior and dissocial disorders (Chapter 14).

The *ICD* is the diagnostic system for mental disorders most widely used by mental health professionals around the world in their day-to-day clinical practice (Evans et al., 2013; First et al., 2018; Reed et al., 2011). From the perspective of the Department of Mental Health and Substance Use, the most important goal in producing a new version of the *ICD* was to provide a better tool for reducing the global burden of mental disorders (GBD 2019 Mental Disorders Collaborators, 2022; Rehm & Shield, 2019). As an extension of this goal, the Department adopted an explicit focus on clinical utility and global applicability in developing the *CDDR* (Reed, 2010). The idea was that a diagnostic system experienced by clinicians around the world as more useful would be implemented more faithfully, leading to better and earlier identification of mental disorders and more effective treatment (International Advisory Group for the Revision of *ICD-10* Mental and Behavioural Disorders, 2011). A more clinically useful and globally applicable system would also help improve the quality and validity of data based on aggregated clinical encounters that are used as a basis for making major policy and resource decisions at the level of the health system, the country, and the world (Reed et al., 2013), in turn resulting in further improvements in a virtuous cycle.

GLOBAL PARTICIPATION IN THE DEVELOPMENT AND TESTING OF THE *ICD-11 CDDR*

The public health and clinical objectives just outlined directly informed the department's commitment to a process for developing the *CDDR* that was global, multilingual, and multidisciplinary at every level. For more than a decade, the WHO Department of Mental Health and Substance Use coordinated an intensive, systematic, international process that involved a wide range of key stakeholder groups including scientific and public health experts, clinicians, service users and those caring for them, representatives of WHO member states, scientific and professional societies, and other nongovernmental organizations. In 2007, the department appointed the International Advisory Group for the Revision of *ICD-10* Mental and Behavioural Disorders. The Advisory Group's primary responsibility was to provide scientific oversight for the development of the *ICD-11* classification of mental disorders, including advising the department on guiding principles, goals, and steps involved in the revision; identification of other groups of relevant consultants and stakeholders; and facilitating the implementation of global field studies to assess and further improve the *ICD-11* and the *CDDR*.

The department specified that the group must include scientific experts from all WHO-designated global regions: the African region, region of the Americas (subdivided into Latin America/Caribbean and North America), the Eastern Mediterranean region, the European region, the South-East Asian region, and the Western Pacific region (subdivided into Asia and Oceania), with substantial representation from low- and middle-income countries. The Advisory Group also included representatives of the main international professional societies for psychology (the International Union of Psychological Science), psychiatry, social work, nursing, and primary care. The Advisory Group also advised the department on the appointment of more than a dozen working groups responsible for reviewing the relevant evidence and making proposals for changes to the structure and content of the *ICD-10* classification of mental, behavioral, and neurodevelopmental disorders. The working groups also included experts from all WHO global regions with enhanced representation of low- and middle-income countries. These working groups developed the core material for both the MMS and the *CDDR*. (For a detailed description of this process, see First et al., 2015.) Many of the authors of the chapters of this book were members of working groups or had other significant roles in the development of the *ICD-11* and the *CDDR*.

The draft *CDDR* were tested in a systematic and innovative program of field studies, incorporating novel study designs and psychological methodologies (Evans et al., 2015; Keeley, Reed, Roberts, Evans, Medina-Mora, et al., 2016; Reed et al., 2019). Global participation was a defining characteristic of these studies, which were conducted in multiple languages and engaged multidisciplinary clinicians working in diverse contexts across the world. Scientific oversight for the field studies was provided by the Field Studies Coordination Group (FSCG; Guler et al., 2018), made up of global leaders in clinical care, scientific research, and public health, with similar regional and country income level composition as other groups. The FSCG members lent their expertise to the design, analysis, and interpretation of the field studies but also were essential in facilitating the engagement of clinicians from across the world in the *ICD-11* field studies. Many members directed International Field Study Centers, which tested the *CDDR* in routine clinical settings with real patients (see Reed, Sharan, Rebello, Keeley, Gureje, et al., 2018; Reed, Sharan, Rebello, Keeley, Medina-Mora, et al., 2018). On the basis of the results of the field studies, the FSCG worked with relevant working groups to propose changes and refinements to the *CDDR* (Keeley, Reed, Roberts, Evans, Medina-Mora, et al., 2016; Keeley, Reed, Roberts, Evans, Robles, et al., 2016).

There were two main types of *CDDR* field studies: case-controlled (Internet-based) and ecological implementation (clinic-based) field studies. Participants in the case-controlled field studies were members of WHO's Global Clinical Practice Network, which now consists of more than 18,500 mental health professionals from 163 countries (see https://gcp.network/) who joined the network specifically to contribute to the development of the *ICD-11* (Reed et al., 2015). Most case-controlled studies compared the accuracy and consistency of clinicians' diagnostic formulation using the proposed *CDDR* compared with the *ICD-10* diagnostic guidelines for a given diagnostic area, using a scientifically rigorous vignette-based methodology (e.g., Claudino et al., 2019; Keeley, Reed, Roberts, Evans, Robles, et al., 2016; Kogan et al., 2020). All case-controlled field studies were conducted in at least three and up to six of the following languages: Chinese, English, French, Japanese, Russian, and Spanish; some additional studies were conducted in German. Overall, the case-controlled field studies found that the *ICD-11 CDDR* were superior to the *ICD-10* diagnostic guidelines (WHO, 1992) in terms of diagnostic accuracy and clinical utility, depending on the disorder grouping. Analyses of global applicability were also conducted by comparing results across global region, country income level, and language, finding few systematic or meaningful differences.

The first ecological implementation (clinic-based) field study tested the proposed *CDDR* diagnostic material when applied by practicing clinicians to adult patients receiving care in the types of clinical settings in which the *CDDR* would be implemented (Reed, Sharan, Rebello, Keeley, Gureje, et al., 2018; Reed, Sharan, Rebello, Keeley, Medina-Mora, et al., 2018). The study was conducted in 14 countries—Brazil, Canada, China, Egypt, India, Italy, Japan, Lebanon, Mexico, Nigeria, Russia, South Africa, Spain, and Tunisia—via a network of International Field Study Centers. The study assessed the reliability and clinical utility of the *CDDR* for disorders that account for the highest percentage of global disease burden and use of services in adult clinical mental health setting: schizophrenia and other psychotic disorders, mood disorders, anxiety and fear-related disorders, and disorders specifically associated with stress.

Participating clinicians received a similar level of training on the *CDDR* to what might be realistically expected in routine clinical settings during *ICD-11* implementation (one 4-hour session). Clinicians were given no instructions on how to conduct their diagnostic interviews other than to assess the areas that were required as part of the study protocol. The study employed a joint rater design using pairs of clinicians, with one randomly assigned to interview the patient and the other assigned to observe, with each separately recording their diagnostic formulation and responding to questions about clinical utility. The reliability of the *ICD-11 CDDR* was found to be superior to that previously reported for equivalent *ICD-10* diagnostic guidelines, with intraclass kappa coefficients for diagnoses weighted by site and study prevalence ranging from 0.45 (dysthymic disorder, which was difficult for clinicians to differentiate from recurrent depressive disorder) to 0.88 (social anxiety disorder). Clinician ratings of the clinical utility of the *ICD-11 CDDR* were highly positive. The *CDDR* were perceived as easy to use, accurately reflecting patients' presentations (i.e., goodness of fit), clear and understandable, and taking about the same amount or even less time than clinicians' standard practice.

A separate study of common child and adolescent diagnoses was conducted in four countries—China, India, Japan, and Mexico—with children and adolescents from 6 to 18 years of age (Medina-Mora et al., 2019). The study focused on attention deficit hyperactivity disorder, disruptive behavior and dissocial disorders, mood disorders, anxiety or fear-related disorders, and disorders specifically associated with stress, using a design analogous to that of the adult study. Kappa estimates indicated substantial agreement for most categories, with moderate agreement for generalized anxiety disorder and adjustment disorder. No differences were found between younger (6–11 years) and older (12–18 years) age groups or between outpatient and inpatient samples. Clinical utility ratings were positive and consistent across the domains assessed, although somewhat lower for adjustment disorder. Taken together, the results of the ecological implementation supported the implementation of the *ICD-11 CDDR* in clinical settings and suggested that the results of the case-controlled studies were generalizable to clinical settings.

Another study conducted in Italy, India, and Sri Lanka assessed the reliability and clinical utility of behavioral indicators (BIs) for assessing the severity of impairments of intellectual and adaptive functioning among individuals with disorders of intellectual development (Lemay et al., 2022). The BIs are intended to provide a basis for making a valid diagnosis when standardized and appropriately normed test of intellectual and adaptive functioning are not available, as is the case in many settings and parts of the world (see Chapter 3). The BIs were shown to have excellent interrater reliability (intraclass correlations ranging from 0.91 to 0.97) and good to excellent concurrent validity (intraclass correlations ranging from 0.66 to 0.82) across sites. The BIs were rated as quick and easy to use and applicable across severities; clear and understandable; and useful for treatment selection, prognosis assessments, communication with other health care professionals, and education efforts.

A separate field studies program to test the section of the *ICD-11 CDDR* on disorders due to substance use and addictive behaviors involved field testing centers in 11 countries: Australia, Brazil, China, France, India, Indonesia, Iran, Malaysia, Mexico, Switzerland, and Thailand. The main aim of the studies was to explore the public health and clinical utility and feasibility of the proposed *CDDR* for disorders due to the use of psychoactive substances (Chapter 15) as well as the newly designated subgrouping of disorders due to addictive behaviors (gambling and gaming disorders; see Chapter 16). These mixed-methods studies involved more than 1,000 health professionals and included key informant surveys and interviews, focus groups, and consensus conferences at each study site. Overall, this section of the *ICD-11* was judged to be a major step forward compared with *ICD-10* in terms of utility for meeting clinical and public health needs and its feasibility for implementation. At the same time, a need for enhanced training was noted due to the increased the complexity of this part of the classification. The field studies also yielded specific suggestions for improving the material in the *CDDR* (e.g., better delineation of the boundaries among some diagnostic categories; improved descriptions of new categories).

Development of the *CDDR* also included the involvement of mental health service users through two studies in 15 countries representing diverse clinical contexts in multiple global regions (Askevis-Leherpeux et al., 2022; Hackmann et al., 2019). These studies were the first instance of a systematic research program studying mental health service users' perspectives during the revision of a major diagnostic classification system. The studies employed participatory research methodologies to examine service user perspectives on key *CDDR* diagnoses, including schizophrenia, depressive episode, bipolar type 1 disorder, generalized anxiety disorder, and personality disorder. Findings from these studies provided an understanding of how mental health service users responded to the diagnostic content of the *CDDR*. They served as a basis for recommendations to WHO about potential enhancements of *CDDR* diagnostic material that could enhance its clinical utility (e.g., usefulness in communicating with service users) and mitigate potential unintended negative consequences of the diagnostic material, including stigmatization of diagnosed individuals. They have also provided important perspectives on how the diagnostic process in health systems might be reformed to improve service user experience and outcomes as a part of the implementation of the *ICD-11*.

CULTURAL FACTORS IN THE *CDDR*

The development and testing of the *ICD-11 CDDR* was the "most global, multilingual, multidisciplinary and participative revision process ever implemented for a classification of mental disorders" (Reed et al., 2019, p. 4). On the basis of this methodology, it is appropriate to state that a wide range of regional, linguistic, and cultural perspectives are intrinsic to the *CDDR* because they were substantially represented throughout the process and as a part of the authority structure responsible for making decisions and recommendations. This is also reflected in the broadly international authorship of the chapters of this book.

As discussed, the development of the *CDDR* emphasized the principle of global applicability—the need for the diagnostic manual to function well across global regions, countries, and languages. The *ICD-11* diagnostic requirements were not designed to emphasize the particularities of different cultural contexts but rather their commonalities, which were found to be substantial. For example, an early *ICD-11* field study examined how clinicians in eight countries (Brazil, China, India, Japan, Mexico, Nigeria, Spain, and the United States) conceptualized the taxonomical structure of mental disorders, with the goal of informing the structure of the *ICD-11* mental disorders classification (Reed et al., 2013). One study finding was that correlations among the structures of "natural taxonomies" of mental disorders produced by clinicians in different countries were extremely high (all > .90), and much higher than the correlation between the structures of the *ICD-10* and the fourth edition of the *Diagnostic and Statistical Manual of Mental Disorders* (*DSM-IV*).

Although the essential purpose of an international classification system is conveying information across diverse boundaries, it was also important to incorporate locally relevant material on clinically important cultural variations in presentation (Gureje et al., 2019) to enhance the clinical utility and global applicability of the *CDDR*. Culture is a fundamental part of conceptualizations of what constitutes normality and deviation from it; it influences coping and help-seeking, as well as the presentation and course of mental disorders (Gureje et al., 2020). Cultural factors also influence social policies that mitigate or exacerbate risks for mental disorders and influence access to care and where and from whom people seek it. Information that makes the diagnostic system more relevant and acceptable to clinicians and service users around the world can enhance the *CDDR*'s usefulness as a tool for identifying those who require care and connecting them to services.

The WHO Department of Mental Health and Substance Use appointed an *ICD-11* Working Group on Cultural Considerations. This working group formulated a series of questions to guide its inquiry and eventually provide a structure for the material on cultural considerations in the *CDDR*:

- Is there evidence that culture exerts a strong influence on the presentation of the disorder? For example, is there notable cross-cultural variation? Is a mechanism known for how culture might influence the symptoms or presentation of the disorder?

- Is there evidence that the prevalence of the disorder is particularly high or low in specific populations? What caveats should be considered in interpreting these data (e.g., misattribution of symptoms by clinicians unfamiliar with cultural expressions of distress)? Is it possible to link prevalence variation to information on mechanisms (e.g., available data suggesting that prevalence of anorexia nervosa is higher in societies where thinness is idealized)?

- What are the cultural concepts of distress (idioms, syndromes, explanations/causes) identified in various cultural groups that are related to the disorder? (Gureje et al., 2019, p. 357)

To address these questions, the working group systematically reviewed the literature on cultural influences on diagnosis and psychopathology for each diagnostic category, as well as relevant material on culture from *ICD-10* and the fifth edition of the *DSM*. It also conducted extensive consultations with experts from around the world. On this basis, the working group developed a section titled "Culture-Related Features" for all diagnostic categories in the *CDDR* for which sufficient evidence was available. The working group's focus was to provide pragmatic and actionable material to assist clinicians in using the *CDDR* to evaluate patients in a culturally informed manner and reduce bias in clinical decision-making. The guidance on culture-related features was intended to be of practical use in engagement, diagnosis, evaluation, and treatment selection. It supports more informed decisions likely to foster more contextually applicable patient-centered care that is sensitive to the cultural and social context of the clinical encounter (Gureje et al., 2019, 2020). The authors of the chapters of this book were asked not to replicate information from the *CDDR*, but many chapters provide substantial additional information about cultural factors in presentation, assessment, and diagnosis.

THE *CDDR* AND GLOBAL MENTAL HEALTH

Global mental health "aims to alleviate mental suffering through the prevention, care and treatment of mental and substance use disorders, and to promote and sustain the mental health of individuals and communities around the world" (Collins, 2020, p. 265). As a field, global mental health prioritizes equity, and is particularly focused on "disparities in provision of care and respect for human rights of people living with mental disorders between rich and poor countries" (Patel & Prince, 2010, p. 1976). Global mental health is an interdisciplinary field, and particularly encompasses the work of many psychologists in prevention, treatment, research, and policy. Advocacy is a central element of global mental health, particularly in terms of translating evidence to actionable and scalable policies and plans for communities, health systems, and policymakers (Collins, 2020).

This way of thinking about global mental health is completely aligned with the WHO's public mental health strategy, of which the *ICD-11* and *CDDR* are important parts. The *CDDR* facilitate early and accurate diagnosis of mental disorders, helping to reduce the still enormous gap between the number of people who need treatment and the number who receive it (Alonso et al., 2018; Degenhardt et al., 2017; Kohn et al., 2004; Thornicroft et al., 2017). In describing the conceptual foundations for developing the *ICD-11* classification of mental, behavioral, and neurodevelopmental disorders, the International Advisory Group (2011) stated, "People are only likely to have access to the most appropriate mental health services when the conditions that define eligibility and treatment selection are supported by a precise, valid, and clinically useful classification system" (p. 89).

The WHO's (2021) *Comprehensive Mental Health Action Plan*, recently updated and extended to 2030, identifies mental health services as an essential component of health care and universal health coverage. The action plan specifically refers to mental disorders as they are defined and described in the *CDDR* as the focus of the services that must be covered, along with evidence-based interventions to prevent or mitigate the progression of incipient disorders (e.g., for dementia, disorders due to substance use, and suicide). These areas are consistent with the work of most mental health professionals. Moreover, the action plan addresses mental health, "conceptualized as a state of well-being in which the individual realizes his or her own abilities, can cope with the normal stresses of life, can work productively and fruitfully, and is able to make a contribution to his or her community" (p. 1). Finally, the action plan specifically mentions "social, cultural, economic, political and environmental factors such as national policies, social protection, living standards, working conditions, and community social supports" (p. 1) as determinants of mental health, drawing particular attention to exposure to adversity at a young age as an established preventable risk factor. Strategies for enhancing mental health and addressing structural inequities that contribute to mental health outcomes are generally not the focus of interventions by mental health professionals, although many are involved in education and advocacy to advance these causes. The action plan has four objectives, all of which are aligned with the *CDDR*: strengthening leadership and governance; providing integrated community-based mental health and social care; implementing strategies for promotion and prevention; and strengthening information systems, evidence, and research. The scope of the action plan makes clear that although the *CDDR* do not address the entire range of population mental health needs, they are extremely important as a framework for those who need treatment for mental disorders.

The action plan also identifies six cross-cutting principles and approaches that are intrinsic to the plan. Each of these can be linked to the innovations and improvements in the *CDDR* (Reed et al., 2019):

1. The *ICD-11 CDDR* support *universal health coverage* by defining and describing in objective and replicable terms the conditions that define eligibility and treatment selection for mental disorders.

2. The *ICD-11 CDDR* support *human rights* through the adoption of new approaches. For example, in the *ICD-11*, remaining *ICD-10* disorder categories related to sexual orientation have been eliminated (Cochran et al., 2014), and transgender identity is no longer defined as a mental disorder (Reed et al., 2016). Diagnostic specifiers for schizophrenia and other primary psychotic disorders place emphasis on current status and needs for treatment in ways that are more consistent with recovery-based approaches (Gaebel, 2012).

3. The *ICD-11 CDDR* incorporate substantial advances in *evidence-based practice* based on extensive reviews by the working groups, as described earlier in this chapter, and taking cultural considerations into account (Gureje et al., 2019, 2020).

4. The *ICD-11 CDDR* take a *life-course approach* to the diagnosis of mental disorders. The material provided for each disorder category—to the extent possible based on available evidence—describes its manifestations in early and middle childhood, adolescence, and older adulthood. Information about adult presentations of categories previously characterized as childhood disorders (e.g., attention deficit hyperactivity disorder; separation anxiety disorder) is also provided.

5. The WHO Department of Mental Health and Substance Use adopted a *multisectoral approach* to the development of the *ICD-11 CDDR*, as described earlier in this chapter.

6. The *ICD-11 CDDR* support *empowerment of persons with mental disorders and psychosocial disabilities* by systematically incorporating, for the first time, service user perspectives in the development of a major classification of mental disorders (Askevis-Leherpeux et al., 2022; Hackmann et al., 2019).

THE IMPORTANCE OF A GLOBAL APPROACH TO PSYCHOLOGICAL PRACTICE

Psychology is central to the global mental health movement. According to WHO's (2016) *Global Mental Health Gap Action Programme Guidelines*, psychological treatments are recommended as the first-line treatments for the majority of mental and substance use disorders and for many are the only recommended treatment. In summarizing the evidence for these psychological treatments, Vikram Patel (2019) wrote that there is

> impressive evidence of (their) acceptability and effectiveness for a range of mental health problems across the life course and in diverse contexts and for a range of goals from promotion and prevention, to the treatment of acute phases of illness, to rehabilitation and recovery. The effect sizes from a range of meta-analyses for these interventions often range from moderate to large, and the occurrence of side effects is rare. (p. xv)

In most countries, however, access to these treatments is limited, covering less than 10% of the population. It is critical for psychologists to know these treatments, not only to deliver them personally where this is possible but also to be able to train and supervise less specialized providers to implement them through task-sharing arrangements. A description of psychotherapy approaches is beyond the scope of this book; however, their sophisticated application depends in part on an understanding of the diagnostic framework, including the psychological characteristics and mechanisms of specific disorders and disorder groupings described in subsequent chapters of this book, as well as an understanding of the common factors in their effective treatment (Wampold, 2015).

Another reason that a global approach is essential relates to steady increases in global international migration over the past two decades (United Nations, 2021). Forced displacement across international borders of people fleeing conflict, persecution, violence, or human rights violations has also continued to rise. Whereas most refugees are hosted in low- and middle-income countries, international migrants made up 15% of the population of high-income countries in 2020. Although the pattern of migration varies substantially by region and country income level, mental health professionals must have the skills to evaluate, diagnose, and treat individuals with national, ethnic, and linguistic backgrounds different from their own.

In this context, a global approach, combined with cultural humility, is essential for assessment, diagnosis, case conceptualization, and treatment. Although this has long been apparent to people in many regions of the world, the American Psychological Association (APA) has also affirmed an international perspective as a basic requirement for competent psychological practice. One of the core guidelines of APA's (2017) multicultural guidelines states: "Psychologists endeavor to examine the profession's assumptions and practices within an international context, whether domestically or internationally based, and consider how this globalization has an impact on the psychologist's self-definition, purpose, role, and function" (p. 5). A global approach has also been increasingly discussed, if not yet fully implemented, in psychology education and training (Khoury & De Castro Pecanha, 2023; Silbereisen et al., 2014).

CONCLUSIONS

The chapters of this book lay out how the *ICD-11* classification of mental, behavioral, and neurodevelopmental disorders and its accompanying manual for implementation by mental health professionals in clinical settings—the *CDDR*—meet the moment as a global classification system that is consistent with a psychological approach. It was developed by the world's foremost public health agency as a global public good through a multidisciplinary and multilingual process that involved hundreds of experts and thousands of clinicians from around the world. It was approved by a governing body comprising the ministers/secretaries of health from 194 WHO member countries.

The *CDDR* were developed and field tested based on the goal of providing mental health professionals with a comprehensive, clinically useful guide to implementation of the *ICD-11* classification of mental, behavioral, and neurodevelopmental disorders that is more clinician-friendly, less concretely algorithmic, and less pseudo-precise in its operationalizations with the explicit goal of leaving room for cultural variation and clinical judgment in the context of individual needs and local circumstances. Some authors have expressed concern that due to this approach the *CDDR* are inherently less reliable (see Stein et al., 2020), but the reliability results from our clinic-based field studies challenge this assertion (Reed, Sharan, Rebello, Keeley, Medina-Mora, et al., 2018). Rather than continuing to devote attention and resources to introducing greater precision in operationalization as a part of successive refinements in diagnostic criteria, we suggest that further gains in reliability among clinicians could best be obtained by focusing greater attention on appropriate training in diagnostic concepts, skills, and interviewing techniques. We believe that this volume will help to advance the field toward that goal.

REFERENCES

Alonso, J., Liu, Z., Evans-Lacko, S., Sadikova, E., Sampson, N., Chatterji, S., Abdulmalik, J., Aguilar-Gaxiola, S., Al-Hamzawi, A., Andrade, L. H., Bruffaerts, R., Cardoso, G., Cia, A., Florescu, S., de Girolamo, G., Gureje, O., Haro, J. M., He, Y., de Jonge, P., . . . the WHO World Mental Health Survey Collaborators. (2018). Treatment gap for anxiety disorders is global: Results of the World Mental Health Surveys in 21 countries. *Depression and Anxiety, 35*(3), 195–208. https://doi.org/10.1002/da.22711

American Psychological Association. (2017). *Multicultural guidelines: An ecological approach to context, identity, and intersectionality.* https://www.apa.org/about/policy/multicultural-guidelines.pdf

Askevis-Leherpeux, F., Hazo, J. B., Agoub, M., Baleige, A., Barikova, V., Benmessaoud, D., Brunet, F., Carta, M. G., Castelpietra, G., Crepaz-Keay, D., Daumerie, N., Demassiet, V., Fontaine, A., Grigutyte, N., Guernut, M., Kishore, J., Kiss, M., Koenig, M., Laporta, M., . . . Roelandt, J. L. (2022). Accessibility of psychiatric vocabulary: An international study about schizophrenia essential features. *Schizophrenia Research, 243*, 463–464. https://doi.org/10.1016/j.schres.2022.03.001

Claudino, A. M., Pike, K. M., Hay, P., Keeley, J. W., Evans, S. C., Rebello, T. J., Bryant-Waugh, R., Dai, Y., Zhao, M., Matsumoto, C., Herscovici, C. R., Mellor-Marsá, B., Stona, A. C., Kogan, C. S., Andrews, H. F., Monteleone, P., Pilon, D. J., Thiels, C., Sharan, P., . . . Reed, G. M. (2019). The classification of feeding and eating disorders in the *ICD-11*: Results of a field study comparing proposed *ICD-11* guidelines with existing *ICD-10* guidelines. *BMC Medicine, 17*(1), 93. https://doi.org/10.1186/s12916-019-1327-4

Cochran, S. D., Drescher, J., Kismödi, E., Giami, A., García-Moreno, C., Atalla, E., Marais, A., Vieira, E. M., & Reed, G. M. (2014). Proposed declassification of disease categories related to sexual orientation in the *International Statistical Classification of Diseases and Related Health Problems* (*ICD-11*). *Bulletin of the World Health Organization, 92*, 672–679. https://doi.org/10.2471/BLT.14.135541

Collins, P. Y. (2020). What is global mental health? *World Psychiatry, 19*(3), 265–266. https://doi.org/10.1002/wps.20728

Degenhardt, L., Glantz, M., Evans-Lacko, S., Sadikova, E., Sampson, N., Thornicroft, G., Aguilar-Gaxiola, S., Al-Hamzawi, A., Alonso, J., Andrade, L. H., Bruffaerts, R., Bunting, B., Bromet, E. J., Caldas de Almeida, J. M., de Girolamo, G., Florescu, S., Gureje, O., Maria Haro, J., Huang, Y., . . . the World Health Organization's World Mental Health Surveys Collaborators. (2017). Estimating treatment coverage for people with substance use disorders: An analysis of data from the World Mental Health Surveys. *World Psychiatry, 16*(3), 299–307. https://doi.org/10.1002/wps.20457

Evans, S. C., Reed, G. M., Roberts, M. C., Esparza, P., Watts, A. D., Correia, J. M., Ritchie, P., Maj, M., & Saxena, S. (2013). Psychologists' perspectives on the diagnostic classification of mental disorders: Results from the WHO-IUPsyS global survey. *International Journal of Psychology, 48*(3), 177–193. https://doi.org/10.1080/00207594.2013.804189

Evans, S. C., Roberts, M. C., Keeley, J. W., Blossom, J. B., Amaro, C. M., Garcia, A. M., Stough, C. O., Canter, K. S., Robles, R., & Reed, G. M. (2015). Vignette methodologies for studying clinicians' decision-making: Validity, utility, and application in *ICD-11* field studies. *International Journal of Clinical and Health Psychology*, *15*(2), 160–170. https://doi.org/10.1016/j.ijchp.2014.12.001

First, M. B., Rebello, T. J., Keeley, J. W., Bhargava, R., Dai, Y., Kulygina, M., Matsumoto, C., Robles, R., Stona, A.-C., & Reed, G. M. (2018). Do mental health professionals use diagnostic classifications the way we think they do? A global survey. *World Psychiatry*, *17*(2), 187–195. https://doi.org/10.1002/wps.20525

First, M. B., Reed, G. M., Hyman, S. E., & Saxena, S. (2015). The development of the *ICD-11* clinical descriptions and diagnostic guidelines for mental and behavioural disorders. *World Psychiatry*, *14*(1), 82–90. https://doi.org/10.1002/wps.20189

Gaebel, W. (2012). Status of psychotic disorders in the *ICD-11*. *Schizophrenia Bulletin*, *38*(5), 895–898. https://doi.org/10.1093/schbul/sbs104

GBD 2019 Mental Disorders Collaborators. (2022). Global, regional, and national burden of 12 mental disorders in 204 countries and territories, 1990–2019: A systematic analysis for the Global Burden of Disease Study 2019. *The Lancet Psychiatry*, *9*(2), 137–150. https://doi.org/10.1016/S2215-0366(21)00395-3

Guler, J., Roberts, M. C., Medina-Mora, M. E., Robles, R., Gureje, O., Keeley, J. W., Kogan, C., Sharan, P., Khoury, B., Pike, K. M., Kulygina, M., Krasnov, V. N., Matsumoto, C., Stein, D., Min, Z., Maruta, T., & Reed, G. M. (2018). Global collaborative team performance for the revision of the *International Classification of Diseases*: A case study of the World Health Organization Field Studies Coordination Group. *International Journal of Clinical and Health Psychology*, *18*(3), 189–200. https://doi.org/10.1016/j.ijchp.2018.07.001

Gureje, O., Lewis-Fernandez, R., Hall, B. J., & Reed, G. M. (2019). Systematic inclusion of culture-related information in *ICD-11*. *World Psychiatry*, *18*(3), 357–358. https://doi.org/10.1002/wps.20676

Gureje, O., Lewis-Fernandez, R., Hall, B. J., & Reed, G. M. (2020). Cultural considerations in the classification of mental disorders: Why and how in *ICD-11*. *BMC Medicine*, *18*(1), 25. https://doi.org/10.1186/s12916-020-1493-4

Hackmann, C., Balhara, Y. P. S., Clayman, K., Nemec, P. B., Notley, C., Pike, K., Reed, G. M., Sharan, P., Rana, M. S., Silver, J., Swarbrick, M., Wilson, J., Zeilig, H., & Shakespeare, T. (2019). Perspectives on *ICD-11* to understand and improve mental health diagnosis using expertise by experience (INCLUDE Study): An international qualitative study. *The Lancet Psychiatry*, *6*(9), 778–785. https://doi.org/10.1016/S2215-0366(19)30093-8

International Advisory Group for the Revision of *ICD-10* Mental and Behavioural Disorders. (2011). A conceptual framework for the revision of the *ICD-10* classification of mental and behavioural disorders. *World Psychiatry*, *10*(2), 86–92. https://doi.org/10.1002/j.2051-5545.2011.tb00022.x

Keeley, J. W., Reed, G. M., Roberts, M. C., Evans, S. C., Medina-Mora, M. E., Robles, R., Rebello, T., Sharan, P., Gureje, O., First, M. B., Andrews, H. F., Ayuso-Mateos, J. L., Gaebel, W., Zielasek, J., & Saxena, S. (2016). Developing a science of clinical utility in diagnostic classification systems field study strategies for *ICD-11* mental and behavioral disorders. *American Psychologist*, *71*(1), 3–16. https://doi.org/10.1037/a0039972

Keeley, J. W., Reed, G. M., Roberts, M. C., Evans, S. C., Robles, R., Matsumoto, C., Brewin, C. R., Cloitre, M., Perkonigg, A., Rousseau, C., Gureje, O., Lovell, A. M., Sharan, P., & Maercker, A. (2016). Disorders specifically associated with stress: A case-controlled field study for *ICD-11* mental and behavioural disorders. *International Journal of Clinical and Health Psychology*, *16*(2), 109–127. https://doi.org/10.1016/j.ijchp.2015.09.002

Khoury, B., & De Castro Pecanha, V. (2023). Transforming psychology education to include global mental health. Cambridge Prisms. *Global Mental Health*, *10*, e17. https://doi.org/10.1017/gmh.2023.11

Kogan, C. S., Stein, D. J., Rebello, T. J., Keeley, J. W., Chan, K. J., Fineberg, N. A., Fontenelle, L. F., Grant, J. E., Matsunaga, H., Simpson, H. B., Thomsen, P. H., van den Heuvel, O. A., Veale, D., Grenier, J., Kulygina, M., Matsumoto, C., Domínguez-Martínez, T., Stona, A. C., Wang, Z., & Reed, G. M. (2020). Accuracy of diagnostic judgments using *ICD-11* vs. *ICD-10* diagnostic guidelines for obsessive-compulsive and related disorders. *Journal of Affective Disorders, 273*, 328–340. https://doi.org/10.1016/j.jad.2020.03.103

Kohn, R., Saxena, S., Levav, I., & Saraceno, B. (2004). The treatment gap in mental health care. *Bulletin of the World Health Organization, 82*(11), 858–866.

Lemay, K. R., Kogan, C. S., Rebello, T. J., Keeley, J. W., Bhargava, R., Sharan, P., Sharma, M., Kommu, J. V. S., Kishore, M. T., de Jesus Mari, J., Ginige, P., Buono, S., Recupero, M., Zingale, M., Zagaria, T., Cooray, S., Roy, A., & Reed, G. M. (2022). An international field study of the *ICD-11* behavioural indicators for disorders of intellectual development. *Journal of Intellectual Disability Research, 66*(4), 376–391. https://doi.org/10.1111/jir.12924

Medina-Mora, M. E., Robles, R., Rebello, T. J., Domínguez, T., Martínez, N., Juárez, F., Sharan, P., & Reed, G. M. (2019). *ICD-11* guidelines for psychotic, mood, anxiety and stress-related disorders in Mexico: Clinical utility and reliability. *International Journal of Clinical and Health Psychology, 19*(1), 1–11. https://doi.org/10.1016/j.ijchp.2018.09.003

Patel, V. (2019). Foreword. In D. J. Stein, J. K. Bass, & S. G. Hofmann (Eds.), *Global mental health and psychotherapy: Adapting psychotherapy for low- and middle-income countries* (pp. xv–xvii). Academic Press. https://doi.org/10.1016/B978-0-12-814932-4.09999-7

Patel, V., & Prince, M. (2010). Global mental health: A new global health field comes of age. *JAMA, 303*, 1976–1977. https://doi.org/10.1001/jama.2010.616

Reed, G. M. (2010). Toward *ICD-11*: Improving the clinical utility of WHO's International Classification of mental disorders. *Professional Psychology, Research and Practice, 41*(6), 457–464. https://doi.org/10.1037/a0021701

Reed, G. M., Drescher, J., Krueger, R. B., Atalla, E., Cochran, S. D., First, M. B., Cohen-Kettenis, P. T., Arango-de Montis, I., Parish, S. J., Cottler, S., Briken, P., & Saxena, S. (2016). Disorders related to sexuality and gender identity in the *ICD-11*: Revising the *ICD-10* classification based on current scientific evidence, best clinical practices, and human rights considerations. *World Psychiatry, 15*(3), 205–221. https://doi.org/10.1002/wps.20354

Reed, G. M., First, M. B., Kogan, C. S., Hyman, S. E., Gureje, O., Gaebel, W., Maj, M., Stein, D. J., Maercker, A., Tyrer, P., Claudino, A., Garralda, E., Salvador-Carulla, L., Ray, R., Saunders, J. B., Dua, T., Poznyak, V., Medina-Mora, M. E., Pike, K. M., . . . Saxena, S. (2019). Innovations and changes in the *ICD-11* classification of mental, behavioural and neurodevelopmental disorders. *World Psychiatry, 18*(1), 3–19. https://doi.org/10.1002/wps.20611

Reed, G. M., Mendonça Correia, J., Esparza, P., Saxena, S., & Maj, M. (2011). The WPA-WHO global survey of psychiatrists' attitudes towards mental disorders classification. *World Psychiatry, 10*(2), 118–131. https://doi.org/10.1002/j.2051-5545.2011.tb00034.x

Reed, G. M., Rebello, T. J., Pike, K. M., Medina-Mora, M. E., Gureje, O., Zhao, M., Dai, Y., Roberts, M. C., Maruta, T., Matsumoto, C., Krasnov, V. N., Kulygina, M., Lovell, A. M., Stona, A. C., Sharan, P., Robles, R., Gaebel, W., Zielasek, J., Khoury, B., . . . Saxena, S. (2015). WHO's Global Clinical Practice Network for mental health. *The Lancet Psychiatry, 2*(5), 379–380. https://doi.org/10.1016/S2215-0366(15)00183-2

Reed, G. M., Roberts, M. C., Keeley, J., Hooppell, C., Matsumoto, C., Sharan, P., Robles, R., Carvalho, H., Wu, C., Gureje, O., Leal-Leturia, I., Flanagan, E. H., Correia, J. M., Maruta, T., Ayuso-Mateos, J. L., de Jesus Mari, J., Xiao, Z., Evans, S. C., Saxena, S., & Medina-Mora, M. E. (2013). Mental health professionals' natural taxonomies of mental disorders: Implications for the clinical utility of the *ICD-11* and the *DSM-5*. *Journal of Clinical Psychology, 69*(12), 1191–1212. https://doi.org/10.1002/jclp.22031

Reed, G. M., Sharan, P., Rebello, T. J., Keeley, J. W., Gureje, O., Ayuso-Mateos, J. L., Kanba, S., Khoury, B., Kogan, C. S., Krasnov, V. N., Maj, M., de Jesus Mari, J., Stein, D. S., Zhao, M., Akiyama, T., Andrews, H. F., Asevedo, E., Cheour, M., Domínguez-Martínez, T., . . . Medina-Mora, M. E. (2018). Clinical utility of *ICD-11* diagnostic guidelines for high-burden mental disorders: Results from mental health settings in 13 countries. *World Psychiatry, 17*(3), 306–315. https://doi.org/10.1002/wps.20581

Reed, G. M., Sharan, P., Rebello, T. J., Keeley, J. W., Medina-Mora, M. E., Gureje, O., Ayuso-Mateos, J. L., Kanba, S., Khoury, B., Kogan, C. S., Krasnov, V. N., Maj, M., de Jesus Mari, J., Stein, D. J., Zhao, M., Akiyama, T., Andrews, H. F., Asevedo, E., Cheour, M., . . . Pike, K. M. (2018). The *ICD-11* developmental field study of reliability of diagnoses of high-burden mental disorders: Results among adult patients in mental health settings of 13 countries. *World Psychiatry, 17*(2), 174–186. https://doi.org/10.1002/wps.20524

Rehm, J., & Shield, K. D. (2019). Global burden of disease and the impact of mental and addictive disorders. *Current Psychiatry Reports, 21*(2), 10. https://doi.org/10.1007/s11920-019-0997-0

Silbereisen, R. K., Ritchie, P. L.-J., & Pandey, J. (Eds.). (2014). *Psychology education and training: A global perspective.* Psychology Press/Routledge. https://doi.org/10.4324/9781315851532

Stein, D. J., Szatmari, P., Gaebel, W., Berk, M., Vieta, E., Maj, M., de Vries, Y. A., Roest, A. M., de Jonge, P., Maercker, A., Brewin, C. R., Pike, K. M., Grilo, C. M., Fineberg, N. A., Briken, P., Cohen-Kettenis, P. T., & Reed, G. M. (2020). Mental, behavioral and neurodevelopmental disorders in the *ICD-11*: An international perspective on key changes and controversies. *BMC Medicine, 18*(1), 21. https://doi.org/10.1186/s12916-020-1495-2

Thornicroft, G., Chatterji, S., Evans-Lacko, S., Gruber, M., Sampson, N., Aguilar-Gaxiola, S., Al-Hamzawi, A., Alonso, J., Andrade, L., Borges, G., Bruffaerts, R., Bunting, B., de Almeida, J. M., Florescu, S., de Girolamo, G., Gureje, O., Haro, J. M., He, Y., Hinkov, H., . . . Kessler, R. C. (2017). Undertreatment of people with major depressive disorder in 21 countries. *The British Journal of Psychiatry, 210*(2), 119–124. https://doi.org/10.1192/bjp.bp.116.188078

United Nations. (2021). *International migration 2020 highlights.* https://www.un.org/development/desa/pd/content/international-migration-2020-highlights

Wampold, B. E. (2015). How important are the common factors in psychotherapy? An update. *World Psychiatry, 14*(3), 270–277. https://doi.org/10.1002/wps.20238

World Health Organization. (1992). *The* ICD-10 *classification of mental and behavioural disorders: Clinical descriptions and diagnostic guidelines.* https://www.who.int/publications/i/item/9241544228

World Health Organization. (2016). *mhGAP intervention guide for mental, neurological and substance use disorders in non-specialized health settings: Mental health Gap Action Programme (mhGAP)—version 2.0.* https://www.who.int/publications/i/item/9789241549790

World Health Organization. (2019, May 25). *World Health Assembly update* [Press release]. https://www.who.int/news/item/25-05-2019-world-health-assembly-update

World Health Organization. (2020). *Basic documents* (49th ed., amended effective May 31, 2019). https://apps.who.int/gb/bd/

World Health Organization. (2021). *Comprehensive mental health action plan: 2013–2030.* https://www.who.int/publications/i/item/9789240031029

World Health Organization. (2022). *International statistical classification of diseases and related health problems (ICD).* https://www.who.int/standards/classifications/classification-of-diseases

World Health Organization. (2023). *ICD-11 for mortality and morbidity statistics* (Version: 01/2023). https://icd.who.int/browse11/l-m/en#/

World Health Organization. (2024). *Clinical descriptions and diagnostic requirements for ICD-11 mental, behavioural and neurodevelopmental disorders.* https://www.who.int/publications/i/item/9789240077263

DIAGNOSIS OF MENTAL AND BEHAVIORAL DISORDERS

3

Disorders of Intellectual Development and Developmental Learning Disorder

Ashok Roy and Cary S. Kogan

OVERARCHING LOGIC

The 11th revision of the *International Classification of Diseases* (*ICD-11*; World Health Organization [WHO], 2023) neurodevelopmental disorders grouping encompasses behavioral and cognitive disorders that have their onset during the developmental period and involve significant difficulties in the acquisition and execution of specific intellectual, motor, language, or social abilities. In the 10th revision of the *ICD* (*ICD-10*; WHO, 1992), these disorders were classified in a variety of groupings. This chapter focuses on two commonly diagnosed disorder categories included in the *ICD-11* grouping of neurodevelopmental disorders: disorders of intellectual development and developmental learning disorder. These disorders are treated together in a single chapter of this book because both rely on the analysis and synthesis of findings from standardized measures such as intelligence tests for their diagnosis. This is an important aspect of the practice of psychology.

Disorders of intellectual development in the *ICD-11* replace mental retardation in *ICD-10*. The change in terminology reflects the view that mental retardation is an unacceptably stigmatizing term (Salvador-Carulla et al., 2011). In contrast to the *ICD-10*, in which mental retardation was defined based on intellectual functioning and primarily assessed through the use of standardized intelligence tests (IQ), in *ICD-11* disorders of intellectual development are characterized by significant impairments in both intellectual and adaptive behavior

https://doi.org/10.1037/0000392-003
A Psychological Approach to Diagnosis: Using the ICD-11 as a Framework, G. M. Reed, P. L.-J. Ritchie, and A. Maercker (Editors)

functioning. That is, they are defined not only by significant limitations in intellectual functioning across various domains (e.g., perceptual reasoning, working memory, processing speed, and verbal comprehension) but also require that equal weight be given to adaptive behavior, which refers to the set of *conceptual, social,* and *practical* skills that are performed by people in their everyday lives.

Developmental learning disorder is characterized by limitations in acquiring academic skills—typically of reading, writing, or arithmetic—that result in a skill level markedly below what would be expected given the person's age, despite opportunities for appropriate academic instruction. These learning difficulties are not explained by a disorder of intellectual development, another neurodevelopmental disorder, or another condition such as a motor disorder or a sensory disorder of vision or hearing. They may affect academic skills narrowly (e.g., inability to master basic numeracy or to decode single words accurately and fluently) or may affect all of reading, writing, and arithmetic. In the *ICD-10,* these disorders were called specific developmental disorders of scholastic skills. The most important shift in conceptualization from the *ICD-10* to the *ICD-11* is that rather than describing each type of learning difficulty as a distinct disorder, the *ICD-11* recognizes that impairments in various underlying psychological processes are presumed to underlie a child's difficulty in learning academic skills. However, the precise relationship between these psychological processes and outcomes related to learning capacity is not yet sufficiently understood to form the basis for a clinically useful classification. Specific areas of academic difficulty (e.g., reading, mathematics, written expression) represent manifestations of the underlying psychological processes rather than discrete disorders. These specific areas are therefore treated as specifiers in the *ICD-11* and as many may be included as necessary to characterize the individual's presentation.

The presumptive etiologies for both disorders of intellectual development and developmental learning disorder are complex and varied. Both conditions are presumed to be primarily due to genetic or other factors that are present from birth. Disorders of intellectual development may also arise from injury, disease, or other insult to the central nervous system when this occurs during the developmental period. However, in many individual cases, the etiology is unknown; the *ICD-11* disorders of intellectual development and developmental learning disorder are still diagnosed in such cases. Indeed, these diagnoses are often needed for eligibility for numerous educational, social, and health services. If it is known, the presumptive causing condition should also be diagnosed (e.g., fragile X syndrome). The following sections address disorders of intellectual development first, followed by developmental learning disorder.

A PSYCHOLOGICAL APPROACH TO DISORDERS OF INTELLECTUAL DEVELOPMENT

As noted, the diagnosis of disorders of intellectual development is based on equal consideration of intellectual and adaptive functioning. *Adaptive functioning* refers to the set of skills that an individual acquires to negotiate their environment successfully, including their relationships. Adaptive functioning is operationalized as falling into three broad categories: conceptual skills, social skills, and practical skills. This model offers a more individualized and psychological approach to a relatively heterogeneous group of people with varied needs by prompting clinicians to consider strengths and weaknesses in the context of the individual's environment as a basis for determining needed supports and appropriate interventions (Salvador-Carulla et al., 2011; WHO, 2024). The consideration of contextual factors that may facilitate or impede an individual's functioning emphasizes inclusiveness and participation in society for affected individuals. It is also consistent with the United Nations Convention on the Rights of Persons with Disabilities that recognizes "the equal right of all persons with disabilities to live in the community, with choices equal to others, and shall take effective and appropriate measures to facilitate full enjoyment by persons with disabilities of this right and their full inclusion and participation in the community" (UN General Assembly, 2007).

The *ICD-11* also includes consideration of the implications of a diagnosis with respect to eligibility for services based on the individualized approach articulated earlier. Disorders of intellectual development are classified according to their severity (mild, moderate, severe, profound). In assigning a severity level, the clinician balances the consideration of both intellectual and adaptive functioning according to the nature and purpose of the assessment as well as the importance of the specific areas of assessment in relation to the individual's overall functioning (WHO, 2024). Consistent with the *ICD-11* approach, the American Association on Intellectual and Developmental Disabilities (AAIDD) has developed a multidimensional theoretical model in which disorders of intellectual development are placed on a continuum within the full spectrum human functioning (Luckasson & Schalock, 2013). The model includes health, participation, and context in relation to intellectual and adaptive behavior functioning in an effort to improve ideographic characterization of individual needs and the provision of appropriate supports to maximize inclusion and participation. The *ICD-11 Clinical Descriptions and Diagnostic Requirements for ICD-11 Mental, Behavioural and Neurodevelopmental Disorders* (*CDDR*; WHO, 2024) incorporate principles from the AAIDD model to improve matching needs with resources for affected individuals.

In the *ICD-10*, the severity of mental retardation was defined based solely on intellectual functioning, primarily assessed by using standardized intelligence tests. When the sole focus of the diagnosis is intellectual functioning, some individuals with greater deficits in adaptive functioning are likely to be denied access to mainstream and specialized services including educational, employment, and financial benefits. Moreover, specific types of behavior problems (e.g., aggression, self-injurious behavior, sexually inappropriate behavior) are the most common reason for referral to health care services for people with disorders of intellectual development, and many are prescribed psychoactive medications to control them (Cooray et al., 2015). A consideration of adaptive behavior skills and limitations can help identify contextual factors in behavior problems and develop tailored psychosocial interventions that may reduce the reliance on pharmacotherapy and their potential for adverse effects (Alexander et al., 2016; Tyrer et al., 2014).

The *ICD-11* emphasizes the importance of using standardized and appropriately normed tests to assess both intellectual and adaptive behavior functioning. However, in some settings, such measures are not available—for example, due to lack of resources or appropriately trained personnel to administer them or linguistic issues. In these circumstances, clinicians can use a set of behavioural indicators included in the *ICD-11* to assess the severity of intellectual and adaptive behavior functioning (Lemay et al., 2022; Tassé et al., 2019; WHO, 2024). The behavioural indicators tables are organized by developmental stage (i.e., early childhood, childhood/adolescence, and adulthood) and describe the behavioral manifestations of different levels of intellectual functioning as well as conceptual, social, and practical skills that are most commonly observed across cultures. Psychologists have particular training and expertise in psychological assessment, behavioral observation, and in understanding the relationship between environmental factors and behavior that can provide the basis for making major contributions to the health and well-being of people with disorders of intellectual development.

SEVERITY SPECIFIERS IN DISORDERS OF INTELLECTUAL DEVELOPMENT

Clinicians should assign the level of severity of a disorder of intellectual development (i.e., mild, moderate, severe, profound) according to the level at which the majority of the domains of the individual's intellectual ability and adaptive behavior skills fall. *ICD-11* defines a mild disorder of intellectual development as one in which the preponderance of intellectual and adaptive behavior functioning fall within 2 to 3 standard deviations of the mean, moderate as within 3 to 4 standard deviations of the mean, and severe and profound as 4 or more standard deviations below the mean. The differentiation between severe and profound disorders of intellectual development is based solely on adaptive behavior functioning because tests of intellectual functioning are not sufficiently sensitive at the lower end of the distribution to make this distinction. A provisional category is also available when reliable assessment of severity is not possible due to age (i.e., younger than 4 years old) or for other reasons (e.g., sensory/motor impairments).

In addition to test scores, the clinician should consider the nature and purpose of the assessment as well as the importance of specific areas of assessment in relation to the individual's overall functioning in assigning severity. For example, it may be appropriate to place greater emphasis on one domain of adaptive behavior skills if that skill is critical to determining eligibility of services for improving occupational functioning. This may occur in an individual with a history of a disorder of intellectual development who, with supports, has developed practical and conceptual skills in the average range but continues to have significant impairments in social functioning.

ASSESSMENT OF DISORDERS OF INTELLECTUAL DEVELOPMENT

Comprehensive assessment includes considering information from genetic testing if available; physical examination; and interviews of the patient, along with family and other caretakers, as well as professionals involved in providing care and treatment. Any problem behaviors that may be present can have a variety of functions such as gaining attention or avoiding a task, or may be a response to a noisy environment, pain, or low mood. A functional behavioral assessment that examines the relationship between antecedent factors, challenging behaviors, and consequences can help in formulating effective management strategies and provides a rational basis for treatment planning. Formulation and implementation of a treatment plan, even one aimed at reducing or eliminating disruptive behaviors, should be undertaken with the goal of improving affected individuals' quality of life. Ideally, intellectual functioning should be assessed using appropriately normed and standardized tests administered in an environment that ensures an accurate reflection of true abilities. Assessment of adaptive behavior functioning should also be assessed with standardized normed instruments and complemented with reports from caregivers and clinical observation.

Where appropriately normed and standardized tests are not available, diagnosis of disorders of intellectual development require greater reliance on clinical judgment based on appropriate evidence and assessment of behavioural indicators. The behavioural indicators tables were developed primarily to assist nonspecialists to determine the level of severity of a disorder of intellectual development as well as to help differentiate severe and profound levels of severity (Lemay et al., 2022; Tassé et al., 2019). In practice, the behavioural indicators tables can guide the clinical interview with a reliable informant (parent, caregiver, or teacher) in determining which level of functioning best fits the profile of the individual. This allows for a balanced and individualized assessment and judgment that can be reviewed longitudinally and with subsequent development of new skills and response to intervention.

The clinical assessment should also include determining whether any co-occurring mental and comorbid medical conditions are present, as well as information about current psychosocial stressors and behavior problems. Along with severity and etiology (if known), this additional information is important as a basis for the treatment and management plan. Behavior problems that may be relevant to a mental health evaluation include aggression toward others, self-injurious behavior, property destruction, and stereotyped behavior. These problems may be of sufficient intensity and severity to have a negative impact on social and academic performance as well as employment.

Depending on the setting, assessment may involve coordination of services across multiple disciplines including psychology, psychiatry, occupational therapy, speech and language therapy, and nursing. This approach is enhanced by working in partnership with parents, teachers, supervisors, and other caregivers to gain an understanding of the individual's functioning in a wide range of settings and the impact of interventions. Modification of the individual's environment should be considered and may have a major positive impact on problem behavior.

SCREENING FOR DISORDERS OF INTELLECTUAL DEVELOPMENT

Identifying people with disorders of intellectual development using population-based screening tools can be expensive and time-consuming. Lakhan and Mawson (2016) showed a high correlation between cases identified through focus group interviews in the communities where the young people lived and cases detected by using a standardized survey. They suggest that early engagement of communities tends to accelerate acceptance of subsequent support. In a systematic review, Fischer et al. (2014) found locally developed screening tools were feasible in early identification of developmental disabilities in low- and middle-income countries. These tools had acceptable sensitivity and specificity and were also feasible in terms of cost, access, and necessary training time and health worker time in daily use. The focus that *ICD-11* provides on both intellectual and adaptive behavior functioning with supporting behavioural indicators tables is anticipated to improve identification and appropriate severity rating.

DIFFERENTIAL DIAGNOSIS IN DISORDERS OF INTELLECTUAL DEVELOPMENT

Special care should be taken in differentiating disorders of intellectual development from normality when evaluating persons with communication, sensory, or motor impairments as well as those exhibiting behavioral disturbances; immigrants who may not yet have mastered the local language; persons with low literacy levels; persons with other mental disorders; persons undergoing health treatments (e.g., chemotherapeutic drugs); and persons who have experienced severe social or sensory deprivation. If not adequately addressed during the evaluation, these factors may reduce the validity of scores obtained on standardized or behavioral measures of intellectual and adaptive functioning. Sensory functioning should be assessed by a qualified practitioner to ensure that a deficit in acquisition of skills is not because of any sensory limitation (e.g., impaired visual or auditory acuity).

Another important differential diagnosis is with developmental learning disorder, which is distinguished from disorders of intellectual development by the presence of normal or near normal intellectual functioning alongside selective and specific areas of low academic achievement (see subsequent section on developmental learning disorder). Unlike disorders of intellectual development, the impairments observed in developmental learning disorder are not generalized across all areas of achievement. People with autism spectrum disorder are also sometimes misidentified as having a disorder of intellectual development based on significant impairments in social functioning including pragmatic language. Pragmatic language refers to the understanding and use of language in social contexts—for example, making inferences, understanding verbal humor, and resolving ambiguous meaning. The differentiation between these two disorders can be aided by using tests of intellectual functioning that do not rely on skills directly affected by autism spectrum disorder (e.g., nonverbal compared with verbal tests). Considering whether the core features of autism spectrum disorder (persistent deficits in social communication and social interaction; and repetitive stereotyped patterns of behaviors and interests) are present across multiple contexts is also important in making this distinction. Developmental speech and language disorders may co-occur with disorders of intellectual development but should only be diagnosed if speech and language abilities are significantly below what would be expected based on the individual's level of intellectual and adaptive behavior functioning.

CO-OCCURRING DISORDERS IN DISORDERS OF INTELLECTUAL DEVELOPMENT

Co-occurrence of other mental disorders is often underdetected in individuals with disorders of intellectual development. When mental disorders are suspected in this population, it is typically because the individual is exhibiting changes in behavior, particularly disruptive behavior. However, in many cases, changes in behavior may be due to physical illness, difficulties in communication, environmental changes, or can be a reaction to stressful circumstances or frustration rather than a co-occurring mental disorder.

Individuals with autism spectrum disorder frequently present with limitations in intellectual and adaptive behavior functioning, and when the diagnostic requirements are met, a diagnosis of a disorder of intellectual development at the corresponding level of severity along with a diagnosis of autism spectrum disorder is assigned. In these circumstances, the *ICD-11 CDDR* indicate that determination of the level of severity of the disorder of intellectual development should be more reliant on the conceptual and practical domains of adaptive behavior functioning, giving less weight to social skill abilities, because social communication deficits are a characteristic feature of autism spectrum disorder (WHO, 2024). Rates of co-occurring attention deficit hyperactivity disorder (ADHD) in individuals with a disorder of intellectual development diagnosis are significantly higher than in the general population. When inattention and/or hyperactivity–impulsivity are significantly beyond what would be expected based on age and the level of intellectual functioning in an individual with a disorder of intellectual development, a co-occurring diagnosis of ADHD may be considered.

A variety of other mental disorders are known to occur at higher rates among individuals affected by disorders of intellectual development compared with the general population (e.g., anxiety or fear-related disorders, depressive disorders, schizophrenia and other primary psychotic disorders, impulse control disorders, dementia). Schizophrenia, for example, is 3 times more common among people with a disorder of intellectual development compared with the general population (Morgan et al., 2008). The *ICD-11 CDDR* emphasize that assessments should be conducted with methods that are appropriate to the individual's level of intellectual functioning. Self-report may be less reliable among affected individuals because it can lead to under-reporting of symptoms of other mental disorders. Therefore, observable signs or reports by caregivers or individuals close to the person being assessed may provide a more accurate understanding.

Medical conditions that occur more frequently in people with a disorder of intellectual development than in the general population include problems related to poor dental and oral hygiene, epilepsy, gastrointestinal problems, respiratory disease, sensory and motor impairments, and feeding and eating problems. Clinicians assessing and managing mental disorders in people with disorders of intellectual development should guard against diagnostic over-shadowing where symptoms and signs of other mental disorders or medical conditions are wrongly attributed to the disorder of intellectual development rather than a separate condition. This can deprive the affected individual of effective and sometimes lifesaving treatment.

PREVALENCE OF DISORDERS OF INTELLECTUAL DEVELOPMENT

Maulik et al. (2011) estimated the global prevalence of disorders of intellectual development to fall between 0.9% to 1%. The prevalence in low- and middle-income countries is almost double that of high-income countries, though some prevalence figures may not be reliable. Higher prevalence in low- and middle-income countries is likely due to exposure to greater adversity and fewer resources to prevent or treat perinatal health conditions that may be associated with disorders of intellectual development.

CULTURAL AND OTHER CONTEXTUAL ISSUES IN DISORDERS OF INTELLECTUAL DEVELOPMENT

Changing terminology used to describe disorders of intellectual development over time has resulted in inconsistent identification of those meeting diag-nostic requirements across settings and countries (Maulik et al., 2011). Diag-nosis of disorders of intellectual development in low-resource settings is influenced by characteristics including accessibility to educational opportuni-ties and cultural differences that influence measurement of intellectual and adaptive behavior functioning. Socioenvironmental factors influence peoples' adaptive capacity, making the assessment of people with mild and moderate disorder of intellectual development particularly challenging (Odiyoor & Jaydeokar, 2019). This is because access to fewer resources in the form of educational, psychological, and medical supports contributes to greater severity of the disorder. In evaluating adaptive functioning—that is, the individual's conceptual, social, and practical skills—the expectations of the individual's culture and social environment should be taken to account.

The cultural appropriateness of tests and norms used to assess these key diagnostic elements should be considered for each person being assessed. Cultural biases in test-item construction have been shown to affect performance on tests of intelligence and adaptive behavior functioning (e.g., reference in test items to terminology or objects not common to a culture or minority group within the population). Moreover, translation of standardized measures without appropriate norms limits the validity of test results. Finally, an individual's proficiency in the language of the test must be considered when interpreting test results, in terms of both whether the individual understood the instructions as well as its impact on verbal performance. The behavioural indicators tables included in the *ICD-11* were developed with these limitations in mind and aim to reduce cultural loading of items for universal applicability in cases where standardized, normed tests are not available.

DIFFERENCES BETWEEN *ICD-11* DISORDER OF INTELLECTUAL DEVELOPMENT AND *DSM-5* INTELLECTUAL DISABILITY

Kishore et al. (2019) produced clinical practice guidelines that describe the key differences between the main diagnostic systems, including the fifth edition of the *Diagnostic and Statistical Manual of Mental Disorders* (*DSM-5*) and *ICD-11*. The *DSM-5* category intellectual disability is equivalent to disorders of intellectual development in the *ICD-11*. A critically important difference between the *ICD-11* and the *DSM-5* relates to how the level of severity is determined. Specifically, whereas *ICD-11* incorporates information about both intellectual functioning and adaptive behavior, *DSM-5* relies solely on adaptive behavior functioning. This may result in certain individuals with average intellectual functioning inappropriately receiving a diagnosis of intellectual disability under *DSM-5*. Furthermore, the *ICD-11* provides separate behavioural indicators tables according to the age of the individual. These tables also offer much more detail than the table included in *DSM-5* for determining severity. The *ICD-11* tables provide consistent information about the behaviors expected to be observed at different stages of development for each of the four severity levels, whereas the *DSM-5* table provides only general guidance for some levels of severity. The *ICD-11* behavioural indicators tables have been shown to have a high level of clinical utility as well as excellent psychometric properties (Lemay et al., 2022).

A PSYCHOLOGICAL APPROACH TO DEVELOPMENTAL LEARNING DISORDER

As mentioned in the chapter overview, developmental learning disorder is defined by significant and persistent limitations in learning academic skills that arise during the developmental period despite adequate opportunities to acquire these skills. Early identification of developmental learning disorder is essential for providing appropriate supports to children and their families to improve learning trajectories and socioemotional well-being. However, some individuals with developmental learning disorder are able to overcome these limitations through significant additional effort and, as a result, may only be identified later in life when demands exceed their capacity to compensate.

In *ICD-11*, developmental learning disorder is conceptualized as a single disorder in which the affected specific areas of academic skill(s) are described using one or more of several possible specifiers (i.e., reading, mathematics, written expression, other specified; see the subsequent specifiers section). In the *ICD-10*, separate disorder categories were available for each affected academic skill, which suggested distinct underlying pathologies. The rationale for consolidating multiple *ICD-10* disorders under a single overarching disorder construct is based on evidence for high rates of co-occurrence of affected skill areas, especially when tracked across development (Tannock, 2013) as well as genetic studies demonstrating shared variance of skill-based subtypes (e.g., Willcutt et al., 2010). The conceptualization of developmental learning disorder as a single disorder with overlapping manifestations influenced by an underlying shared set of psychological processes is more consistent with the available evidence. Moreover, emphasizing the current manifestation of the disorder at the time of assessment using specifiers imparts greater clinical utility for planning immediate interventions because targeted interventions for specific academic skills appear to produce better outcomes than general approaches (see Tannock, 2013).

Historically, learning disorders have been diagnosed based of the presence of a discrepancy between ability on the one hand, as measured by tests of intelligence, and achievement on the other, based on tests of scholastic skills or academic achievement. However, this approach has been demonstrated to have poor diagnostic validity (Stanovich, 2005). Ability–achievement discrepancies are poor predictors of impairment (e.g., Lovett et al., 2009) and of learning outcomes (e.g., Flowers et al., 2001). There are also practical, statistical, and psychometric limits to measuring the ability–achievement gap that results in high levels of both false positives and false negatives (e.g., Cotton et al., 2005; Francis et al., 2005). Discrepancies in ability–achievement are subject to normal variability in test scores, regression to the mean, and measurement error across development, leading to poor differentiation between typically developing individuals and those with a developmental learning disorder (e.g., Brooks, 2011). Finally, there is no established empirical basis for setting a specific threshold for the magnitude of the discrepancy.

Another feature that had previously been considered important in diagnosis was whether a child had failed to respond to educational interventions targeting gaps in achievement. The rationale was that children who improve with intervention were considered to have likely not been receiving appropriate educational instruction rather than being affected by a developmental learning disorder, whereas those who did not respond were the true cases. However, there is no consensus on the specific content of evidence-based instructional programs for developmental learning disorder that would constitute an adequate intervention trial, and such programs are not universally available. In addition, failure to respond to intervention results in unacceptably high false-positive rates because factors other than a developmental learning disorder potentially explain continuing difficulties in acquiring academic skills (e.g., attentional problems, inadequate intervention; Fuchs & Vaughn, 2012). Finally, there is a lack of evidence for what constitutes a sufficient response to instructional intervention that would allow one to preclude a developmental learning disorder diagnosis.

Therefore, although the *ICD-11 CDDR* indicate that developmental learning disorder should only be diagnosed if adequate opportunities to acquire academic skills have been provided, the diagnostic requirements focus on significant and persistent limitations in skill acquisition, resulting in a skill level that is markedly below what would be expected for age. This provides a clinically useful starting point for developing a comprehensive individualized psychological case formulation. Typically, an individual comes to clinical attention because of repeated underperformance in a particular subject at school (e.g., failing grades in mathematics), with average performance in other subjects. The *ICD-11* requirements are intended to ensure that underperformance is not limited to a particular context (e.g., a given teacher). Examination of school records can assist in determining persistence of difficulties with skill acquisition.

Whether significant limitations in academic skills exist is determined using normed, standardized measures of academic achievement (e.g., the Wechsler Individual Achievement Test). The Additional Clinical Features section of the *ICD-11 CDDR* acknowledge that psychological processes (e.g., phonological awareness, executive functions, perceptual motor integration) likely underlie observed academic skill deficits. However, current evidence does not yet allow for an accurate and clinically useful classification of developmental learning disorder based on these processes (Tannock, 2013). Therefore, caution is advised not to assume a one-to-one correspondence between psychological processes and any given deficit in learning. For example, in individuals with reading difficulties, the presence or absence of cognitive processing deficits (i.e., phonological awareness, language skill, and processing or naming speed) may not be predictive of reading deficits (Pennington et al., 2012). Furthermore, impairments in psychological (e.g., cognitive) processes are often found to be shared with other neurodevelopmental disorders (e.g., processing speed deficits are also observed in ADHD; Willcutt et al., 2005). Valid measures intended to assess a particular cognitive ability often rely on intact functioning in other psychological processes, making it difficult to infer the exact nature of the deficit based on test scores.

Even though the precise mechanisms through which underlying psychological processes are linked to learning difficulties are not fully understood, in many settings assessment of psychological processes is important for developing individualized case formulations for those diagnosed with developmental learning disorder (see Hale et al., 2010). Understanding which psychological processes are affected can assist in selecting effective interventions, learning strategies, and accommodations. Examples of psychological processes that may underlie different subtypes of developmental learning disorder are provided in Table 3.1.

TABLE 3.1. Psychological Mechanisms and Academic Impairment Associated With the Three Specifiers for Developmental Learning Disorder

Specifier	Psychological mechanisms presumed to be affected	Impairments in academic skills
With impairment in reading (dyslexia)	Auditory/language processing (e.g., listening comprehension), phonological processing (e.g., segmenting words into syllables or individual sounds), speech sound difficulties, and auditory working memory	Word recognition, reading fluency, reading comprehension, as well as understanding and following written directions; individuals may also manifest difficulties in other areas of academic learning where reading is required
With impairment in mathematics (dyscalculia)	Working memory, spatial processing, sequential processing, visual-spatial-motor integration, numerical reasoning, number sense, representation of numerical magnitude, retrieval of facts from long-term memory, general fluency of processing, and processing speed	Mathematical competency, including numerical facility, mathematical reasoning, and understanding of number-related concepts such as time, speed, distance, measurement, and geometry
With impairment in written expression (dysgraphia)	Retrieval and production of alphabet letters, orthographic coding, ability to form mental representations of written words, graphomotor planning for sequential finger movements, handwriting, phonological and orthographic coding, vocabulary knowledge, working memory, processing speed, and executive functions Underlying difficulties with language processing that affect the content of written language may be present	Handwriting, spelling, composition, organization and production of assignments, and completing tests within a given time frame

PRESENTATIONS AND SYMPTOM PATTERNS

Developmental learning disorder typically affects one or more academic skills of reading, mathematics, or written expression but can also impact acquisition of other academic skills (e.g., history, science) reliant on these basic abilities. Symptom expression and functioning—namely, performance on academic tasks—varies across time according to numerous factors such as external demands on deficient skills, severity of the impairment, co-occurring disorders (e.g., ADHD), and, importantly, the interventions, learning strategies, and accommodations provided to the individual. In some cases, a developmental learning disorder may only become evident later during a person's academic trajectory when efforts to compensate for limitations are overwhelmed by academic demands.

The breadth of impairment within a skill area can vary significantly across affected individuals. For example, impairment in reading may be restricted to phonological awareness deficits or be found to be more pervasive, affecting, for example, phonological awareness, phonological memory, oral language, and listening comprehension. In all the latter cases, the developmental learning disorder is specified as "with impairment in reading." Most individuals with learning difficulties exhibit deficits that are persistent despite efforts to provide additional pedagogical support in the relevant subject area.

Developmental learning disorder may be preceded by attentional difficulties or speech and language impairments before formal schooling. Developmental learning disorder also typically persists into adulthood, presumably because the affected underlying psychological processes remain impaired even with adequate intervention.

DEVELOPMENTAL LEARNING DISORDER SPECIFIERS

Specifiers for developmental learning disorder are used to describe the current academic area(s) affected, which is important for planning appropriate interventions, strategies, and accommodations. These areas include reading, mathematics, and written expression and can be applied independently or in combination. The specifier "with other specified impairment in learning" can also be applied to capture significant impairments in learning of other subject matter (e.g., science). These specifiers are helpful in directing the clinician to develop hypotheses about which psychological processes might exhibit weaknesses as well as selecting appropriate psychoeducational or neuropsychological assessment measures. See Table 3.1 for a brief description of the psychological processes and abilities that may be part of a comprehensive assessment of developmental learning disorder.

ASSESSMENT OF DEVELOPMENTAL LEARNING DISORDER

Assessment of developmental learning disorder is best understood as a multi-step process (Ontario Psychological Association, 2018). Individuals suspected of developmental learning disorder have a history of academic impairment in one or more areas of academic skills. Clinicians should determine whether there is evidence of the presence of risk factors known to be associated with learning difficulties, including developmental, medical, educational, or contextual factors (e.g., cultural or linguistic). Next, academic achievement and psychological processes should be assessed on the basis of the results of appropriately normed, validated, and standardized tests. At least 1 standard deviation below the mean on achievement tests is a reasonable approximation of limitation in achievement provided that other diagnostic requirements are met, although different cut points may be appropriate given the clinical situation (e.g., if an individual comes from a marginalized community where access to educational opportunities is limited, a lower cut point may be more appropriate).

The *CDDR* also consider the importance of the global applicability of the diagnostic guidance in settings where valid tests in the local language may not be available. In these circumstances, it is anticipated that clinical judgment will be exercised which is similarly based on a comprehensive approach that includes a thorough history of academic problems and integration of information obtained from clinical interview with parents/caregivers and educators, school reports, and observation of the child's behavior while engaging with academic materials. Academic achievement limitations may need to be estimated by proxies such as consistent failing grades in school, the need for excessive effort to maintain achievement compared with same-age peers, a history of remedial services, or notable impairments in specific areas of performance (e.g., inability to complete homework assignments or take adequate notes).

Cognitive and academic profiles suggestive of a developmental learning disorder then need to be differentiated from other disorders and factors such as insufficient effort or noncompliance (see Differential Diagnosis section). Furthermore, the presence of socioemotional difficulties (e.g., low self-esteem) or co-occurring mental disorders (e.g., a depressive disorder, ADHD) should be identified and included in the case formulation.

DIFFERENTIAL DIAGNOSIS FOR DEVELOPMENTAL LEARNING DISORDER

Differential diagnosis for developmental learning disorder should begin with a determination of whether inadequate effort or poor compliance in the academic setting might better explain low achievement. Lack of effort or noncompliance should be formally assessed (e.g., through classroom observation or collateral reports from teachers and parents; DeRight & Carone, 2015) because these factors will also affect the validity of results of psychological measures used to diagnose and characterize a developmental learning disorder. Performance validity can be assessed in various ways, including with standalone measures (e.g., Test of Memory Malingering; Silver et al., 2011) or measures that are embedded in tests administered to assess cognitive or other psychological processes (e.g., reliable digit span subtest of the Wechsler Intelligence Scale for Children). Conclusions regarding the influence of effort or noncompliance should also consider convergent information from other sources such as teacher and parent reports.

Sensory impairments such as those affecting vision and hearing impact learning and should be ruled out with appropriate assessment in primary or specialized care (e.g., audiological examination). Similarly, developmental speech and language disorders can affect the ability to decode or produce language but do not directly affect the capacity for learning academic skills. History of traumatic brain injury and, if positive, the temporal relationship of the emergence of learning difficulties with the injury should also be assessed.

In general, profiles of strengths and weaknesses on normed, standardized instruments of cognitive and achievement functioning assist in differentiating developmental learning disorder from other neurodevelopmental disorders that commonly also affect learning. For example, developmental learning disorder is not a consequence of generalized intellectual deficits, which is characteristic of a disorder of intellectual development. Although many children with a developmental learning disorder exhibit uneven profiles on tests of intellectual functioning, globally, intellectual functioning is typically found to be in the average range. Nonetheless, the *ICD-11* does allow for the co-occurring diagnosis of a developmental learning disorder and a disorder of intellectual development when unexpected academic underachievement is observed in the context of intellectual functioning that is found to be significantly below the average range.

ADHD commonly co-occurs in people with developmental learning disorder (DuPaul et al., 2013). Differentiation can be challenging because the disorders share impairments in executive functioning (e.g., lack of focus). However, in ADHD, executive functioning impairments affect the ability to focus across contexts, not just those related to academic skill acquisition. Furthermore, in circumstances where a person with ADHD is able to focus on academic material, they are typically able to acquire new academic skills. In contrast, people with developmental learning disorder demonstrate consistent difficulties acquiring specific academic skills, presumably due to inefficient processing in selective psychological mechanisms (e.g., phonological awareness). Formal assessment measures of attention in addition to standard cognitive measures can help differentiate ADHD from developmental learning disorder. It is important to identify co-occurring ADHD because it often suggests greater severity of impairment and requires separate interventions.

Mood disorders and anxiety or fear-related disorders can affect cognitive functioning and motivation that disrupt learning, which should be differentiated from developmental learning disorder. However, the persistent underachievement characteristic of developmental learning disorder often leads to reductions in self-esteem among affected individuals and is an ancillary target of intervention strategies.

CULTURAL AND OTHER CONTEXTUAL ISSUES

Given the importance of formal psychoeducational or neuropsychological testing in diagnosing and characterizing developmental learning disorder, it is imperative that cultural, language, and literacy skills be taken into account. Performance on many measures of intellectual functioning is affected by cultural and linguistic factors (Geva & Wiener, 2015). Academic underachieve-ment may also be influenced by disenfranchisement of certain (often minori-tized) communities.

Measures administered to assess developmental learning disorder should be culturally appropriate, in the language of the individual to whom they are given (whether as originally developed or as a validated translation; typically, in the language of the preponderance of the child's schooling), and any stan-dardization (e.g., *t* scores, clinical cutoffs) should be appropriately normed for the local population to which the child belongs. When these conditions are not met, test results must be interpreted with caution. Furthermore, a diag-nosis of developmental learning disorder should not be made based on any single test result but rather based on an integration of multiple data sources.

KEY POINTS

- Disorders of intellectual development and developmental learning disorder are common neurodevelopmental disorders. These disorders are treated together in this chapter because both rely on the analysis and synthesis of findings from standardized measures for their diagnosis.

- People with disorders of intellectual development have significant limita-tions in intellectual and adaptive behavior functioning. Ideally, limitations are assessed with standardized, appropriately normed measures. *ICD-11* also includes behavioural indicators tables in cases when such measures are unavailable.

- Assessment of disorders of intellectual development must account for exist-ing supports and understand the nature of associated behavior problems, co-occurring mental disorders, and comorbid health conditions to obtain a holistic picture.

- This holistic approach of diagnosis reflects greater individualization for a relatively heterogeneous group of people with varied needs. Consistent with the UN Convention on the Rights of Persons with Disabilities (UN General Assembly, 2007), the *ICD-11*'s consideration of contextual factors that may facilitate or impede an individual's functioning emphasizes inclusiveness and participation in society.

- Developmental learning disorder is characterized by consistent impairment in achievement of academic skills that emerges during the developmental period. The *ICD-11* provides specifiers that allow for description of the cur-rent difficulties including reading, mathematics, written expression, and other areas of impairment. As many of these specifiers as necessary may be applied to describe the clinical presentation.

- Assessment of developmental learning disorder includes establishing the pres-ence of low achievement—ideally using standardized, normed measures—but should also focus on a comprehensive, individualized formulation that differentiates low achievement from disorders of intellectual development, sensory or motor impairments, lack of access to adequate educational opportunities, sociocultural factors, and language proficiency. Identification of impairments in underlying psychological mechanisms that logically relate to the observed impairment in achievement are crucial in formulating a coherent individualized case conceptualization.

REFERENCES

Alexander, R., Devapriam, J., Branford, D., Roy, A., Sheehan, R., Anand, E., Mccarthy, J., & Bhaumik, S. (2016). *Psychotropic drug prescribing for people with intellectual disability, mental health problems and/or behaviours that challenge: Practice guidelines*. Royal College of Psychiatrists. https://www.rcpsych.ac.uk/docs/default-source/members/faculties/intellectual-disability/id-faculty-report-id-09.pdf?sfvrsn=55b66f2c_6

Brooks, B. L. (2011). A study of low scores in Canadian children and adolescents on the Wechsler Intelligence Scale for Children, Fourth Edition (WISC-IV). *Child Neuropsychology, 17*(3), 281–289.

Cooray, S. E., Bhaumik, S., Roy, A., Devapriam, J., Rai, R., & Alexander, R. (2015). Intellectual disability and the *ICD-11*: Towards clinical utility? *Advances in Mental Health and Intellectual Disabilities, 9*(1), 3–8. https://doi.org/10.1108/AMHID-10-2014-0036

Cotton, S. M., Crewther, D. P., & Crewther, S. G. (2005). Measurement error: Implications for diagnosis and discrepancy models of developmental dyslexia. *Dyslexia, 11*(3), 186–202. https://doi.org/10.1002/dys.298

DeRight, J., & Carone, D. A. (2015). Assessment of effort in children: A systematic review. *Child Neuropsychology, 21*(1), 1–24. https://doi.org/10.1080/09297049.2013.864383

DuPaul, G. J., Gormley, M. J., & Laracy, S. D. (2013). Comorbidity of LD and ADHD: Implications of *DSM-5* for assessment and treatment. *Journal of Learning Disabilities, 46*(1), 43–51. https://doi.org/10.1177/0022219412464351

Fischer, V. J., Morris, J., & Martines, J. (2014). Developmental screening tools: Feasibility of use at primary healthcare level in low- and middle-income settings. *Journal of Health, Population and Nutrition, 32*(2), 314–326.

Flowers, L., Meyer, M., Lovato, J., Wood, F., & Felton, R. (2001). Does third grade discrepancy status predict the course of reading development? *Annals of Dyslexia, 51*(1), 49–71. https://doi.org/10.1007/s11881-001-0005-2

Francis, D. J., Fletcher, J. M., Stuebing, K. K., Lyon, G. R., Shaywitz, B. A., & Shaywitz, S. E. (2005). Psychometric approaches to the identification of LD: IQ and achievement scores are not sufficient. *Journal of Learning Disabilities, 38*(2), 98–108. https://doi.org/10.1177/00222194050380020101

Fuchs, L. S., & Vaughn, S. (2012). Responsiveness-to-intervention: A decade later. *Journal of Learning Disabilities, 45*(3), 195–203. https://doi.org/10.1177/0022219412442150

Geva, E., & Wiener, J. (2015). *Psychological assessment of culturally and linguistically diverse children and adolescents: A practitioner's guide*. Springer Publishing Company.

Hale, J., Alfonso, V., Berninger, V., Bracken, B., Christo, C., Clark, E., Cohen, M., Davis, A., Decker, S., Denckla, M., Dumont, R., Elliott, C., Feifer, S., Fiorello, C., Flanagan, D., Fletcher-Janzen, E., Geary, D., Gerber, M., Gerner, M., . . . Yalof, J. (2010). Critical issues in response-to-intervention, comprehensive evaluation, and specific learning disabilities identification and intervention: An expert white paper consensus. *Learning Disability Quarterly, 33*(3), 223–236. https://doi.org/10.1177/073194871003300310

Kishore, M. T., Udipi, G. A., & Seshadri, S. P. (2019). Clinical practice guidelines for assessment and management of intellectual disability. *Indian Journal of Psychiatry, 61*(8, Suppl. 2), 194–210. https://doi.org/10.4103/psychiatry.IndianJPsychiatry_507_18

Lakhan, R., & Mawson, A. R. (2016). Identifying children with intellectual disabilities in the tribal population of Barwani district in state of Madhya Pradesh, India. *Journal of*

Applied Research in Intellectual Disabilities, 29(3), 211–219. https://doi.org/10.1111/jar.12171

Lemay, K. R., Kogan, C. S., Rebello, T. J., Keeley, J. W., Bhargava, R., Sharan, P., Sharma, M., Kommu, J. V. S., Kishore, M. T., de Jesus Mari, J., Ginige, P., Buono, S., Recupero, M., Zingale, M., Zagaria, T., Cooray, S., Roy, A., & Reed, G. M. (2022). An international field study of the *ICD-11* behavioural indicators for disorders of intellectual development. *Journal of Intellectual Disability Research, 66*(4), 376–391. https://doi.org/10.1111/jir.12924

Lovett, B. J., Gordon, M., & Lewandowski, L. J. (2009). Measuring impairment in a legal context: Practical considerations in the evaluation of psychiatric and learning disabilities. In J. Naglieri & S. Goldstein (Eds.), *Assessing impairment* (pp. 93–103). Springer US. https://doi.org/10.1007/978-1-387-87542-2_8

Luckasson, R., & Schalock, R. L. (2013). Defining and applying a functionality approach to intellectual disability. *Journal of Intellectual Disability Research, 57*(7), 657–668. https://doi.org/10.1111/j.1365-2788.2012.01575.x

Maulik, P. K., Mascarenhas, M. N., Mathers, C. D., Dua, T., & Saxena, S. (2011). Prevalence of intellectual disability: A meta-analysis of population-based studies. *Research in Developmental Disabilities, 32*(2), 419–436. https://doi.org/10.1016/j.ridd.2010.12.018

Morgan, V. A., Leonard, H., Bourke, J., & Jablensky, A. (2008). Intellectual disability co-occurring with schizophrenia and other psychiatric illness: Population-based study. *The British Journal of Psychiatry, 193*(5), 364–372. https://doi.org/10.1192/bjp.bp.107.044461

Odiyoor, M. M., & Jaydeokar, S. (2019). Intellectual disability in rural backgrounds: Challenges and solutions. In S. Chaturvedi (Ed.), *Mental health and illness in rural world* (pp. 1–21). Springer. https://doi.org/10.1007/978-981-10-0751-4_28-1

Ontario Psychological Association. (2018). *Ontario Psychological Association guidelines for diagnosis and assessment of children, adolescents, and adults with learning disabilities: Consensus statement and supporting documents.*

Pennington, B. F., Santerre-Lemmon, L., Rosenberg, J., MacDonald, B., Boada, R., Friend, A., Leopold, D. R., Samuelsson, S., Byrne, B., Willcutt, E. G., & Olson, R. K. (2012). Individual prediction of dyslexia by single versus multiple deficit models. *Journal of Abnormal Psychology, 121*(1), 212–224. https://doi.org/10.1037/a0025823

Salvador-Carulla, L., Reed, G. M., Vaez-Azizi, L. M., Cooper, S.-A., Martinez-Leal, R., Bertelli, M., Adnams, C., Cooray, S., Deb, S., Akoury-Dirani, L., Girimaji, S. C., Katz, G., Kwok, H., Luckasson, R., Simeonsson, R., Walsh, C., Munir, K., & Saxena, S. (2011). Intellectual developmental disorders: Towards a new name, definition and framework for "mental retardation/intellectual disability" in *ICD-11*. *World Psychiatry, 10*(3), 175–180. https://doi.org/10.1002/j.2051-5545.2011.tb00045.x

Silver, J. M., McAllister, T. W., & Yudofsky, S. C. (Eds.). (2011). *Textbook of traumatic brain injury* (2nd ed.). American Psychiatric Publishing. https://doi.org/10.1176/appi.books.9781585624201

Stanovich, K. E. (2005). The future of a mistake: Will discrepancy measurement continue to make the learning disabilities field a pseudoscience? *Learning Disability Quarterly, 28*(2), 103–106. https://doi.org/10.2307/1593604

Tannock, R. (2013). Rethinking ADHD and LD in *DSM-5*: Proposed changes in diagnostic criteria. *Journal of Learning Disabilities, 46*(1), 5–25. https://doi.org/10.1177/0022219412464341

Tassé, M. J., Balboni, G., Navas, P., Luckasson, R., Nygren, M. A., Belacchi, C., Bonichini, S., Reed, G. M., & Kogan, C. S. (2019). Developing behavioural indicators for intellectual functioning and adaptive behaviour for *ICD-11* disorders of intellectual development. *Journal of Intellectual Disability Research, 63*(5), 386–407. https://doi.org/10.1111/jir.1258

Tyrer, P., Cooper, S.-A., & Hassiotis, A. (2014). Drug treatments in people with intellectual disability and challenging behaviour. *BMJ, 349*, g4323. https://doi.org/10.1136/bmj.g4323

UN General Assembly. (2007, January 24). *Convention on the Rights of Persons with Disabilities: Resolution adopted by the General Assembly* (A/RES/61/106). https://www.refworld.org/docid/45f973632.html

Willcutt, E. G., Pennington, B. F., Duncan, L., Smith, S. D., Keenan, J. M., Wadsworth, S., Defries, J. C., & Olson, R. K. (2010). Understanding the complex etiologies of developmental disorders: Behavioral and molecular genetic approaches. *Journal of Developmental and Behavioral Pediatrics, 31*(7), 533–544. https://doi.org/10.1097/DBP.0b013e3181ef42a1

Willcutt, E. G., Pennington, B. F., Olson, R. K., Chhabildas, N., & Hulslander, J. (2005). Neuropsychological analyses of comorbidity between reading disability and attention deficit hyperactivity disorder: In search of the common deficit. *Developmental Neuropsychology, 27*(1), 35–78. https://doi.org/10.1207/s15326942dn2701_3

World Health Organization. (1992). *International statistical classification of diseases and related health problems* (10th rev.).

World Health Organization. (2023). *ICD-11 for mortality and morbidity statistics* (Version: 01/2023). https://icd.who.int/browse11/l-m/en#/

World Health Organization. (2024). *Clinical descriptions and diagnostic requirements for ICD-11 mental, behavioural and neurodevelopmental disorders*. https://www.who.int/publications/i/item/9789240077263

4

Autism Spectrum Disorder

David Skuse, Kirstin Greaves-Lord, Graccielle Rodrigues da Cunha, and Gillian Baird

OVERARCHING LOGIC

Autism spectrum disorder (ASD) is characterized by deficits in social communication and social interaction together with restrictive, repetitive, and inflexible patterns of behavior including routines, rituals, and overfocused interests, sensory sensitivities, and motor stereotypies (e.g., hand flapping when excited or anxious). Until just a few years ago, it was thought that the prototypic individual with autism was a male with intellectual impairment. We now recognize that disabling—although less explicit—features characterize many children and adults with ASD with normal to high IQ. Unfortunately, most standardized methods of diagnosing ASD are still subject to diagnostic bias against the identification of higher functioning individuals, especially females. The apparent prevalence of ASD varies worldwide, but it is higher in countries with greater experience of diagnosing the condition. Within Europe and North America, the proportion of children with a diagnosis is at least 1.5% (Fombonne, 2020).

ASD is classified in the 11th revision of the *International Classification of Diseases* (*ICD-11*; World Health Organization [WHO], 2023) as a neurodevelopmental disorder because the condition results from dysregulation of the brain's development. The use of the term *spectrum* is based on increasing evidence that the biological substrate of the condition is highly variable and features of the condition are heterogeneous (Robinson et al., 2016), in part reflecting gender and the age at presentation as well as the severity of any associated disorder

https://doi.org/10.1037/0000392-004
A Psychological Approach to Diagnosis: Using the ICD-11 as a Framework, G. M. Reed, P. L.-J. Ritchie, and A. Maercker (Editors)

of intellectual development. ASD is not an acquired condition, except in very rare circumstances, such as prenatal exposure to toxins, extreme prematurity, or postnatal infections of the brain. It is not caused by environmental pollutants, parenting, or vaccines. The precise cause of the conditions remains unknown in the great majority of cases, but they certainly have a strong but complex biological/genetic foundation (Lord et al., 2018). Multimorbidity with other neurodevelopmental disorders is common, and there is increasing evidence that biological susceptibility to a range of neurodevelopmental disorders is shared. For that reason, most individuals with ASD exhibit characteristics of other conditions as well (Gillberg, 2010).

A PSYCHOLOGICAL APPROACH TO ASD

As described in the *Clinical Descriptions and Diagnostic Requirements for ICD-11 Mental, Behavioural and Neurodevelopmental Disorders* (*CDDR*; WHO, 2024), a core feature of ASD is a failure to recognize another person's social cues and respond appropriately. Clinicians used to believe that people with ASD were characteristically uninterested in having close friendships, but this is wrong. Many want social relationships with their peers but are unable to build such relationships successfully. People with ASD lack social competence due to abnormal social cognition, and this deficiency cannot be explained by general impairment in intellectual functioning. A relative lack of social competence may also be associated with a range of other conditions (e.g., blindness, deafness, attention deficit hyperactivity disorder [ADHD]), but, in these cases, compensatory behaviors often develop over time and the skills to build social relationships are not fundamentally lacking; they just take longer to develop. Although ASD has a clear biological, largely genetic substrate (Taylor et al., 2020), available treatments are almost exclusively behavioral and psychological. A detailed assessment of its psychological and behavioral manifestations in an individual case is therefore essential to treatment planning.

PRESENTATIONS AND SYMPTOM PATTERNS

Preschool Child (0–5 years)

Most children with ASD do not present with marked abnormalities of behavior in the first year of life, although parents often report some delay in smiling, poor gaze focus on faces, and distress provoked by changes of state or place. Infants later identified as having ASD are sometimes exceptionally quiet and rarely babble; they may appear to be "good" babies, and undemanding. Social monitoring by the infant is often absent or reduced, and nonverbal communication skills may be delayed, or even absent; they use few if any spontaneous nonverbal gestures such as waving goodbye or pointing to express shared interest. Comprehension may be restricted to single words or simple phrases, but a delayed onset of spoken language is not necessary to make the diagnosis;

distinguishing between the language deficits of ASD and language impairments due to a disorder of intellectual development or a developmental speech or language disorder requires the evaluation of other developmental skills (e.g., acquisition of gross motor skills, such as sitting, crawling, and walking). Unlike those with an ASD, children with a primary language disorder do not show impaired play, disinterest in social interaction, or limited nonverbal communication skills; they typically try to compensate for their failure to make their needs known verbally by using nonverbal means of communication.

Some infants later diagnosed with ASD avoid eye contact, do not like to be held, and if held may demand to face away. They do not mirror facial expressions and rarely actively engage in social games such as pat-a-cake or peek-a boo (although they may passively be amused by them). They do not explore their parent's face with their eyes or hands. Eye contact in social interactions (especially with unfamiliar people) is usually transient or absent. They have limited interest in physical contact (especially hugging), except when they initiate it. They may persistently ignore their name being called but have normal hearing (which should be confirmed by audiometry). However, screening for ASD traits in infancy should be undertaken with caution because of the danger of false-positive findings, which can be detrimental to parent–child relationships in the longer term.

Toddlers with ASD typically do not seek their parents' attention or praise for their achievements, nor do they engage in age-typical persistent enquiries (e.g., a lack of "why?" questions). In preschool group settings, there is little if any social play, and the friendly approaches of other children evoke disinterest or aversion. Social rules in group play (e.g., turn-taking, sharing) are not followed. They may isolate themselves from their peers, there is little or no "social chat," and preschool children with ASD rarely share interests with or seek praise from an adult. Identifying differences in play can be difficult because so many preschool children have access to electronic media such as phones and tablets, which appeal to both typically developing children and those with ASD. Play with objects is often stereotyped, and lacks a social element; for instance, a child with ASD may like to stroke soft toys but does not talk to them or name them. Persistent lining up of objects commonly takes the place of other play; typically developing children may do this also but will usually tolerate them being moved. Construction toys are used by both boys and girls with ASD but novel assemblies, beyond the creation of objects outlined in the instructions provided with the toy, are rarely observed. Rarely, there are unusual interests in numbers or letters from an early age.

Difficulties in breastfeeding (inability to suckle efficiently), resistance to the introduction of solids, and increasing sensitivity to food textures (often with gagging) are characteristic of early infancy, although children with other neurodevelopmental disorders may have feeding difficulties due to immature or uncoordinated lip, tongue, and swallowing movements. Some children with ASD develop unusually strong food preferences—for example, based on brand, color or other aspect of appearance, or texture. Occasionally, such preferences are persistent and severe enough to cause weight loss or failure to gain weight or have some other impact on physical health or related functional impairment;

avoidant and restricted food intake disorder may also be diagnosed. Although many children with ASD learn bladder and bowel control at the same age as typically developing children, some have difficulty recognizing and responding appropriately to internal sensations of bladder or bowel fullness or exhibit behavioral problems related to toileting (e.g., insistence on using diapers for bowel actions or refusal to use toilet facilities outside the home).

There may be both negative and positive responses to sensory experiences. Distress caused by specific sensations is common, most frequently loud or unusual sounds. Typical children at this age dislike loud noises such as fireworks, but children with ASD have more extreme reactions. Other sounds they dislike may be idiosyncratic, and they do not develop tolerance to them. Those with strong sensory sensitivities experience extreme anxiety in anticipation of the triggering sound. Some preschool children with ASD become preoccupied with favored sensations, such as smells, textures, or visual stimuli.

During the preschool years, there are the beginnings of rigid routines, such as an insistence on following familiar routes. Resistance to change begins at this age, with distress at unanticipated events even if they are pleasurable. The anticipation of a novel event raises anxiety, and that anxiety can manifest as anger. Although tantrums are not unexpected in preschool children, they can be exceptionally severe and protracted in children with ASD.

Even without specific treatment, traits and behaviors do not stabilize until at least 6 years of age, and amelioration is common as children develop. There is no convincing evidence to support the view that very early treatment can rectify an abnormal developmental trajectory (Paynter et al., 2020). Although psychological treatment can modify the overt expression of the condition, it cannot reverse the underlying atypical neurodevelopmental process.

In a small proportion of children with ASD (between 5% and 20%), parents or caretakers report that a period of normal development (usually about 18 months but sometimes much longer) was followed by the loss of previously acquired skills, including language. Skill regression can be gradual or sudden (e.g., within a few weeks). Parents often attribute the cause to an external event, such as a vaccination, birth of a new baby, or a house move, for example, although there is no evidence for any such causal connection. Although this pattern of development is a marker for possible ASD, some children make a full recovery. Rarely, regression of skills (verbal, social, and adaptive functions including bowel/bladder control and emotional distress) occurs in later childhood, in which case, recovery is unlikely (Pearson et al., 2018).

Middle Childhood

Many school-age children with ASD exhibit a continuing failure to make appropriate eye contact and a limited use of spontaneous gestures, such as beckoning or waving to attract attention. There are limited spontaneous facial emotions, especially subtler emotions such as guilt or embarrassment. Reduced social smiling is prominent; for instance, the child may not smile when greeting people with whom they are familiar. Children with ASD at this age will avoid or fail to recognize individuals they know well (e.g., teachers, friends) when seeing them out of context (e.g., at the shopping mall). There are reduced or absent nonverbal head movements in conversation (e.g., nodding to agree or acknowledge turn-taking, shaking head to disagree). Conversations are rarely initiated or sustained; children with ASD will respond to direct questions but tend to redirect social conversation to their own interests or needs. Echolalia (repeating words or phrases spoken by other people) is rare in children without co-occurring disorders of intellectual development, but if present, it may be either immediate or delayed. Some children with ASD continue to misuse pronouns. Their literal interpretation of language can be a major issue, and common idioms are often misunderstood. Unlike same-age peers with equivalent verbal intelligence, there is often a failure to follow hints, understand jokes, or cope with sarcasm or teasing.

Children with ASD in middle childhood do not usually develop close friendships. At school, they can often be observed in the playground standing on the periphery of groups, or they may completely avoid unstructured social situations and refuse to go and play outside. Some are intolerant of others encroaching on their personal space yet are unaware of other people's personal space, and so they make overfriendly approaches. Girls with ASD in mainstream schools often become skilled at feigning social engagement. Many children with ASD resist engaging in social events such as children's birthday parties, and most do not like to share, sometimes demonstrating extreme possessiveness. Although it is often said that children with ASD lack empathy, this is not usually an appropriate description (Fletcher-Watson & Bird, 2020). Most affected children are not callous and unfeeling, but when faced with another person's emotional distress, they do not respond in an appropriate way. This is in part because when other people express high levels of negative emotion, youth with ASD experience intense anxiety, which can trigger irritable behavior and tantrums. Dealing with unregulated emotions can lead them to respond to other people's negative emotional states inappropriately, such as laughing at distress, ignoring it, or becoming angry.

Social and emotional development is less mature than other areas of development. Parents may describe an excessive naiveté and a lack of common sense and express concern that the child is less independent than same-age peers. During this period of development, many children with ASD prefer to play with younger children to control social interactions (e.g., the rules of a game). They may more easily sustain conversations with unfamiliar adults who are accepting of the child's self-centered style. Many girls with ASD who have normal or high IQ practice social scripts and can "act normal" for limited periods of time (Dean et al., 2017). Functional rather than symbolic play is typical but differs substantially by gender. A preoccupation with construction toys is more typical of boys, although novel constructions are not usual. Girls may become focused on collections of figures, including dolls, but they do not act out social scenarios with those toys. There is typically little if any imaginative, social, or role play unless it is led by other children with the child with ASD acting as a passive participant.

Sensory preoccupations and aversions may become more apparent during middle childhood. These include a wish to wear the same clothes, or type of material, every day. Oversensitivity to touch can mean that labels must be removed from all clothing. Sensitivity to sounds may persist, and some children wear earplugs in school because the background noise in a classroom is so distressing to them. A high pain threshold is commonly associated with limited self-awareness of internal senses, such as feeling hungry, full, hot, cold, or thirsty. Continuing sensitivity to mixed textures in food is common, and many children demand that foods are separated on a plate, so that they do not touch or blend together. Children with ASD may have an obsessive interest in watching objects that spin.

Restricted interests are increasingly apparent during middle childhood. There are difficulties distinguishing this from typical behavior if it involves media such as computer games. Many children with ASD make collections of objects, often of no value. They tend to resist new experiences for which they have not been prepared, even if these are pleasurable, and this can have a major impact on family life and education. Cognitive rigidity can also lead to insistence on routines and rituals (e.g., taking the same route to school and demanding to leave the house at the same time each day), with great distress if a routine is altered. Overt tantrums, which may include aggression or violence, are a common response to challenges to their resistance to change. Another manifestation of cognitive rigidity is an insistence on fairness and rule following, which are more often applied to others rather than to self, with a lack of flexibility and no ability to compromise or change a decision once made.

Many children with ASD in middle childhood have impaired control of both gross motor skills (e.g., ungainly running, poor hand–eye coordination) and fine motor skills (e.g., exceptionally slow and untidy handwriting). Dyspraxia, the inability to perform a coordinated planned motor task with ease, is also common (e.g., difficulties tying shoelaces, fastening buttons). Clinically, problems in motor planning are often overlooked, but they can have far-reaching social and functional consequences, affecting educational progress and social acceptance by peers (Gowen & Hamilton, 2013). Some attainments such as reading competence or vocabulary skills may be advanced for the child's chronological or mental age, but specific learning difficulties in literacy and numeracy may co-occur and often go unidentified. Many children with ASD find it difficult to remember more than one instruction at a time, even if they have above-average IQ, making it hard for them to follow lessons efficiently; slow processing speed, together with a poor verbal working memory, can lead to educational underachievement.

Adolescence

Although all children develop new skills in social communication during adolescence, especially after puberty, the gap between individuals with ASD and typically developing peers tends to widen at this time. In some, especially girls, the increased social demands of adolescence may reveal difficulties that were previously hidden. Symptoms reflecting limited social skills can emerge at this time, even though ASD was not previously diagnosed; on careful enquiry, a history of autistic characteristics of behavior going back to early childhood is likely to be found.

Adolescents on the autism spectrum who do not have co-occurring disorders of intellectual development may superficially appear to communicate well, with an extensive vocabulary that is used without grammatical errors, but the pattern of stress and intonation of their language is often monotonous, pedantic, or exaggerated. Many adolescent girls with ASD speak quietly, and their speech is excessively fast or slow. Some adolescents with otherwise good formal language skills do not use associated emphatic gestures while talking, so they appear to be stiff and awkward. These communication differences may contribute to increasing social alienation from their peers.

Adolescents with ASD typically find it hard to adjust to an increasingly complex social world, in which insight into other people's motivations, the hidden meanings in their communications, and appropriate responses to social hierarchies are required to be socially accepted, especially in the school context. Boys with co-occurring ADHD often exhibit impulsive disruptive behaviors and are at risk of being manipulated by more socially skilled peers who take advantage of their naiveté. Disruptive behaviors can lead to school exclusion, often without recognition of the underlying disorder (Kaat & Lecavalier, 2013). Girls are vulnerable because of social naiveté too, especially in terms of sexual relationships. At this age, social communication difficulties are rarely the proximal reason for presentation to clinical services. Rather, underlying ASD may be masked by acts of self-harm, disordered eating, drug and alcohol abuse, and depressive symptoms. Due to their distinctive cognitive style (e.g., eye/ear for detail, unconventional associative thinking), many adolescents with ASD have a capacity to be creative in the arts and music and may be highly talented. Nurturing their capacity to focus attention and to practice skills can lead to success and can offer entry into a social milieu.

Some sensory sensitivities (such as extreme aversion to certain sounds) are less pronounced than at a younger age, but those related to touch or temperature tend to persist. There is often a need to wear clothes that have certain tactile qualities (usually loose fitting), a requirement for removal of clothing labels, and a tendency to dress in inappropriate clothing for the weather. Certain food textures continue to be avoided, and many have a very limited range of preferred foods. Repetitive stereotyped behaviors are less obvious in adolescence than in earlier childhood, and focused and restricted interests may appear to be socially acceptable or even desirable, especially if linked to educational pursuits. Poor motor skills are associated with an avoidance of, or exclusion from, team sporting activities, as well as impaired educational progress. However, the capacity for intense practice can sometimes lead to excellence in more individual sporting activities.

Adulthood

By the time they reach adulthood, many people with ASD who do not have co-occurring disorders of intellectual development have developed compensatory strategies for their lack of social communication skills and have intentionally suppressed motor stereotypies. Adult outcome for most people diagnosed with ASD in recent years is uncertain because the characteristics of individuals given the diagnosis of autism 20 years ago were quite different from those receiving the diagnosis today; in the past, a much higher proportion had generalized difficulties in intellectual functioning (Steinhausen et al., 2016). Most adults receiving a first diagnosis will have functioned reasonably well in situations that are familiar to them, even though they have typically placed a strong emphasis on routine. Given the increased societal demands in work and early-family settings, considerable effort is required to pass as "normal" in everyday life, but this is less of a problem when communicating electronically or by social media, which allows the timing of responses to be determined by the receiver; typically, adults with ASD who use textual modes of communication appear more fluent than they would in real-time discourse.

Emotional distress, which often has its roots in social alienation, is clinically important, and presentations to services may be prompted by depression, self-harm, substance misuse, social anxiety, or disruptive behaviors that are sometimes a reaction to conflict in the workplace or in intimate relationships (Hollocks et al., 2019). Expressive language skills are usually well developed among those with normal to high IQs, but some use pedantic, arcane vocabulary and complex grammatical constructions to compensate for, or to camouflage, other limitations. It is important to observe adults with suspected ASD on several occasions in different social contexts to determine whether what appear to be socially attuned, flexible behaviors are in fact imitative or preconceived routines.

Similar issues may apply to nonverbal behaviors; even though a wide variety of facial expressions and associated patterns of stress and intonation of language may give the appearance of social adeptness, on further observation, it becomes apparent that these responses were rehearsed. (Many individuals will admit to practicing them if asked.) Of course, rehearsing appropriate social behavior is not an invariable sign of autism, but if such practiced behavior is necessary in everyday life, it can become emotionally exhausting. The stress of keeping up appearances can lead to anxiety and depression. Both males and females with ASD in adulthood find informal social events, in which social conversation (or chat) is expected, very challenging; some compensate with alcohol, risking exacerbation of the problem and socially inappropriate behavior. With the increasing use of social media, which is often the preferred mode of communication, a lack of social awareness and associated naiveté can lead to people with ASD being exploited by others who contact them online. They are vulnerable to being manipulated into detrimental social, sexual, or financial situations.

Creative activities offer an important route by which adults with ASD can increase their social inclusion and gain better emotional regulation. Loss of engagement in creative activities can impact negatively on mental health. It is important to ask about these activities, and to learn how successfully the adult balances their day-to-day interests and commitments. Sensory sensitivities can become increasingly disabling in adulthood because sensitivities to certain sounds, smells, and lights are distracting, interfere with work, and potentially lead to irritated or aggressive behavior that could result in conflict with coworkers or even to job loss.

By adulthood, routines and rituals have often become habitual, and resistance to change is even stronger than in childhood. Motor issues are not very different in adulthood than during previous developmental periods; clumsiness and poorly coordinated fine and gross motor skills may emerge or be exacerbated when the individual is under stress or exhausted.

Adults with ASD sometimes come to clinical attention because they become aware of their differences with others and may even diagnose themselves. Events that lead to their seeking treatment include bullying, social exclusion, or difficulty coping with unexpected life events. A diagnosis of ASD may have been overlooked when they were younger because at that time the predominant symptoms were related to ADHD or anxiety. Adults with ASD usually experience ongoing social communication difficulties, as well as routines and rituals, and resistance to new experiences, although many form relationships with partners and children, an outcome that is probably more common for females than males. Adults with ASD are employed in a range of settings; those with high nonverbal intelligence are in demand for tasks that require attention to detail and logical planning, such as computer programming. The greatest threat to their employability arises from difficulties in their social relationships in the work environment, conflict arising from their preference to repeatedly do tasks the same way, their distress if their routine is changed, and their absorption in detail, which can lead to the neglect of important contextual information. Typically, they do not enjoy and do not wish to participate in social activities, so they avoid social events relating to work. Most importantly, they find it exceptionally hard to manage other people, which means that promotion can lead to a breakdown of their working relationships and even to the termination of their employment.

SPECIFIERS

The *ICD-11* provides a range of specifiers to describe aspects of the presentation of ASD that may be especially relevant to treatment selection (WHO, 2024). First, a specifier is used to indicate the presence or absence of a co-occurring disorder of intellectual development ("with disorder of intellectual development" and "without disorder of intellectual development"). If a co-occurring disorder of intellectual development is identified, that diagnosis should also be assigned together with the severity designation corresponding to the degree of impairment in intellectual and adaptive functioning (mild, moderate, severe, or profound). The *CDDR* indicate that because deficits in social communication are a core feature of ASD, in determining the severity of the co-occurring disorder of intellectual development, assessment of adaptive functioning should emphasize the intellectual, conceptual, and practical domains rather than social skills.

The *ICD-11* also provides specifiers to indicate the degree of functional language impairment, which is prognostically important in individuals with ASD. It is most often, although not exclusively, relevant for individuals with co-occurring disorders of intellectual development. For the purpose of this specifier, functional language refers to the individual's ability to use spoken or signed language to express personal needs and desires, not to the social communication deficits that are a core feature of ASD. Specifiers are provided for "mild or no impairment of functional language," "impaired functional language" (i.e., not able to use more than single words or simple phrases), and "complete, or almost complete, absence of functional language."

DIFFERENTIAL DIAGNOSIS

A different pattern of differential diagnoses is found at each developmental stage. The distinction from disorders of intellectual development, developmental speech or language disorders, and hearing impairment is particularly relevant during the preschool period. The differential diagnosis between ASD and disorders of intellectual development can be difficult, although they often co-occur, as indicated by a provision of a specifier for this situation. In practical terms, the distinction may rest on a clinical decision about which is the more prominent and disabling condition. Disorders of intellectual development encompass aspects of language, motor skills, and adaptive functions including social communication skills. Diagnostically, it is useful to conceptualize the core deficit in ASD as being a failure to interpret other people's social cues accurately and respond appropriately (for developmental age). Social interest and associated skills are often maintained in individuals with disorders of intellectual development relative to other adaptive functions. In those with ASD, the opposite is generally true. If intellectual limitations are so severe that there is no verbal or nonverbal communication beyond basic expressions of need, the ability to gather supportive evidence for an associated diagnosis of ASD may be so compromised as to be clinically meaningless.

A careful developmental history is of critical importance in distinguishing ASD from developmental speech sound disorder or developmental speech fluency disorder because these can also result in social withdrawal, and social anxiety is often a prominent symptom. In these disorders, inquiring about early (preschool) development should reveal a history of social responsiveness that gradually diminishes over time. The distinction between ASD and developmental language disorder, especially with pragmatic language impairment, is even more challenging. Both are associated with impaired social communication, but ASD is, by definition, characterized by additional evidence of cognitive rigidity and often by pervasive sensory sensitivities. A history of marked regression in language skills occurs in some cases of ASD (usually in the second or third year of life) but never in developmental language disorder. ASD can also co-occur with developmental speech and language disorders if the speech and language difficulties are not better explained by ASD or by a disorder of intellectual development.

By middle childhood, it should be clear whether the child has significant intellectual impairment, but the relative weighting of ASD and a disorder of intellectual development as components of the clinical presentation continues to be challenging. Other neurodevelopmental disorders need to be evaluated, especially ADHD, which is clinically significant in more than a third of ASD cases (Visser et al., 2016). Some children with selective mutism may be almost impossible to assess for underlying ASD. In adolescence, the initial presentation of ASD in boys is often disruptive behavior but, in girls, it is more commonly precipitated by an emotional crisis with anxiety and depressive symptoms, or an eating disorder. A differential diagnosis in such cases requires careful assessment of social communication difficulties, which are not characteristic symptoms of other disorders. in adulthood, the distinction from personality disorder can present a challenge; the key distinguishing feature is evidence of an abnormal trajectory of early neurodevelopment in ASD (requiring, ideally, an independent informant).

ASSESSMENT

Preliminary evaluation of suspected ASD can be done in a primary care setting, but a full diagnostic workup requires specialist assessment. There are several screening questionnaires that can assist, but they are no substitute for personal evaluation by direct observation of the child (or adult) in social interaction with the clinician as well as a developmental history. A diagnosis of ASD is a clinical judgment, ideally based on consensual agreement between members of a multidisciplinary team (e.g., psychologists, psychiatrists, and speech and language therapists). They should come to a decision about the severity of symptoms and their impact on the individual's social adjustment in relationship to family, education, and broader social interactions (i.e., daily functioning).

Diagnostic assessment of children and adolescents—and, if possible, even adults—should include an interview with a parent or caregiver who can describe in detail a lifelong pattern of developmental difficulties in social communication and social interaction skills. Identifying the relatively subtle symptoms that indicate restricted interests, resistance to change, and sensory sensitivities in children with ASD whose IQ is in the normal to high range requires considerable clinical expertise because they cannot reliably be assessed by observation alone. When assessing females, clinicians should be mindful that their focused interests are more likely to be socially unexceptional (e.g., animals, celebrities, clothes) than those of boys, but they are equivalently restricted and of similar intensity. The obsessional interests of boys differ with age but typically involve the collection of unusual facts or objects that have no value or use. The severity and quality of individual symptoms is likely to vary over the lifespan; in many cases, the diagnosis is not made until the social limitations of the condition are outweighed by social demands.

The assessment should combine and integrate several sources of information. There should be independent observations of the individual's behavior in different social contexts, such as within the family, in nursery, in school, or during unstructured leisure (social) activities. Making such personal observations of adolescents or adults is difficult, but even secondary observations (e.g., reports by teachers or coworkers) can provide clinically useful information. Because families usually adapt to their autistic child's unusual behaviors, subjective family reports can underestimate the degree of impairment; it is often more productive to approach this in terms of the disruptive impact of the child's behavior on family life.

Many subtle traits and individual symptoms consistent with ASD can be observed in children who are not clinically on the autism spectrum. No single behavior (e.g., presence or lack of sustained eye contact) or symptom cluster either confirms or rules out the diagnosis. Children without intellectual impairment may try to disguise or compensate for their autistic traits. For instance, they may suppress motor stereotypies such as hand flapping and learn to avoid situations that are associated with subjectively unpleasant sensory experiences. The impact of ASD traits on educational progress often depends on how tolerant the educational establishment is of unusual or disruptive behaviors; some children respond well to the rules and structure of schools.

Because children with ASD often have both strengths and weaknesses in their verbal or nonverbal skills, a formal evaluation of their cognitive profile is of value (Mandy et al., 2015). Specific characteristics, including executive skills, should be quantified by psychometric testing. Educational progress can be compromised without remedial attention to areas of weakness. Superior verbal intelligence does not equate to the appropriate use of language in everyday social discourse; expressive language skills can exceed comprehension and speed of processing, causing teachers, parents, and peers to overestimate the language skills of their student, child, or classmate with autism. Common areas of specific weakness include working memory and processing speed, which have functional consequences because affected individuals have great difficulty in, for example, remembering instructions, following rapid changes in conversation topics, or conversing with several people at once. Executive functions in which deficits are often observed include sustained attention, planning, shifting attention from one task to another, emotional regulation, and initiating tasks. Many individuals with ASD show an excessive focus on detail at the expense of the "bigger picture." They also tend to introduce subjects into a conversation without setting a context, which induces confusion in the listener. Both traits reflect the autistic individual's lack of appreciation that other people's perspective on, and knowledge about, the world is different from their own.

A clinical assessment of ASD should also inquire about the individual's range of sensory sensitivities. Many people have both a maximum and minimum tolerance of sensory stimulation. We are often more aware of their response to excessive sensory stimulation, but people with ASD are also at risk of becoming understimulated, which can lead to passivity, depression, and a sense of meaninglessness. Both positive and negative sensory sensitivities should be explored to formulate a "window of tolerance" within which they function optimally.

For adolescents with ASD, an assessment of their knowledge of psychosexual functioning is important to guide them into a healthy period of sexual development. Parents and adolescents often have quite different perspectives on the issues under discussion, and adolescents with ASD will tend to be surprisingly concrete in their understanding of social and sexual relationships. Notions of companionship and emotional involvement are not easy for them to comprehend, and they may see such relationships in purely functional terms.

People with ASD can develop long-term, stable sexual and loving relationships. There are also many adults with ASD who struggle to find a partner, but their single status can be wrongly interpreted as a lack of motivation or desire; many adults with ASD say that they do have romantic and sexual desires, but they find it difficult to initiate contact with potential partners. It is important to ask about these desires in a concrete and explicit way. Follow-up questions are needed to ensure that the subject matter and its implications have been correctly understood.

It is important to assess suicidality and violence when interviewing adolescents and adults with suspected ASD. Although clinicians prefer to use avoidant or polite language, they should be explicit and concrete, asking "Do you want to be dead?" rather than "Do you have suicidal thoughts?" and "Do you ever hit someone?" rather than "Are you ever physically violent?" Moreover, it is important to ask follow-up questions to make sure that the question was understood correctly, and not take no for an answer too easily, especially if the individual's nonverbal behavior is at odds with their verbal response.

CO-OCCURRING DISORDERS

It is important to inquire about a history of co-occurring mental health conditions and whether the individual has suffered any traumatic life experiences. Anxieties are often present during the preschool period, including separation anxiety and a variety of specific phobias, which may be severe. Phobias commonly involve sensory sensitivities, flying insects, dogs, and people dressed up in costumes (e.g., as clowns). ADHD is difficult to diagnose with confidence in the preschool period, especially if the child is developmentally delayed. Developmental speech or language disorders and developmental motor coordination disorder may co-occur and require specific intervention. Some degree of oppositional and defiant behavior and emotional volatility is to be expected in typically developing preschoolers, but in those with ASD, it is often more severe. In middle childhood and adolescence, multimorbidity is common, including ADHD, tic disorders, anxiety or fear-related disorders, oppositional defiant disorder, and eating disorders (Simonoff et al., 2008). As social exclusion often increases steadily throughout adolescence and adulthood, anxiety or fear-related disorders and depressive disorders are increasingly common, and suicidal thoughts or attempts may occur. Some individuals become aggressive toward themselves or others.

Medical conditions that predispose to ASD include various genetic disorders that are associated with intellectual disability, certain intrauterine exposures (e.g., to sodium valproate or alcohol), perinatal factors such as prematurity, and infections such as encephalopathy. A family history of ASD suggests there could be an identifiable genetic risk to other family members; therefore, genetic testing of the affected individual and their first-degree relatives may be indicated (DeThorne & Ceman, 2018).

CULTURAL CONSIDERATIONS

Apparent rates of ASD vary among cultures, but these are likely to reflect differences in recognition and diagnosis rather than underlying population characteristics (de Leeuw et al., 2020). Recognition of the disorder may reflect, for example, parental reluctance to endorse symptoms that are regarded as socially undesirable or reflect cultural attitudes toward disability, such as difficulties in self-care tasks or instrumental activities of daily living (Liao et al., 2019). When parents do express a concern about their children's behavior, they may focus on symptoms that have a particular cultural salience for them. For example, in Latino cultures, parental concern during the preschool period may be more likely to focus on difficult temperament, irritability, hyperactivity, and impaired psychomotor development rather than unusual social behavior. In contrast, White North American parents may be particularly watchful of any delay or other abnormality in language development. Alternatively, ASD-like characteristics can be culturally congruent, such as avoidance of eye gaze or a limited range of publicly expressed facial expressions in some Asian cultures. Conversational conventions, such as forms of greeting, turn-taking, intonation, the use of humor, and associated nonverbal gestures during conversation also vary widely between cultures. In countries where access to specialist services is limited, individuals with ASD without intellectual impairment often go undiagnosed until adulthood, and other cases may be incorrectly considered to have only a disorder of intellectual development.

GENDER-RELATED FEATURES

For many years, the widely accepted figure for the male-to-female ratio in the prevalence of ASD was 4:1, but this has changed with greater awareness that ASD affects girls of normal-range intellectual functioning (Halladay et al., 2015). There is still relatively little identification of girls with ASD in the preschool years, unless they have associated severe developmental or language delay. Social behavior may appear to be less detrimentally affected in girls than boys at this age, in part because compensatory behavior (e.g., mimicking the behavior of typical girls) usually commences in the preschool years and continues through middle childhood. Compensatory strategies are probably secondary to greater social motivation in females, and their social communication difficulties are usually more obvious to families than to teachers. By the time they reach adolescence, girls with ASD generally find it increasingly difficult to conform to the social norms of their peer group (Mandy et al., 2012).

Motor stereotypies are generally more evident in boys than girls with IQs in the normal range. Preoccupations with facts, numbers, spinning objects, and the collection and categorization of unusual objects are also more male-typical in this age group. Preoccupations in girls are more likely to be socially acceptable (e.g., obsessions with celebrities, music, animals, clothes, or makeup) and are therefore harder to differentiate from normal-range behaviors. Girls may also be very different in their behavior at home versus at school. Their social relationships at school may superficially appear to be appropriate, and teacher reports may be at variance with the parental account of their daughter's pervasively challenging behavior. Girls typically try to keep up a more "normal" persona at school, but they become exhausted by the end of the school day. At home they can appear completely different, sometimes including confrontational and aggressive behavior. Clinicians may erroneously attribute the emotional manifestations of ASD in these families to family dysfunction.

Presentations of emotional disturbance in girls with ASD, possibly related to the onset of puberty, are characterized by generalized anxiety disorder or depressive disorders. There is unlikely to be the same risk of antisocial behavior as seen in boys, in part because girls with ADHD traits tend to be inattentive rather than overtly hyperactive and impulsive. As the compensatory strategies employed by girls with normal-range IQ become relatively less effective because of increasing social environment complexity, there is a risk they will internalize their distress, leading to eating disorders, depressive disorders, or self-harm.

In adolescence, affected boys may have conduct problems, especially if there is associated ADHD, but girls are more vulnerable than boys to romantic/sexual exploitation during adolescence. They tend to behave in the way they believe is appropriate or that they think other people expect of them. A minority experience gender dysphoria at this time, a period when typical children focus on their individual gender identity, romantic relationships, and sexual preferences. There are also gender differences in autistic features exhibited in adulthood. An absorbing interest in categorization, numbers, and in logical sets of information is much more characteristic of males. Both genders are at risk for stalking people of interest to them.

Gender-role issues may rise in adult females with ASD who become mothers. Some such women do not feel comfortable in a cultural role of motherhood because that involves a caring and emotionally engaged relationship with their child and because many do not enjoy close physical contact. Consequently, such women feel unfit to be a mother or struggle to combine motherhood with other responsibilities or activities.

KEY POINTS

- Diagnostic requirements for ASD have evolved over the past 40 years. There is now far greater awareness of the prevalence of the symptoms among individuals of all ages whose verbal and nonverbal intelligence lie within the normal range.

- ASD is associated with a range of associated mental health and behavioral issues, as well as specific and generalized learning difficulties and impairments of motor development.

- The majority of affected individuals have other clinically significant mental, behavioral, or neurodevelopmental disorders, which require a separate diagnosis and tailored management.

- Common co-occurring internalizing mental health conditions include generalized anxiety disorder, specific phobias, and depressive disorders, with characteristics of withdrawal, irritability, and emotional dysregulation.

- Externalizing characteristics can include oppositionality, excessive tantrums, reactive aggression, and other issues that may predominate in the individual's initial clinical presentation, which may meet diagnostic requirements for a co-occurring diagnosis of ADHD or oppositional defiant disorder.

REFERENCES

Dean, M., Harwood, R., & Kasari, C. (2017). The art of camouflage: Gender differences in the social behaviors of girls and boys with autism spectrum disorder. *Autism, 21*(6), 678–689. https://doi.org/10.1177/1362361316671845

de Leeuw, A., Happé, F., & Hoekstra, R. A. (2020). A conceptual framework for understanding the cultural and contextual factors on autism across the globe. *Autism Research, 13*(7), 1029–1050. https://doi.org/10.1002/aur.2276

DeThorne, L. S., & Ceman, S. (2018). Genetic testing and autism: Tutorial for communication sciences and disorders. *Journal of Communication Disorders, 74*, 61–73. https://doi.org/10.1016/j.jcomdis.2018.05.003

Fletcher-Watson, S., & Bird, G. (2020). Autism and empathy: What are the real links? *Autism, 24*(1), 3–6. https://doi.org/10.1177/1362361319883506

Fombonne, E. (2020). Epidemiological controversies in autism. *Swiss Archives of Neurology, Psychiatry and Psychotherapy, 171*(01). https://doi.org/10.4414/sanp.2020.03084

Gillberg, C. (2010). The ESSENCE in child psychiatry: Early symptomatic syndromes eliciting neurodevelopmental clinical examinations. *Research in Developmental Disabilities, 31*(6), 1543–1551. https://doi.org/10.1016/j.ridd.2010.06.002

Gowen, E., & Hamilton, A. (2013). Motor abilities in autism: A review using a computational context. *Journal of Autism and Developmental Disorders, 43*(2), 323–344. https://doi.org/10.1007/s10803-012-1574-0

Halladay, A. K., Bishop, S., Constantino, J. N., Daniels, A. M., Koenig, K., Palmer, K., Messinger, D., Pelphrey, K., Sanders, S. J., Singer, A. T., Taylor, J. L., & Szatmari, P. (2015). Sex and gender differences in autism spectrum disorder: Summarizing evidence gaps and identifying emerging areas of priority. *Molecular Autism, 6*(1), 36–40. https://doi.org/10.1186/s13229-015-0019-y

Hollocks, M. J., Lerh, J. W., Magiati, I., Meiser-Stedman, R., & Brugha, T. S. (2019). Anxiety and depression in adults with autism spectrum disorder: A systematic review and meta-analysis. *Psychological Medicine, 49*(4), 559–572. https://doi.org/10.1017/S0033291718002283

Kaat, A. J., & Lecavalier, L. (2013). Disruptive behavior disorders in children and adolescents with autism spectrum disorders: A review of the prevalence, presentation, and treatment. *Research in Autism Spectrum Disorders, 7*(12), 1579–1594. https://doi.org/10.1016/j.rasd.2013.08.012

Liao, X., Lei, X., & Li, Y. (2019). Stigma among parents of children with autism: A literature review. *Asian Journal of Psychiatry, 45*, 88–94. https://doi.org/10.1016/j.ajp.2019.09.007

Lord, C., Elsabbagh, M., Baird, G., & Veenstra-Vanderweele, J. (2018). Autism spectrum disorder. *The Lancet, 392*(10146), 508–520. https://doi.org/10.1016/S0140-6736(18)31129-2

Mandy, W., Chilvers, R., Chowdhury, U., Salter, G., Seigal, A., & Skuse, D. (2012). Sex differences in autism spectrum disorder: Evidence from a large sample of children and adolescents. *Journal of Autism and Developmental Disorders, 42*(7), 1304–1313. https://doi.org/10.1007/s10803-011-1356-0

Mandy, W., Murin, M., & Skuse, D. (2015). The cognitive profile in autism spectrum disorders. In M. Leboyer & P. Chaste (Eds.), *Autism spectrum disorders: Phenotypes, mechanisms and treatments* (pp. 34–45). Karger. https://doi.org/10.1159/000363565

Paynter, J., Luskin-Saxby, S., Keen, D., Fordyce, K., Frost, G., Imms, C., Miller, S., Sutherland, R., Trembath, D., Tucker, M., & Ecker, U. (2020). Brief report: Perceived evidence and use of autism intervention strategies in early intervention providers. *Journal of Autism and Developmental Disorders, 50*(3), 1088–1094. https://doi.org/10.1007/s10803-019-04332-2

Pearson, N., Charman, T., Happé, F., Bolton, P. F., & McEwen, F. S. (2018). Regression in autism spectrum disorder: Reconciling findings from retrospective and prospective research. *Autism Research, 11*(12), 1602–1620. https://doi.org/10.1002/aur.2035

Robinson, E. B., St Pourcain, B., Anttila, V., Kosmicki, J. A., Bulik-Sullivan, B., Grove, J., Maller, J., Samocha, K. E., Sanders, S. J., Ripke, S., Martin, J., Hollegaard, M. V., Werge, T., Hougaard, D. M., Neale, B. M., Evans, D. M., Skuse, D., Mortensen, P. B., Børglum, A. D., . . . the iPSYCH-SSI-Broad Autism Group. (2016). Genetic risk for autism spectrum disorders and neuropsychiatric variation in the general population. *Nature Genetics, 48*(5), 552–555. https://doi.org/10.1038/ng.3529

Simonoff, E., Pickles, A., Charman, T., Chandler, S., Loucas, T., & Baird, G. (2008). Psychiatric disorders in children with autism spectrum disorders: Prevalence, comorbidity, and associated factors in a population-derived sample. *Journal of the American Academy of Child & Adolescent Psychiatry, 47*(8), 921–929. https://doi.org/10.1097/CHI.0b013e318179964f

Steinhausen, H. C., Mohr Jensen, C., & Lauritsen, M. B. (2016). A systematic review and meta-analysis of the long-term overall outcome of autism spectrum disorders in adolescence and adulthood. *Acta Psychiatrica Scandinavica, 133*(6), 445–452. https://doi.org/10.1111/acps.12559

Taylor, M. J., Rosenqvist, M. A., Larsson, H., Gillberg, C., D'Onofrio, B. M., Lichtenstein, P., & Lundström, S. (2020). Etiology of autism spectrum disorders and autistic traits over time. *JAMA Psychiatry, 77*(9), 936–943. https://doi.org/10.1001/jamapsychiatry.2020.0680

Visser, J. C., Rommelse, N. N., Greven, C. U., & Buitelaar, J. K. (2016). Autism spectrum disorder and attention-deficit/hyperactivity disorder in early childhood: A review of unique and shared characteristics and developmental antecedents. *Neuroscience and Biobehavioral Reviews, 65*, 229–263. https://doi.org/10.1016/j.neubiorev.2016.03.019

World Health Organization. (2023). *ICD-11 for mortality and morbidity statistics* (Version: 01/2023). https://icd.who.int/browse11/l-m/en#/

World Health Organization. (2024). *Clinical descriptions and diagnostic requirements for ICD-11 mental, behavioural and neurodevelopmental disorders.* https://www.who.int/publications/i/item/9789240077263

5

Schizophrenia and Other Primary Psychotic Disorders

Tania Lincoln and Paul French

OVERARCHING LOGIC

Schizophrenia and other primary psychotic disorders are characterized by the presence of one or more psychotic experiences, such as aberrations in perception (hallucinations), beliefs (delusions), or visible behavior (disorganized speech, bizarre behavior; World Health Organization [WHO], 2024). A central feature is referred to as loss of touch with reality, in which the person perceives things that others do not (e.g., hearing voices), holds on to extreme beliefs that deviate from the cultural norm without convincing proof (e.g., beliefs about being persecuted), or has difficulties making themself understood. However, it is important to recognize that loss of touch with reality typically only relates to the individual's symptoms and not to a broader or complete breakdown of understanding and orientation.

The grouping of schizophrenia and other primary psychotic disorders in the 11th revision of the *International Classification of Diseases* (*ICD-11*; WHO, 2023) includes six categories: schizophrenia, schizoaffective disorder, schizotypal disorder, acute and transient psychotic disorder, delusional disorder, and other primary psychotic disorder. These categories differ in regard to the intensity of the symptoms (e.g., symptoms in schizotypal disorder are less pronounced than in the other categories), their duration (e.g., symptoms are of shorter duration in acute and transient psychotic disorder), the range of the experiences included (e.g., delusional disorder does not typically involve other psychotic symptoms),

https://doi.org/10.1037/0000392-005

A Psychological Approach to Diagnosis: Using the ICD-11 as a Framework, G. M. Reed, P. L.-J. Ritchie, and A. Maercker (Editors)

79

and their degree of overlap with other disorders (e.g., schizoaffective disorder is characterized by the presence of symptoms of mood disorders). Psychotic experiences can also occur in other *ICD-11* disorders. For example, delusions of guilt can occur in moderate or severe depressive episodes, paranoid symptoms are common in severe personality disorder, and hallucinations can arise in the context of posttraumatic stress disorder (PTSD). However, in these other disorders, psychotic symptoms are not the defining features.

For a long time, psychiatrists and psychologists assumed that psychotic symptoms, especially delusions or hallucinations, were qualitatively different from normal experiences and that they could not be changed using logical reasoning; therefore, psychological interventions were not promoted. We now know that people who do not have a psychotic disorder can also have psychotic experiences. For example, many people admit feeling paranoid at least occasionally, and even auditory hallucinations are not uncommon. Prevalence rates of typical psychotic experiences range from about 5% up to 30% in the general population, depending on the type of phenomenon and how the question is asked. This has led researchers to conclude that these symptoms occur on a continuum from normal to pathological. The continuum view implies that normal processes of reasoning must be involved in the formation and maintenance of psychotic symptoms and has encouraged the systematic development of psychological interventions for schizophrenia and other primary psychotic disorders.

However, the psychotic-like symptoms or unusual subjective experiences that are observed in the general population are usually fleeting in nature, are not accompanied by other symptoms of a psychotic disorder, and do not interfere with functioning. People who fulfill the diagnostic requirements for a psychotic disorder generally rate their psychotic experiences as much more distressing. The experiences tend to occur more frequently, the content of auditory hallucinations tends to be more negative, and the delusional beliefs tend to be more extreme and to be held with stronger conviction. Symptoms in the context of a psychotic disorder are thus more likely to cause impairment in personal, family, social, educational, and occupational or other important areas of functioning.

A PSYCHOLOGICAL APPROACH TO SCHIZOPHRENIA AND OTHER PRIMARY PSYCHOTIC DISORDERS

Taking a psychological approach to schizophrenia and other primary psychotic disorders means going beyond a mere diagnosis and attempting to understand how symptoms have developed and which factors are maintaining them. Due to the complexity of psychoses, there is no "one size fits all" solution. The predisposing (e.g., genetic factors, trauma) or maintaining factors (e.g., ongoing social stress) vary among people. Additionally, predisposing or maintaining factors vary among symptoms. For example, negative symptoms such as constricted affect and paucity of speech may be maintained by social withdrawal, whereas incoherent speech that is characteristic of thought disorder may be maintained by too much interpersonal stress. Psychological approaches to date have tended to focus on understanding specific symptoms (e.g., delusions) rather than the complete disorder (e.g., schizophrenia).

To develop suitable interventions, a detailed assessment and formulation needs to be undertaken with each patient. A formulation-based approach is used to help make sense of the assessment and guide intervention strategies. The formulation will vary depending on whether the focus is on trying, for example, to understand the occurrence of hallucinations as such or on the emotional distress they are causing. Finally, we need to distinguish a macro level of analysis (i.e., Under which circumstances did the symptoms develop in the broader context of a person's life history?) from a micro level (i.e., Which factors are triggering and maintaining symptoms in the person's specific everyday situations?). The concept of *functional analyses* (e.g., Kanfer et al., 2012) offers a helpful framework for this type of assessment and provides an optimal basis for planning individualized interventions. This framework considers the association between situational stimuli such as external or internal triggers and the symptomatic response at the behavioral, emotional, physiological, and cognitive levels. This association is assumed to be influenced by the preexisting differences between individuals resulting from both biological dispositions and a person's experiences, as well as the interaction of the two.

There are several predisposing risk factors for psychotic disorders. One is a significant genetic component: There is about a 67% chance of inheriting a vulnerability to developing schizophrenia (Wray & Gottesman, 2012). No specific genes that "cause" psychotic disorders have been identified, but there are numerous gene variations (polymorphisms) associated with psychoses, some of which appear to be involved in brain structure and neurotransmitter systems relevant to the psychotic experiences (Ripke et al., 2014). Vulnerability to psychotic disorders is also increased by exposure to sexual, physical, and emotional childhood trauma; migration; and discrimination (van Os et al., 2010). For example, people with a psychotic disorder have experienced childhood trauma approximately 3 times more frequently than those without a psychotic disorder (Varese et al., 2012). Other risk factors include prenatal and birth complications (Cannon et al., 2002). Environmental stressors that occur later in life, such as major life events, interpersonal stressors, and urbanicity are also associated with psychosis. These risk factors manifest themselves in *vulnerability characteristics* that can be evidenced at different levels—neurobiological, neurochemical, physiological, cognitive—and are linked to symptom formation and maintenance. For example, compared with healthy control subjects, individuals with psychotic disorders tend to show the following:

- stronger emotional responses to stressors (Myin-Germeys & van Os, 2007);

- higher overall arousal and negative affect, and greater difficulties in emotion regulation and coping (Ludwig et al., 2019);

- neuropsychological impairment in terms of memory-related difficulties, difficulties in maintaining and focusing attention, and difficulties in planning (executive functioning; Jirsaraie et al., 2018);

- biases in reasoning, such as the tendency to use less information before drawing conclusions ("jumping to conclusions"; Dudley et al., 2016) and the tendency to attribute an event to external causes (Murphy et al., 2018);

- difficulties in identifying other people's emotions, feeling connected to others, inferring people's thoughts, and reacting emotionally to others (Green et al., 2015); and

- more fluctuations in self-esteem over time, as well as lower self-esteem and more negative schemas of the self and others (e.g., Beck et al., 2019; Murphy et al., 2018).

Some of these factors are likely to influence the way a patient responds in clinical interactions, and all have been a focus of psychological interventions for psychosis.

Various theoretical models have attempted to link the biological and social risk factors with the resulting vulnerability to explain how psychotic symptoms arise. These models all build on the assumption of an interaction between vulnerability and stress and are often used by clinicians to explain to patients why they may have developed psychosis. The different models stress different aspects. For example, an early model assumed that stress increases neurocognitive deficits and thereby makes it difficult for patients to filter incoming stimuli (Nuechterlein & Dawson, 1984). Biological models have emphasized abnormal physiological stress regulation that is assumed to be linked to an overactivation of dopamine pathways, the neurotransmitter most prominently associated with psychosis (Pruessner et al., 2017). Cognitive models have stressed the relevance of cognitive vulnerability caused by traumatizing experiences or other social adversity (e.g., Garety et al., 2001). These models postulate that psychotic symptoms evolve when stressors cause a vulnerable person to have unusual experiences (e.g., increased arousal, bodily sensations, or hallucinations). The crucial assumption is that it is not the unusual experiences in themselves that cause distress but the way in which the experience is appraised or interpreted by the person. This appraisal is assumed to be influenced by the individuals' affective state, their view of the world and their way of processing information (e.g., the reasoning biases described earlier). There have also been attempts to combine cognitive and neurobiological models. In a model put forward by Howes and Murray (2014), developmental alterations due to genes, early hazards to the brain, and childhood adversity are assumed to sensitize the dopaminergic system, which results in excessive presynaptic dopamine synthesis and release. This dysregulated dopamine is assumed to make it more likely that irrelevant perceptions are perceived as relevant. As in the cognitive models, the way these "unusual experiences" are interpreted are hypothesized to depend on the persons' beliefs and way of processing information.

SCHIZOPHRENIA

Presentations and Symptom Patterns

In the *ICD-11*, the characteristic symptoms of schizophrenia include (a) persistent delusions; (b) persistent hallucinations; (c) disorganized thinking; (d) experiences of influence, passivity, or control (e.g., feeling influenced by devices, feeling under control of external force); (e) negative symptoms (e.g., constricted, blunted, or flat affect; alogia or paucity of speech; avolition, asociality, and anhedonia); (f) grossly disorganized behavior; and (g) psychomotor disturbances. To make a diagnosis of schizophrenia, at least two of the seven characteristic symptoms must be present for a period of 1 month or more, of which one must be a positive symptom (i.e., symptoms a–d; WHO, 2024). The term *positive symptoms* is used if there is an alteration in the normal way of experiencing things, such as if a person starts hearing voices that were not previously heard.

Delusions are the most characteristic and frequent positive symptom in Schizophrenia. They can be defined as strongly held beliefs that are not consistent with reality, not shared by others, and not easily changed when confronted with counterevidence. Although people without delusions can also hold beliefs with strong conviction in the absence of evidence (e.g., religious beliefs, political views), these beliefs tend to be shared by others. They are also less clearly associated with distress or impaired functioning. One of the most frequently reported delusions is the belief that others intend harm. Delusions can cover a broad range of topics that vary by culture and gender but tend to revolve around personally relevant themes, such as relationships, religious beliefs, sexuality, and health issues. Delusions are often easier to understand in the early phases of symptom formation, where they can take on the form of an extreme interpretation (e.g., a person experiencing difficulties at work begins to believe that their coworkers are trying to get rid of them). Later, they can evolve to more complex delusions (e.g., that person begins to believe there is an organized conspiracy against them which goes beyond the immediate work context). The amount of time a person spends thinking about the delusion, the emotional distress associated with it, and even the rate of conviction varies from individual to individual. It can also vary over time within a given individual depending on external stressors and can be used as an indicator of recovery versus deterioration.

Hallucinations are sensory experiences, in any sensory modality, in the absence of corresponding external stimulation. In schizophrenia, they are most commonly auditory (e.g., hearing things) and verbal (i.e., hearing voices, specifically). What the voices say can vary in length (e.g., single words or complete sentences), complexity (e.g., single or several voices), content (e.g., benevolent or malevolent), and mode (e.g., commentary or commands). The content of the voices tends to have a lot in common with the content of automatic thoughts in other mental disorders, such as depression (e.g., voices saying critical things like "you are stupid"). However, in hallucinations, these thoughts are experienced as being heard rather than thought. Many people with psychotic disorders report that voices occurred for the first time in a period of extreme distress. The frequency, intensity, and content of hallucinations can vary over time in an individual, with variation often linked to the person's general mental state (e.g., hearing more negative voices when feeling sad, angry, or stressed).

Disorganized thinking tends to be indicated by the way a person speaks. For example, a person might be unable to answer a question without providing excessive unnecessary detail (circumstantiality), keep losing track of the topic (derailment), or start inventing new words. In extreme cases, a person's speech can become difficult or impossible to understand.

Closely linked to both hallucinations and delusions are what the *ICD-11* describes as *experiences of influence, passivity, or control*, which refer to the experience that ones' feelings, impulses, thoughts, bodily functions, or behavior are under the control of another person or other external force (WHO, 2024). For example, some people with schizophrenia feel that thoughts are being placed in their minds or withdrawn from their mind by others, or that their thoughts are being broadcast to others.

The term *negative symptoms* is used to express that something is missing from the range of normal experiences, such as when a person dramatically reduces their activity or speaks much less and with less expression than was previously the case. With a prevalence of approximately 60%, *negative symptoms* are as frequent as hallucinations among individuals with schizophrenia (Bobes et al., 2010) and are clearly associated with impairment in social functioning and quality of life. Negative symptoms are now widely considered a two-dimensional construct, comprising both motivational and expressive negative symptoms (Strauss et al., 2012). Motivational negative symptoms are defined as a lack of motivation to engage in, or sustain, goal-directed behavior, including avolition (general lack of drive or lack of motivation to pursue meaningful goals), asociality (reduced or absent engagement with others and interest in social interaction), and anhedonia (inability to experience pleasure from normally pleasurable activities). Expressive negative symptoms comprise diminished expression in several domains of nonverbal and verbal communication, such as in expressive movements of the facial muscles, intonation and quantity of spoken words, and gesturing. This does not necessarily mean that people with expressive negative symptoms do not experience strong feelings.

The term *disorganized behavior* is used to describe behavior that appears bizarre or unnecessary to observers. For example, a person might start throwing things out of the window, rearranging furniture in a strange way, or muttering loudly to themselves or may respond to a simple question with an emotional outburst. Most people may behave bizarrely at times. However, people's behavior can usually be explained by a combination of the context and their personality. Whether behavior is considered disorganized is dependent on whether this behavior is outside the norm after considering other factors, such as context, culture, developmental age, and personality. The behavior may also be understandable in the context of other psychotic symptoms. For example, a person's disorganized behavior may occur because they are following commanding voices (auditory hallucinations) or acting on delusions.

Finally, *psychomotor disturbances* include catatonic restlessness or agitation (i.e., extreme restlessness with purposeless or bizarre motor activity to the point of exhaustion), posturing (i.e., spontaneous and active maintenance of a posture against gravity), waxy flexibility (i.e., maintaining a position or posture after being placed in it by another person), negativism (i.e., opposition or no response to instructions or external stimuli), mutism (i.e., no, or very little, verbal response), or stupor (i.e., no psychomotor activity; not actively relating to environment).

Differential Diagnosis

Schizophrenia is the most severe disorder within this grouping in terms of how pronounced the symptoms are (e.g., more pronounced than in schizotypal disorder), their duration and stability (e.g., longer and with less fluctuation than in acute and transient psychotic disorder), and their range (e.g., broader spectrum of symptoms than in delusional disorder). Schizophrenia also includes symptoms that go beyond the realm of positive symptoms, such as negative symptoms and psychomotor disturbances. Negative and psychomotor symptoms may also be present in schizoaffective disorder (discussed later in this chapter) but are not characteristic of other psychotic disorders.

Psychotic symptoms can also occur during moderate or severe depressive episodes or during manic or mixed episodes in bipolar type I disorder. In these cases, however, they are confined to the mood episode. In PTSD, some symptoms, such as severe flashbacks or intrusive images, may have a hallucinatory quality, and hypervigilance may reach proportions that appear to be paranoid, but PTSD diagnosis requires exposure to a traumatic event alongside reexperiencing of the traumatic event in the present and other features that are not characteristic of schizophrenia. However, many people with schizophrenia or other primary psychotic disorders have significant histories of trauma as well as co-occurring PTSD.

Developmental Course

It is rare for the onset of schizophrenia to occur before puberty. Although some signs of vulnerability may be present before the onset of the disorder, schizophrenia symptoms typically begin in late adolescence to early adulthood, with a variable pattern but frequently a nonspecific deterioration in functioning heralding the onset of more specific psychotic symptoms. Women tend to show a slightly later peak of onset (toward the end of their 20s) than men (toward the beginning of their 20s). After this peak, there is a gradual decline in onset, although there is indication of a second peak around age 40, which may have some relation to the menopause, although this requires further investigation. Studies have shown that men are more likely to be assigned a diagnosis of schizophrenia, whereas women are more likely to be assigned a diagnosis of bipolar disorder (Dell'Osso et al., 2021; Li et al., 2022).

The course of the disorder is characterized by several specific phases. A first psychotic episode is often preceded by a *prodromal phase* with nonspecific symptoms, such as worry, rumination, sleep disorder, tension, difficulties concentrating, or irritability. The *acute phase* can begin abruptly or gradually and is dominated by positive symptoms. Negative symptoms are more likely to be present in the postacute phase, which is most often followed by a remission phase. The reports on the long-term course vary considerably across studies, but overall, one can conclude that approximately 20% to 30% of patients only experience one psychotic episode, followed by a complete recovery and another 20% to 30% experience a couple of episodes with no symptoms between the episodes. The remaining patients remain impaired in their psychosocial functioning to a certain degree even between the episodes, with some showing a chronic course. Factors that are more predictive of more positive outcomes include having a high level of social functioning before the disorder begins, an acute onset of the disorder, an absence of negative symptoms, an absence of neuropsychological dysfunctions and brain-structural abnormalities, getting treatment quickly, and having supportive and accepting family members.

In the *ICD-11*, the course of schizophrenia can be characterized using specifiers as "first episode" when the most recent episode is the first manifestation of Schizophrenia. If there has been a previous episode of schizophrenia or schizoaffective disorder with a period of partial or full remission between episodes lasting for at least 3 months, the "multiple episodes" specifier should be used. The "continuous" specifier is used when symptoms have been present for almost the entire course of the disorder since first onset.

SCHIZOAFFECTIVE DISORDER

Presentations and Symptom Patterns

To make a diagnosis of schizoaffective disorder, all diagnostic requirements for schizophrenia need to be met concurrently with mood symptoms that are sufficiently severe to meet the diagnostic requirements of a moderate or severe depressive episode, a manic episode, or a mixed episode (refer to Chapter 6, this volume, on depressive disorders). The onset of psychotic and mood symptoms should not occur more than a few days apart and have a duration of at least 1 month. A *schizodepressive episode* could thus be characterized by depressive symptoms, such as psychomotor retardation, loss of interest, insomnia, slow movements, concentration problems, feelings of guilt, hopelessness, and suicidal ideation, and the person may also have the impression that others may either hear or somehow be aware of their thoughts or that external forces are trying to control them. They may be convinced that people are spying on them, or they may be hearing condemning voices. Similarly, in a *schizomanic episode*, a person may experience elevated mood along with delusions of grandeur or may show symptoms of irritability and agitation along with delusions of persecution and aggressive behavior. They will also likely have increased drive and activity, along with problems concentrating, experiences of influence, passivity or control, and clearly impaired functioning.

Differential Diagnosis

Schizoaffective disorder is distinguished from schizophrenia based on co-occurring mood symptoms that meet the diagnostic requirements for an affective disorder (i.e., a moderate or severe depressive episode, a manic episode, or a mixed episode) and last for at least 1 month. Schizoaffective disorder is distinguished from mood disorders with psychotic symptoms because the symptom requirements for schizophrenia are fully met. The diagnosis of schizoaffective disorder thus should be considered only when a diagnosis of schizophrenia and a mood disorder are both substantiated and occur either together or within a few days of each other. It is possible for an individual to meet the diagnostic requirements for schizoaffective disorder, schizophrenia, moderate or severe depressive episodes, manic episodes, and mixed episodes during different periods as they are all intended to describe the *current* episode of the disorder. This conceptualization in *ICD-11* differs from previous ones, in which a person retained the diagnosis for all future episodes, regardless of symptom presentation.

Developmental Course

The onset of schizoaffective disorder can be characterized by serious disturbance, which becomes apparent within a few days (acute) or by a gradual development of signs and symptoms. A prodromal phase characterized by loss of interest in work or social activities, neglect of personal appearance or hygiene, inversion of the sleep cycle, attenuated psychotic symptoms, and/or anxiety and depressive symptoms can precede the onset of psychotic symptoms. As with schizophrenia, the course of schizoaffective disorder tends to be episodic with periods of remission and can be further described using the *ICD-11* specifiers. Overall, the course for this disorder is somewhat better than that for schizophrenia (both in terms of age of onset and in terms of remission between episodes) but somewhat poorer than that for mood disorders. Schizodepressive episodes tend to be less dramatic than schizomanic episodes but last longer and are associated with a poorer prognosis (Brieger et al., 2017).

SCHIZOTYPAL DISORDER

Schizotypal disorder is characterized by an enduring pattern of unusual speech, perceptions, beliefs, and behaviors that are not of sufficient severity or duration to meet the diagnostic requirements for other psychotic disorders. There must be several symptoms that are similar in nature to the symptoms of schizophrenia but milder or more transitory. For example, the diagnosis of schizotypal disorder might apply to people who find it hard to make close friends because they are perceived as slightly awkward in communication (e.g., avoiding eye contact, smiling inappropriately, remaining vague on matters of importance, pronouncing sentences in an unusual way) and slightly odd in appearance and behavior, while also feeling distrustful of other people's intentions. At the same time, such individuals may have a fascination for topics that seem eccentric to others, such as ghosts or supernatural powers, be superstitious, and have occasional odd perceptions, such as seeing their surroundings change color or hearing a frightening voice that says their name at night. There may be occasional transient psychotic episodes, perhaps with intense illusions where people process information in a way that does not align with reality, auditory or other hallucinations, and delusion-like ideas. Because people with schizotypal disorder often do not "fit in" in mainstream school or other social contexts, they tend to spend a lot of time alone, which can cause great loneliness. Emotional distress can also result from the symptoms themselves, such as anxiety due to having strange perceptual experiences. To make a diagnosis, the symptoms must have been present for at least 2 years and cause distress or impairment in important areas of functioning, which is an essential boundary with normality.

The differential diagnosis with schizophrenia is important in schizotypal disorder. Symptoms of schizotypal disorder may be qualitatively similar to those of schizophrenia without meeting the diagnostic requirements for schizophrenia in terms of severity or duration. For example, the speech disturbance in schizotypal disorder is without gross incoherence, and magical thinking and paranoid ideation do not reach the diagnostic requirements for a delusion. The severity of symptoms can also guide the differential diagnosis with other related disorders (e.g., obsessive ruminations without a sense that the obsession is unwanted, as it would be in obsessive-compulsive disorder). Interpersonal difficulties in schizotypal disorder may share features of autism spectrum disorder, such as poor rapport and social withdrawal. However, individuals with schizotypal disorder do not exhibit other core features of autism spectrum disorder, such as restricted, repetitive, and stereotyped patterns of behavior, interests, or activities.

Schizotypal disorder typically begins in late adolescence or early adulthood, without a definite onset. The disorder may persist over years with fluctuations of intensity and symptom expression but rarely evolves into schizophrenia.

ACUTE AND TRANSIENT PSYCHOTIC DISORDER

This diagnosis applies to cases in which psychotic symptoms begin acutely within 2 weeks, with the symptoms changing rapidly in nature and intensity. The disorder remits quickly, and most commonly lasts from a few days to 1 month; once psychotic symptom duration extends beyond 1 month, a diagnosis of schizophrenia would be considered. Along with prominent psychotic symptoms of hallucinations and/or delusions, there are often other symptoms such as disturbances of mood, transient states of perplexity or confusion, or impairment of attention and concentration. The disorder has been observed to follow stressors, such as loss of job or loss of significant others, but this is not obligatory to make the diagnosis.

The most characteristic differentiating factor from other psychotic disorders is the acute onset and the short duration. The fluctuations of symptoms and the absence of negative symptoms during the psychotic episode also distinguish the disorder from schizophrenia and schizoaffective disorder. In contrast to depressive disorders, mood symptoms that may occur are transient and do not meet the required duration or associated symptoms to qualify for a mood disorder. In contrast to delirium, the person maintains a regular level of alertness and relatively clear sense of consciousness.

Similar to schizophrenia and schizoaffective disorder, the course is episodic and can be described in *ICD-11* both in terms of the number of episodes and of the current remission status. The short-duration episodes are associated with deterioration in functioning, although this is generally regained after the episode has remitted. Risk of relapse is high, although a chronic course is excluded by definition.

DELUSIONAL DISORDER

Delusional disorder is characterized by distinct and enduring delusional beliefs in the absence of any other psychotic symptoms. In these cases, symptoms may not be apparent as long as the delusional topic(s) are not discussed. Common forms of delusions relate to persecution, somatic delusions (e.g., a belief that organs are rotting or malfunctioning), grandiose delusions, delusions related to jealousy (e.g., the unjustified belief that one's spouse is unfaithful), and love (i.e., the belief that another person, usually a famous or high-status stranger, is in love with the person experiencing the delusion). Delusions may be accompanied by actions directly related to their content. For example, a person with the delusion of being the loved one of a famous singer writes letters to the singer. The delusions need to persist for at least 3 months to make a diagnosis, but typically persist much longer. The content of delusions varies across individuals, while showing remarkable stability within individuals.

Delusional disorder can be differentiated from other psychotic disorders because the delusions occur in the absence of additional characteristic psychotic symptoms. For example, in contrast to other psychotic disorders, mood, speech, and behavior are typically unaffected. When hallucinations do occur, they tend to be related to the content of the delusions (e.g., tactile hallucinations in delusions of being infected by parasites).

Delusional disorder typically has a later onset and greater stability of symptoms than other psychotic disorders with delusional symptoms. In contrast to schizophrenia or schizoaffective disorder the overall functioning is less impaired, even in cases that take a more chronic course.

ASSESSMENT

The diagnosis of schizophrenia or another primary psychotic disorders can have serious negative implications and should not be given lightly. To obtain a more reliable diagnosis, not only of the psychotic disorder but also of relevant co-occurring disorders, standardized procedures such as structured interviews or diagnostic checklists are recommended. Symptom assessment can be based on an individual's report or through observation by the clinician or other informants.

The *Clinical Descriptions and Diagnostic Requirements for ICD-11 Mental, Behavioural and Neurodevelopmental Disorders* (*CDDR*; WHO, 2024) provides specifier scales to indicate the level of severity of positive symptoms, negative symptoms, depressive mood symptoms, manic mood symptoms, psychomotor symptoms, and cognitive symptoms. These symptom domains can be rated as mild, moderate, or severe, based on their severity during the past week. Although the *CDDR* provide diagnostic descriptions for each symptom domain specifically, the general rule is that a domain is rated as mild when only one or two of the symptoms in the domain have been present, everyday functioning is not or is only minimally affected, and no significant negative social or personal consequences of symptoms have occurred. A rating of moderate severity is given when three or four symptoms in the domain have been present (or fewer if they have shown a substantial degree of impact), everyday functioning is moderately affected, negative social or personal consequences of the symptoms are not severe, and most of the symptoms are present the majority of the time. A domain is rated as severe when many symptoms of the domain have been present (or fewer with severe impact), everyday functioning is persistently impaired, and there are serious negative social or personal consequences. For the positive symptoms domain, there are descriptions for each of the individual symptoms within the domain (i.e., delusions, hallucinations, experiences of passivity and control, disorganized thinking, and disorganized behavior). For example, delusions would be rated as mild if the person holds a delusion but does not feel pressure to act on it and the delusion leads to minimal distress; as moderate if behavior is clearly affected by the delusion but functioning is not significantly impaired (e.g., a person with persecutory delusions is watchful of their surroundings but continues to venture outside); and as severe if the person is preoccupied with delusional beliefs that have a strong impact on that person's behavior and impair functioning (e.g., a person with persecutory delusions refuses to eat most food because of a conviction that food has been poisoned). In this case, where multiple symptoms fall within a particular domain, the rating should reflect the most severe symptom within that domain.

As a basis for diagnosis and also for assigning the *ICD-11* symptom domain specifier scales, there are validated self- and observer-rated instruments available in numerous languages. The use of such measures with predefined questions and anchors for qualifying the severity of different symptoms (from not present to severe) is recommended and can be particularly helpful for less experienced clinicians. All these measures include prompts related to frequency, duration, and impact on functioning to aid in accurate diagnosis. The use of standardized measures can also be a normalizing process for the patient by demonstrating that other people also experience these types of symptoms. Frequently used measures include the Positive and Negative Syndrome Scale (Kay et al., 1987), the Psychotic Symptoms Rating Scales (Haddock et al., 1999), and the Brief Negative Symptom Scale (Kirkpatrick et al., 2011). Of course, a diagnosis cannot be made based on any single test result, and measures used should be culturally and linguistically appropriate for the individual being tested. Any standardization of measures (e.g., *t*-scores, clinical cutoffs) should be appropriately normed for the local population.

For therapy planning, it is also important to assess the triggering and maintaining conditions of the symptoms and the way the patient appraises them alongside any coping strategies they may have developed. The clinician should also bear in mind the psychosocial risk and vulnerability factors for schizophrenia described in the first section of this chapter. These can guide the collaborative development of a formulation of why an individual's symptoms may have developed and how they are being maintained. This type of formulation-based approach can also be applied to individuals who present with distressing symptoms in the absence of a diagnosable psychotic disorder. Recently there has been a great deal of research and clinical service development around early intervention in psychosis. This approach allows for treatments to commence at the earliest opportunity but without the need for definitive diagnoses and recognizes that diagnoses may change over time.

PREVALENCE

The prevalence of schizophrenia and other primary psychotic disorders is fairly consistent across different countries. However, starting with studies carried out by WHO (e.g., Jablensky et al., 1992), several studies have found the course to be better in some non-Western, less industrialized countries. Different reasons have been discussed for this, including differences in family support, stigmatization, integration into social and occupational activities that are associated with differences in culture, or economic status of countries. Schizophrenia has a lifetime prevalence of about 0.3% to 0.7%. Men and women are affected equally often in most epidemiological studies, but women tend to show a better long-term course (fewer episodes, more complete recovery, and better long-term functioning). Schizoaffective disorder has a lifetime prevalence of about 0.3% with women affected more frequently than men. The prevalence for schizotypal disorder is about 4% with high variation across studies. Estimates for acute and transient psychotic disorder also vary around approximately 0.1%, with some studies finding women to be affected more frequently than men. The prevalence of delusional disorder is estimated at about 0.2% to 0.4%.

CO-OCCURRING DISORDERS

Schizophrenia and other primary psychotic disorders often co-occur with disorders due to substance use, anxiety and fear-related disorders, and mood disorders. It is important to attend to these diagnoses because they can affect treatment success and adherence. It is also relevant to keep in mind the high rate of attempted and completed suicides in psychotic disorders. The rate of completed suicides at approximately 5% (Hor & Taylor, 2010), and similar rates have been reported for schizoaffective disorder and acute and transient psychotic disorder. Risk factors for later suicide include being young; being male; having a high level of education, depressive symptoms, active hallucinations, and/or delusions; acknowledgment of having a severe mental disorder; a family history of suicide; and co-occurring substance misuse. Furthermore, individuals with schizophrenia tend to die significantly earlier than healthy control individuals. Reasons for this include adverse effects of medication, comorbidity with other medical conditions, suboptimal treatment of other medical conditions, and suboptimal lifestyle, including smoking and reduced activity. These factors also interact and enhance each other's effects. For example, increased weight may be due to antipsychotic medication and inactivity. The impact of being overweight subsequently increases the risk of the metabolic disorders. Significantly, most of the weight gain happens in the early course of the disorder, which provides an opportunity for intervention.

VALIDITY AND OTHER KEY SCIENTIFIC ISSUES

There has been some controversy regarding whether the distinction between psychotic and affective disorders is meaningful. Critics of this distinction point to the strong overlap between these groupings (van Os & Reininghaus, 2016). For example, negative symptoms resemble depression, and depression can also occur with psychotic symptoms. The overlap has created the necessity for "overlap diagnoses," such as schizoaffective disorder. There is also controversy about maintaining the label schizophrenia, which is associated with stigmatization and poses a further barrier to recovery because it is associated with continued social stress and less willingness to seek and accept help. Finally, there has been controversy about whether or not a "high risk of psychosis" status (which resembles the prodromal phase in patients before a first episode of schizophrenia) should have been included in the *ICD-11* as a diagnostic entity. A reason to include it is that people who meet the diagnostic requirements for an at-risk mental status have high levels of mental distress along with a substantially increased likelihood of transitioning to a full psychotic episode over time. The transition rate varies between approximately 20% and 40% depending on how the at-risk state is assessed and the length of the investigated period. The high rate of transition makes it important for clinicians to recognize this at-risk mental state. A diagnosis would increase the likelihood of professional help and the development of interventions to reduce the likelihood of transition to a full disorder. Reasons not to include such a diagnosis are that the majority of the "at-risk" people do not develop a full clinical disorder and that early labeling could trigger stigmatization processes. Also, many of those classified as being "at risk" fulfill diagnostic requirements for other disorders and should have access to mental health services on this basis. Overall, the WHO considered the potential liabilities of including a high risk in the *ICD-11* to outweigh the benefit, but this may change over time with additional research.

KEY POINTS

- Schizophrenia and other primary psychotic disorders are characterized by a loss of touch with reality (although this is milder in schizotypal disorder). These disorders are some of the most disabling in mental health care, and early recognition is vital to ensure that the correct treatment pathway is identified and to maximize the opportunity to promote recovery.

- The *ICD-11* includes six categories in the schizophrenia and other primary psychotic disorders grouping—namely, schizophrenia, schizoaffective disorder, schizotypal disorder, acute and transient psychotic disorder, delusional disorder, and other primary psychotic disorder. The *ICD-11 CDDR* focus on the key clinical aspects useful for identification of each disorder.

- In *ICD-11*, the characteristic symptoms of schizophrenia include (a) persistent delusions; (b) persistent hallucinations; (c) disorganized thinking; (d) experiences of influence, passivity, or control (e.g., feeling influenced by devices, feeling under control of external force); (e) negative symptoms; (f) grossly disorganized behavior; and (g) psychomotor disturbances. Symptoms fall into positive and negative symptom profiles and the intensity and duration of symptoms are key to understanding the disorder boundaries.

- In schizoaffective disorder, symptoms must simultaneously meet the diagnostic requirements for schizophrenia and a mood episode (i.e., a moderate or severe depressive episode, a manic episode, or a mixed episode) and last for at least 1 month.

- Psychotic disorders often co-occur with substance use disorders, anxiety disorders, and mood disorders. It is important to attend to these diagnoses because they can affect treatment success and adherence.

- There are different types of predisposing risk factors that make people vulnerable to developing a psychotic disorder. These include a significant genetic component as well as exposure to significant psychosocial stressors. Vulnerability shows up in varying ways, including increased stress sensitivity, higher overall arousal and negative affect, neuropsychological impairment, and unstable self-esteem that can also be relevant to symptom maintenance.

- Taking a psychological approach to psychosis means contextualizing the symptoms to gain an understanding of how they have developed and are being maintained.

- Assessment from multiple sources, incorporating data from the clinical interview, monitoring of symptoms, and validated questionnaires will help to establish the baseline level of symptoms, enabling accurate diagnosis but also guiding the formulation and understanding of symptom development, which is necessary to derive an evidence-based case conceptualization and treatment plan.

REFERENCES

Beck, A. T., Himelstein, R., & Grant, P. M. (2019). In and out of schizophrenia: Activation and deactivation of the negative and positive schemas. *Schizophrenia Research*, 203, 55–61. https://doi.org/10.1016/j.schres.2017.10.046

Bobes, J., Arango, C., Garcia-Garcia, M., Rejas, J., & the CLAMORS Study Collaborative Group. (2010). Prevalence of negative symptoms in outpatients with schizophrenia spectrum disorders treated with antipsychotics in routine clinical practice: Findings from the CLAMORS study. *The Journal of Clinical Psychiatry*, 71(3), 280–286. https://doi.org/10.4088/JCP.08m04250yel

Brieger, P., Marneros, A., & Jäger, M. (2017). Schizoaffektive störungen, akute vorübergehende psychotische störungen und wahnhafte störungen [Schizoaffective disorders, acute transient psychotic disorders and delusional disorders]. In H.-J. Möller, G. Laux, & H.-P. Kapfhammer (Eds.), *Psychiatrie, psychosomatik, psychotherapie* (pp. 1675–1700). Springer. https://doi.org/10.1007/978-3-662-49295-6_65

Cannon, M., Jones, P. B., & Murray, R. M. (2002). Obstetric complications and schizophrenia: Historical and meta-analytic review. *The American Journal of Psychiatry*, 159(7), 1080–1092. https://doi.org/10.1176/appi.ajp.159.7.1080

Dell'Osso, B., Cafaro, R., & Ketter, T. A. (2021). Has bipolar disorder become a predominantly female gender related condition? Analysis of recently published large sample studies. *International Journal of Bipolar Disorders*, 9(1), 3. https://doi.org/10.1186/s40345-020-00207-z

Dudley, R., Taylor, P., Wickham, S., & Hutton, P. (2016). Psychosis, delusions and the "jumping to conclusions" reasoning bias: A systematic review and meta-analysis. *Schizophrenia Bulletin*, 42(3), 652–665. https://doi.org/10.1093/schbul/sbv150

Garety, P. A., Kuipers, E., Fowler, D., Freeman, D., & Bebbington, P. E. (2001). A cognitive model of the positive symptoms of psychosis. *Psychological Medicine*, 31(2), 189–195. https://doi.org/10.1017/S0033291701003312

Green, M. F., Horan, W. P., & Lee, J. (2015). Social cognition in schizophrenia. *Nature Reviews Neuroscience*, 16(10), 620–631. https://doi.org/10.1038/nrn4005

Haddock, G., McCarron, J., Tarrier, N., & Faragher, E. B. (1999). Scales to measure dimensions of hallucinations and delusions: The psychotic symptom rating scales (PSYRATS). *Psychological Medicine*, 29(4), 879–889. https://doi.org/10.1017/S0033291799008661

Hor, K., & Taylor, M. (2010). Suicide and schizophrenia: A systematic review of rates and risk factors. *Journal of Psychopharmacology*, 24(Suppl. 4), 81–90. https://doi.org/10.1177/1359786810385490

Howes, O. D., & Murray, R. M. (2014). Schizophrenia: An integrated sociodevelopmental-cognitive model. *The Lancet*, 383(9929), 1677–1687. https://doi.org/10.1016/S0140-6736(13)62036-X

Jablensky, A., Sartorius, N., Ernberg, G., Anker, M., Korten, A., Cooper, J. E., Day, R., & Bertelsen, A. (1992). Schizophrenia: Manifestations, incidence and course in different cultures. A World Health Organization ten-country study. *Psychological Medicine Monograph Supplement, 20,* 1–97. https://doi.org/10.1017/S0264180100000904

Jirsaraie, R. J., Sheffield, J. M., & Barch, D. M. (2018). Neural correlates of global and specific cognitive deficits in schizophrenia. *Schizophrenia Research, 201,* 237–242. https://doi.org/10.1016/j.schres.2018.06.017

Kanfer, F. H., Reinecker, H., & Schmelzer, D. (2012). *Selbst-management-therapie: Ein lehrbuch für die klinische praxis* [Self-management therapy: A textbook for clinical practice]. Springer.

Kay, S. R., Fiszbein, A., & Opler, L. A. (1987). The positive and negative syndrome scale (PANSS) for schizophrenia. *Schizophrenia Bulletin, 13*(2), 261–276. https://doi.org/10.1093/schbul/13.2.261

Kirkpatrick, B., Strauss, G. P., Nguyen, L., Fischer, B. A., Daniel, D. G., Cienfuegos, A., & Marder, S. R. (2011). The brief negative symptom scale: Psychometric properties. *Schizophrenia Bulletin, 37*(2), 300–305. https://doi.org/10.1093/schbul/sbq059

Li, X., Zhou, W., & Yi, Z. (2022). A glimpse of gender differences in schizophrenia. *General Psychiatry, 35*(4), e100823. https://doi.org/10.1136/gpsych-2022-100823

Ludwig, L., Werner, D., & Lincoln, T. M. (2019). The relevance of cognitive emotion regulation to psychotic symptoms—A systematic review and meta-analysis. *Clinical Psychology Review, 72,* 101746. https://doi.org/10.1016/j.cpr.2019.101746

Murphy, P., Bentall, R. P., Freeman, D., O'Rourke, S., & Hutton, P. (2018). The paranoia as defence model of persecutory delusions: A systematic review and meta-analysis. *The Lancet Psychiatry, 5*(11), 913–929. https://doi.org/10.1016/S2215-0366(18)30339-0

Myin-Germeys, I., & van Os, J. (2007). Stress-reactivity in psychosis: Evidence for an affective pathway to psychosis. *Clinical Psychology Review, 27*(4), 409–424. https://doi.org/10.1016/j.cpr.2006.09.005

Nuechterlein, K. H., & Dawson, M. E. (1984). A heuristic vulnerability/stress model of schizophrenic episodes. *Schizophrenia Bulletin, 10*(2), 300–312. https://doi.org/10.1093/schbul/10.2.300

Pruessner, M., Cullen, A. E., Aas, M., & Walker, E. F. (2017). The neural diathesis-stress model of schizophrenia revisited: An update on recent findings considering illness stage and neurobiological and methodological complexities. *Neuroscience and Biobehavioral Reviews, 73,* 191–218. https://doi.org/10.1016/j.neubiorev.2016.12.013

Ripke, S., Neale, B. M., Corvin, A., Walters, J. T. R., Farh, K.-H., Holmans, P. A., Lee, P., Bulik-Sullivan, B., Collier, D. A., Huang, H., Pers, T. H., Agartz, I., Agerbo, E., Albus, M., Alexander, M., Amin, F., Bacanu, S. A., Begemann, M., Belliveau, R. A., Jr., . . . the Schizophrenia Working Group of the Psychiatric Genomics Consortium. (2014). Biological insights from 108 schizophrenia-associated genetic loci. *Nature, 511*(7510), 421–427. https://doi.org/10.1038/nature13595

Strauss, G. P., Hong, L. E., Gold, J. M., Buchanan, R. W., McMahon, R. P., Keller, W. R., Fischer, B. A., Catalano, L. T., Culbreth, A. J., Carpenter, W. T., & Kirkpatrick, B. (2012). Factor structure of the Brief Negative Symptom Scale. *Schizophrenia Research, 142*(1–3), 96–98. https://doi.org/10.1016/j.schres.2012.09.007

van Os, J., Kenis, G., & Rutten, B. P. F. (2010). The environment and schizophrenia. *Nature, 468*(7321), 203–212. https://doi.org/10.1038/nature09563

van Os, J., & Reininghaus, U. (2016). Psychosis as a transdiagnostic and extended phenotype in the general population. *World Psychiatry, 15*(2), 118–124. https://doi.org/10.1002/wps.20310

Varese, F., Barkus, E., & Bentall, R. P. (2012). Dissociation mediates the relationship between childhood trauma and hallucination-proneness. *Psychological Medicine, 42*(5), 1025–1036. https://doi.org/10.1017/S0033291711001826

World Health Organization. (2023). *ICD-11 for mortality and morbidity statistics* (Version: 01/2023). https://icd.who.int/browse11/l-m/en#/

World Health Organization. (2024). *Clinical descriptions and diagnostic requirements for ICD-11 mental, behavioural and neurodevelopmental disorders.* https://www.who.int/publications/i/item/9789240077263

Wray, N. R., & Gottesman, I. I. (2012). Using summary data from the Danish National Registers to estimate heritabilities for schizophrenia, bipolar disorder, and major depressive disorder. *Frontiers in Genetics, 3,* 118. https://doi.org/10.3389/fgene.2012.00118

6

Depressive Disorders

Rebeca Robles, Ana Fresán, and José Luis Ayuso-Mateos

OVERARCHING LOGIC

In the 11th revision of the *International Classification of Diseases* (*ICD-11*; World Health Organization [WHO], 2023b), depressive disorders are part of the broader grouping of mood disorders, which also includes bipolar and related disorders. The rationale for placing depressive and bipolar disorders together within the same superordinate grouping is that marked disturbances in mood or affect is the defining feature of both. The shared symptoms and clinical features of these two groups of disorders likely reflect overlap in underlying biological mechanisms, etiology, and risk factors.

Both groups of mood disorders are defined by the presence or absence and pattern over time of four types of mood episodes: depressive, manic, mixed, and hypomanic. If an individual has ever experienced a manic, mixed, or hypomanic episode, this indicates the presence of a bipolar or related disorder and the individual should not be diagnosed with a depressive disorder. A depressive episode, like other type of mood episodes, is not a distinct disorder because mood disorder diagnoses are conceptualized as longitudinal—that is, they account not only for the current clinical presentation (i.e., the current mood episode) but also for past mood episodes. For example, a diagnosis of bipolar type I disorder, current episode depressive indicates that the individual is currently experiencing a depressive episode but also has a history of at least one manic or mixed episode.

https://doi.org/10.1037/0000392-006

A Psychological Approach to Diagnosis: Using the ICD-11 as a Framework, G. M. Reed, P. L.-J. Ritchie, and A. Maercker (Editors)

A person who has experienced one or more depressive episodes but has no history of manic, mixed, or hypomanic episodes can be diagnosed with one of two main depressive disorder diagnoses depending on the number of depressive episodes they have experienced: (a) single episode depressive disorder if the person has only ever had one depressive episode or (b) recurrent depressive disorder if the person has a history of two or more depressive episodes (including a current episode) separated by at least several months without significant mood disturbance.

There are two additional disorders in the *ICD-11* depressive disorders grouping that are characterized by depressive symptoms that do not meet the full diagnostic requirements for a depressive episode. The diagnosis mixed depressive and anxiety disorder (MDAD), which is common in primary care settings, is assigned to individuals exhibiting both depressive and anxiety symptoms but not in a sufficiently severe, frequent, or lasting manner to justify the diagnosis of either single or recurrent depressive disorder or an anxiety or fear-related disorder. The diagnosis of dysthymic disorder is assigned to individuals who exhibit persistent depressive symptoms (2 years or more) that are attenuated or subthreshold in relation to the diagnostic requirements for a depressive episode, although later in its course, dysthymic disorder may be punctuated by periods of more intense depressive symptoms that do meet the diagnostic requirements for a depressive episode, in which case both diagnoses are assigned (so-called double depression). Finally, the *ICD-11* depressive disorders grouping includes a cross-referenced category from the *ICD-11* chapter on diseases of the genitourinary system: premenstrual dysphoric disorder (PMDD). The diagnosis of PMDD may be assigned to women with a distinct characteristic pattern of mood, somatic, and cognitive symptoms that occurs in a specific temporal relationship with most of their menstrual cycles.

A PSYCHOLOGICAL APPROACH TO DEPRESSIVE DISORDERS

The three symptom clusters (neurovegetative, affective, and cognitive-behavioral) that make up the diagnostic requirements for a depressive episode in *ICD-11* (WHO, 2024) are congruent with the conceptualization of depression in at least two of the main psychological approaches to treatment of depressive disorders: the behavioral model and the cognitive model. According to the behavioral model of depression, a lack of positive environmental reinforcers (such as social recognition after accomplishing a task) is the underlying phenomenon that explains the passivity of depressed individuals. Interventions based on this perspective often focus on helping the person to plan systematically and engage in gratifying activities that produce a sense of personal accomplishment or pleasure. This approach, known as behavioral activation, has proven to be an effective tool in managing depression, even without medication (Stein et al., 2021).

Another important psychological approach to depression focuses on the cognitive symptoms of depressive episodes, specifically what is termed the *cognitive triad of depression* (Beck et al., 1979). The cognitive triad refers to the presence of negative or dysfunctional beliefs about (a) oneself (e.g., beliefs of low self-worth or excessive or inappropriate guilt), (b) the world, and (c) the future. In particular, negative beliefs about the future are the central component of hopelessness, which is not only one of the specific diagnostic elements for a depressive episode in the *ICD-11* but is also an important predictor of suicide risk (McGlinchey et al., 2006). Using cognitive techniques to modify these negative or dysfunctional beliefs, usually combined with behavioral activation in cognitive-behavioral treatment approaches, has proven to be highly effective in reducing depressive symptoms compared with treatment with medication alone (Uphoff et al., 2020). This includes significantly reduced levels of hopelessness and improvement in self-concept.

The conceptualization of specific clusters of symptoms in the diagnostic requirements for depressive episode in the *Clinical Descriptions and Diagnostic Requirements for ICD-11 Mental, Behavioural and Neurodevelopmental Disorders* (*CDDR*; WHO, 2024) allows clinicians to develop individualized profiles for targeted psychological interventions. For example, for individuals who present markedly diminished interest or pleasure in activities along with reduced ability to concentrate and sustain attention, behavioral treatment such as behavioral activation may be more effective because certain cognitive strategies may be difficult to implement (Cuijpers et al., 2019). Similarly, the profile of cognitive symptoms may help determine the need for more intensive treatments such as hospitalization, continuous supervision, or additional cautionary measures—for example, to prevent suicide attempts (Perini et al., 2019).

Another psychological feature of the *CDDR* for depressive disorders is the incorporation of a dimensional conceptualization of psychopathology, as opposed to a purely categorical one. This is implied by the provision of severity specifiers for depressive episodes and by the inclusion of attenuated forms of depression (dysthymic disorder, MDAD, and PMDD). Another important conceptual feature of the *ICD-11* diagnostic formulation for depressive disorders, as in other parts of the *CDDR*, is the consideration of the level of associated disability or functional impairment in personal, familial, social, educational, occupational, or other important areas of functioning (e.g., participation in community and civic life). This is consistent with the biopsychosocial model of disability presented in the International Classification of Functioning, Disability and Health (ICF; WHO, 2001), which conceptualizes a person's level of functioning as a dynamic interaction among their health conditions, environment and context, and personal characteristics.

The *ICD-11 CDDR* also recognize that in some cases, individuals are able to maintain functioning even in the face of substantial clinical depression because of personal resources (e.g., a high level of skill or expertise) or particular histories or types of environmental circumstances. The functioning of such people with even moderate or severe depression may not be objectively impaired to the extent that they may continue to work and maintain their relationships, for example, but only with significant additional effort. Although there is a positive correlation between the severity of a disorder and the resulting disability, disability is an outcome of the underlying disorder in a given environment, reflected in the activities in which people can or cannot engage. On this basis, clinical severity and disability can be adequately distinguished, and both should be addressed as a part of evaluation, case conceptualization, and treatment (e.g., via additional psychosocial interventions specifically designed to improve functioning).

SINGLE EPISODE DEPRESSIVE DISORDER AND RECURRENT DEPRESSIVE DISORDER

Presentations and Symptom Patterns

The diagnoses of single episode depressive disorder and recurrent depressive disorder is based on the occurrence of one or more than one depressive episodes, respectively. The diagnostic requirements for a depressive episode represent one of comparatively few instances in the *CDDR* in which precise thresholds in symptom counts and duration are required. The 10 symptoms that make up the diagnostic features of depressive episodes are organized into three clusters: affective (i.e., depressed mood, loss of interest or pleasure), cognitive-behavioral (e.g., difficulty concentrating or sustaining attention, beliefs of low self-worth, hopelessness about the future), and neurovegetative (sleep disruption, appetite disturbance, fatigue). For a depressive episode, at least five of the 10 symptoms are required, including at least one symptom from the affective cluster. Additionally, symptoms must occur most of the day, nearly every day, for a period of at least 2 weeks and result in significant impairment in functioning.

Depression, including both single episode and recurrent depressive disorders, is among the most common mental disorders worldwide. The World Health Organization (2023a) estimated that 5% of adults around the world suffer from depression, and data from many high-income countries indicate substantially higher prevalence (e.g., National Institute of Mental Health, 2022). Prevalence among women is consistently found to be higher than among men. In these statistics, clinical depression is sometimes referred to as major depression, the *Diagnostic and Statistical Manual* term, to distinguish it from subthreshold depressive symptoms. *ICD-11* separates single episode disorder and recurrent depressive disorder because as many as half of people who experience a depressive episode do not experience another after recovery from it (Burcusa & Iocono, 2007). The treatment implications of a single episode are substantially different from those of recurrent episodes (e.g., use of prophylactic medication).

Subtypes and Specifiers

To reflect the clinical heterogeneity of single episode and recurrent depressive disorders, several specifiers can be applied to describe the relevant features of

the clinical presentation or of the course, onset, and pattern of depressive episodes. These specifiers are not mutually exclusive, and as many may be added
as apply. Specifiers include the severity of the current episode, whether the
current episode is persistent (i.e., has been continuously present for 2 or more
years), and the presence of psychotic symptoms, melancholia, panic attacks,
other significant anxiety symptoms, and a seasonal pattern of onset and remission. If the depressive episode is not current but has occurred in the recent
past, another specifier indicating partial or total remission at time of the evaluation may be applied.

Severity and Psychotic Symptoms
Current depressive episodes in the context of single episode or recurrent
depressive disorder are described according to one of three levels of severity:
mild, moderate, or severe. The severity of a depressive episode has important
clinical implications (e.g., consideration of medication as a part of treatment).
Severity level is established by considering the number and intensity of symptoms and the resulting degree of functional impairment.

In a mild depressive episode, none of the symptoms should be present to an
intense degree, and there are no delusions or hallucinations. The individual
is usually distressed by the symptoms and has some difficulty continuing to
function in personal, familial, social, educational, occupational, and other
important domains. In a moderate depressive episode, several symptoms are
present to a marked degree, or a large number of depressive symptoms of
lesser severity are present overall. The individual typically has considerable
difficulty functioning in personal, familial, social, educational, occupational,
and other important domains. In a severe depressive episode, many or most
symptoms of a depressive episode are present to a marked degree, or a smaller
number of symptoms are manifest to an intense degree. The individual has
serious difficulty continuing to function in most domains (personal, family,
social, educational, occupational, or other important domains).

Psychotic symptoms can be a part of the presentation of depressive episodes, and their presence has major clinical implications. In *ICD-11*, specifiers
for "with psychotic symptoms" or "without psychotic symptoms" are applied
to both moderate and severe depressive episodes. In the 10th revision of the
ICD (ICD-10), psychotic symptoms were considered as only occurring in severe
cases of depression, but more recent evidence suggests that they can occur at
varying levels of severity (Dubovsky et al., 2021). The psychotic symptoms
specifier in moderate and severe depressive episodes encompasses only delusions and hallucinations and does not include other types of psychotic symptoms (e.g., disorganized thinking or behavior that would be more suggestive
of schizophrenia or schizoaffective disorder). Delusions during depressive episodes are commonly persecutory or self-referential (i.e., the conviction that
strangers are talking about the individual). However, delusions of guilt, poverty, impending disaster, or other delusions focused on the body (e.g., being
completely convinced there is something medically, physically, or biologically
wrong with one's body) can also occur. Hallucinations in moderate or severe

depressive episodes are more commonly auditory than visual or olfactory. Psychotic symptoms can vary in intensity over the course of a depressive episode or even over the course of the day. Careful assessment of potential psychotic symptoms is important because individuals experiencing a depressive episode are often reluctant to report them.

Persistent Symptoms and Remission

A specifier is also provided to document the presence of a "persistent" depressive episode, in which the diagnostic requirements for a depressive episode are currently met and have been met continuously for at least the past 2 years. Conversely, a specifier for "in partial remission" indicates that the full diagnostic requirements for a depressive episode are no longer met but that some significant mood symptoms remain, and a specifier for "in full remission" indicates that are no longer any significant mood symptoms after a depressive episode. Consideration of persistent and remission presentations in single episode and recurrent depressive disorders can assist clinicians in assessment, treatment selection, evaluation of progress, and determination of prognosis. However, it should be noted that even though an individual may be in partial or full remission in terms of depressive symptoms, they still may not have achieved a level of functioning or well-being similar to what they had experienced before the depressive episode.

Additional Specifiers Describing Symptomatic and Course Presentations

ICD-11 allows the use of six other symptomatic and course specifiers to describe the individual's specific clinical presentation of single episode or recurrent depressive disorder. Multiple specifiers can be applied to as appropriate. These specifiers include (a) "with prominent anxiety symptoms," when clinically significant anxiety symptoms have been present for most of the time during the episode; (b) "with panic attacks," when panic attacks have been present during the past month and occurred specifically in response to depressive ruminations or other anxiety-provoking depressive cognitions; (c) "with melancholia," in which several of the following symptoms have occurred during the worst period of the current episode: anhedonia, lack of emotional reactivity, terminal insomnia, depressive symptoms worse in the morning, marked psychomotor retardation or agitation, and/or marked loss of appetite or loss of weight; and (d) "with seasonal pattern," which is applied to a recurrent depressive disorder if there has been a regular seasonal pattern of onset and remission of a substantial majority of depressive episodes that is not predominantly related to a psychological stress that regularly occurs during a particular season (e.g., seasonal unemployment). In cases where the onset of a depressive episode occurs during pregnancy or within about 6 weeks after delivery, a diagnosis of mental or behavioral disorders associated with pregnancy, childbirth, or the puerperium should be assigned in addition to the applicable depressive disorder diagnosis, using the appropriate category to indicate the presence or absence of psychotic symptoms.

These specifiers are all important for a comprehensive case conceptualization and formulation of a treatment plan. For example, for an individual with a perinatal episode of depression, adaptations should be incorporated in both cognitive therapy and interpersonal therapy for depression, social support during pregnancy and the postnatal period should be offered, and special sessions aimed at processing a difficult or traumatic birth experience should be incorporated into therapy if this has been a part of the individual's experience (National Institute for Health and Care Excellence, 2020).

DIFFERENTIAL DIAGNOSIS

In addition to the distinction between single episode or recurrent depressive disorder from other depressive disorders, which are discussed in later sections of this chapter focusing on those disorders, other important differential diagnoses include the following.

Bereavement and Prolonged Grief Disorder

In diagnosing single episode or recurrent depressive disorder, the symptoms of a depressive episode should not be better accounted for by bereavement. That is, normal grief symptoms should not be interpreted as indicating a depressive episode if the individual has experienced the death of a loved one within the past 6 months, or longer depending on what is considered normative grieving within the individual's religious and cultural context. Depressive symptoms during bereavement do not indicate a subsequent greater risk of depressive episode in individuals who have not previously experienced them (Wakefield & First, 2012). However, a depressive episode can be superimposed on normal grief, particularly in individuals with a prior history of a depressive or bipolar disorder. The *CDDR* indicate that the possibility of a depressive episode during bereavement is suggested by persistence of constant depressive symptoms a month or more following the loss without periods of positive mood or enjoyment of activities, severe depressive symptoms such as extreme beliefs of low self-worth or guilt that are not related to the lost loved one, the presence of psychotic symptoms, suicidal ideation, or psychomotor retardation.

Prolonged grief disorder may also share symptoms of a depressive episode, such as sadness, loss of interest, guilt, withdrawal, or suicidal ideation. However, in prolonged grief disorder, these symptoms are specifically focused on the loss of the loved one, whereas in depressive disorders, the depressive thoughts and emotional reactions typically encompass multiple areas of life. Prolonged grief disorder also includes some features that are not characteristic of a depressive episode, such as difficulty accepting the loss or feeling bitter or angry about the loss. As with normal bereavement, the timing of the onset of the depressive symptoms in relation to the loss should be considered, as well as whether there is a prior history of depressive episodes.

Bipolar and Related Disorders

Depressive episodes occur in the context of bipolar type I and bipolar type II disorders. Single episode and recurrent depressive disorder are distinguished from these disorders by the absence of a history of manic or mixed episodes, which indicate the presence of bipolar type I disorder, or hypomanic episodes indicating the presence of bipolar type II disorder. Cyclothymic disorder is characterized by persistent mood instability including numerous hypomanic and depressive periods, but depressive symptoms are not numerous or long-lasting enough to meet the diagnostic requirements for a depressive episode.

Anxiety and Fear-Related Disorders

Given their high rate of co-occurrence, another major differential diagnosis for single episode and recurrent depressive disorder is with anxiety and fear-related disorders. Generally, there are two possible scenarios. The first is when the diagnostic requirements for a depressive disorder are met, but the individual also presents with panic attacks or other anxiety symptoms that do not meet the diagnostic requirement for a separate anxiety or fear-related disorder. In this case, the specifiers "with panic attacks" or "with prominent anxiety symptoms," as appropriate, should be applied to the depressive disorder diagnosis. The second is when the diagnostic requirements for a depressive episode are met but the individual also presents with anxiety symptoms (including panic attacks) that do meet the diagnostic requirements for an anxiety or fear-related disorder, in which case both diagnoses may be assigned as long as the anxiety symptoms have at times appeared outside of depressive episodes.

Schizophrenia and Other Primary Psychotic Disorders

There are at four main scenarios when considering the boundary between depressive and psychotic symptoms: (a) When the psychotic symptoms only occur during moderate or severe depressive episodes, the "with psychotic symptoms" specifier should be applied to the single episode or recurrent depressive disorder diagnosis; (b) when an individual who meets the diagnostic requirements for schizophrenia or other primary psychotic disorder experiences significant depressive symptoms during psychotic episodes that do not meet the diagnostic requirements for a depressive episode, this should be reflected in the rating for the specifier for "depressive mood symptoms" applied to the primary psychotic disorder diagnosis; (c) when all diagnostic requirements for both a depressive episode and schizophrenia are present concurrently, or within a few days of each other, schizoaffective disorder is the appropriate diagnosis; and (d) when all diagnostic requirements for a depressive episode are met and the person has preexisting diagnosis of schizophrenia or other primary psychotic disorder but does not currently meet the diagnostic requirements for that disorder, an additional diagnosis of single or recurrent depressive disorder may be assigned.

There are several other disorders that should be considered in the differential diagnosis for single or recurrent depressive disorder, especially in children and adolescents. Adjustment disorder is characterized by a maladaptive reaction to identifiable psychosocial stressors that may include depressive symptoms, but symptoms are not sufficient in number or severity to meet the requirements for a depressive episode. Oppositional defiant disorder can co-occur with mood disorders. However, it is also common for children and adolescents to appear to be noncompliant as a result of diminished interest or pleasure in activities, difficulty concentrating, hopelessness, psychomotor retardation, or reduced energy, as well as to present with symptoms of irritability as part of a mood disorder. Attention deficit hyperactivity disorder is characterized by problems with attention and concentration that persist over time and are not temporally linked to changes in mood.

The differential between depressive disorders and neurocognitive disorders is particularly important in older adults. The clinician should consider the possibility that memory difficulties and other cognitive symptoms are explained by single episode or recurrent depressive disorder. If these symptoms occur during a depressive episode, it is generally important to treat the depressive disorder and to reassess memory difficulties and other cognitive symptoms after depressive symptoms have remitted before assigning a diagnosis of dementia or other neurocognitive disorder. However, a depressive episode can be diagnosed together with dementia or another neurocognitive disorder when it is well documented that the memory difficulties and other cognitive symptoms substantially predated or occur outside of depressive episodes.

OTHER DEPRESSIVE DISORDERS

Dysthymic Disorder

Dysthymic disorder is conceptualized as a chronic form of mood disorder that involves the persistent presentation of attenuated depressive symptoms (i.e., more than 2 years without a clear return to normal mood). During the first 2 years of the disorder, and most of the time thereafter, depressive symptoms are not sufficient in number and duration to meet the full diagnostic requirements for a depressive episode. Later in the course of the disorder, depressive episodes may be superimposed on dysthymic disorder, and most people with dysthymia develop at least one diagnosable depressive episode during their lifetime (Klein et al., 2000).

In dysthymic disorder, attenuated depressive symptoms most commonly involve depressed mood, lack of interest or excitement, low self-worth, pessimism, and hopelessness. Importantly, recurrent thoughts of death, suicidal ideation, and suicide attempts are more common in this population than those with single episode or recurrent depressive disorder (Klein et al., 2000). Therefore, suicide risk should be carefully and regularly evaluated, especially when "double depression" is present and feelings of hopelessness intensify (Joiner et al., 2007). More than half of those who have been treated for dysthymic disorder continued to experience suicidal ideation for years afterward (Young et al., 2008).

Differential Diagnosis

Dysthymic disorder should be distinguished from normal sadness or discouragement in response to adverse life events and problems. Several other common conditions should be considered in the differential diagnosis. A diagnosis of a bipolar or related disorders is appropriate when an individual presents with a pattern of depressive symptoms that resembles dysthymic disorder but also has a history of manic, mixed, or hypomanic episodes. Individuals with generalized anxiety disorder focus on potentially negative outcomes that could occur in a variety of aspects in daily life, such as family, finances, and work, which may resemble some of the negative cognitions seen in dysthymic disorder and other depressive disorders, but they do not exhibit chronic low mood or loss of interest or pleasure. In substance-induced mood disorder, a chronic or episodic depressive syndrome may occur as a result of the effect of a substance or medication on the central nervous system (e.g., benzodiazepines), including withdrawal effects (e.g., from stimulants). In secondary mood syndrome, the chronic depressive syndrome is a manifestation of another medical condition (e.g., hypothyroidism). Certain maladaptive patterns of emotional experience in personality disorder may resemble some symptoms of dysthymic disorder (e.g., indecisiveness, low self-worth or excessive guilt, social isolation, limited capacity for self-direction), particularly when traits of negative affectivity, anankastia, or detachment are present, but chronic low mood and loss of interest or pleasure are not features of personality disorder.

Mixed Depressive and Anxiety Disorder

Individuals with MDAD report a mixture of depressive and anxiety symptoms that are subsyndromal in the sense that neither set of symptoms is sufficient in themselves to meet the diagnostic requirements for a depressive episode or for an anxiety or fear-related disorder. In primary care settings, where MDAD is more common than in mental health specialty settings, individuals presenting for care are more likely to complain of somatic symptoms (e.g., back pain, chest pain, heart palpitations, problems with sleep or appetite, and fatigue) than psychological ones (Goldberg et al., 2016).

Although individuals with MDAD present with subsyndromal symptoms of anxiety and depression, their levels of distress and disability, as well as the negative impact on their health and quality of life, are often similar to those of individuals who meet the full diagnostic requirements for single episode or recurrent depressive disorder (Das-Munshi et al., 2008). Moreover, individuals with MDAD are at a high risk of developing a depressive disorder within the next year, and more than 10% of people with MDAD have reported a lifetime suicide attempt (Das-Munshi et al., 2008).

Differential Diagnosis

Given that MDAD is characterized by subthreshold depressive and anxiety symptoms, it is important to consider its boundary with normality. To this end, the *ICD-11* CDDR indicate that if worry or overconcern is the only anxiety symptom and no other sympathetic autonomic or other anxiety symptoms are present, the diagnosis of a MDAD is not appropriate. MDAD is one of four clinical diagnoses reflecting the frequent co-occurrence of depressive and anxiety symptoms. The other three diagnoses to consider for people with co-occurring depressive and anxiety symptoms include (a) single episode or recurrent depressive disorder, using the specifier "with prominent anxiety symptoms" or "with panic attacks" (or both) as appropriate; (b) an anxiety or fear-related disorder, if a person meets criteria for an anxiety disorder with subsyndromal levels of depressive symptoms; and (c) a co-occurring depressive disorder and anxiety or fear-related a depressive disorder, if the presentation meets the full diagnostic requirements of both. Another important differentiation is between MDAD and adjustment disorder. Both may be associated with similar depressive and anxiety symptoms, but if the onset of these symptoms occurs in close association with significant life changes or stressful life events, a diagnosis of adjustment disorder is often more appropriate.

Premenstrual Dysphoric Disorder

PMDD is a syndrome characterized by moderate to severe mood, somatic, and cognitive symptoms that consistently begin several days before the onset of menses and start to improve within a few days after the onset of menses (Pearlstein et al., 2005). PMDD is classified in the grouping of female pelvic pain associated with genital organs or menstrual cycle in the chapter on diseases of the genitourinary system (i.e., it is not considered a mental disorder). It is cross-listed in the grouping of depressive disorders because of the prominence of similar symptoms. PMDD mood symptoms may include depressed mood, anger/irritability, anxiety/tension, and mood swings. Frequent somatic symptoms are lethargy, joint pain, and overeating. The most common cognitive symptoms are concentration difficulties and forgetfulness. The symptoms do not represent the exacerbation of another mental disorder and result in significant distress or significant impairment in personal, family, social, educational, occupational, or other important areas of functioning. To qualify for a diagnosis of PMDD, the nature and timing of the symptoms must characterize a majority of the woman's menstrual cycles within the past year. The temporal relationship of the symptoms and luteal and menstrual phases of the cycle should be confirmed by a prospective symptom diary over at least two symptomatic menstrual cycles.

Differential Diagnosis

Many women experience mild mood changes (e.g., increased emotional lability, irritability, subjective tension) during the late luteal or menstrual phase of the cycle that do not typically cause significant distress or have significant effects on functioning. These experiences should not be labeled as PMDD, which is characterized by considerably more severe symptoms that cause significant distress or disability. PMDD generally involves mood symptoms, such as depressive or irritable mood or mood lability and may also involve symptoms of anxiety. However, PMDD is distinguished from mood disorders and anxiety and fear-related disorders in that the symptoms occur in a specific relationship to the luteal and menstrual phases of the cycle, with symptoms typically absent by 1-week postmenses. However, it is also possible for PMDD to be superimposed on a mood disorder or anxiety or fear-related disorder, in which case, both diagnoses may be assigned. In addition, certain medical conditions (e.g., endometriosis, polycystic ovary disease, adrenal system disorders such as hyperprolactinemia, dysmenorrhea) can cause pain preceding or accompanying menstruation that interferes with daily activities and may be associated with mood changes due to pain. Use of hormone treatments, including for contraceptive purposes, may result in unwanted side effects that include mood, somatic, and cognitive symptoms. If symptoms are absent after cessation of these medications and after the period during which they still may have physiological effects, a diagnosis of PMDD should not be assigned.

DEVELOPMENTAL COURSE OF DEPRESSIVE DISORDERS

The presentation of depressive disorders varies according to the developmental stage of the individual. In young children, depressed mood may present as somatic complaints (e.g., headaches, stomachaches), whining or excessive crying, or increased separation anxiety. Suicidal ideation may be communicated through more indirect or passive statements (e.g., "I don't want to be here anymore") or as themes of death during play. In adolescents, depressed mood may present as pervasive irritability, and suicidality may be communicated more directly with statements regarding a desire to die. Cognitive symptoms of depression can manifest in a child or adolescent's academic performance declining significantly, taking longer to complete or being unable complete school assignments, or decreased ability to concentrate or sustain attention. In children and adolescents, changes in appetite may lead to a failure to gain weight as expected for their age and stage of development rather than weight loss. In addition, hyperphagia (i.e., abnormally increased consumption of food) and hypersomnia (i.e., excessive time spent sleeping or excessive sleepiness) are more common in adolescents than in adults. In all cases, symptoms of a depressive episode should represent a change from previous functioning.

In childhood, depressive episodes that meet the full diagnostic requirements are relatively rare and occur with similar frequency among gender groups. During adolescence, however, single episode and recurrent depressive disorders are among the most frequent mental disorders, with females approximately twice as likely as males to experience a depressive episode. Earlier age of onset of depressive disorders is associated with a longer and more chronic course. For an adolescent, having a depressive disorder can substantially interfere with social, cognitive, and emotional development and limit their ability to make important life decisions (Berenzon et al., 2013). It is important to bear in mind that individuals with bipolar disorders often present initially with one or more depressive episode during adolescence. Factors associated with an increased risk of developing bipolar disorder include earlier age at onset of depressive episodes, a family history of bipolar disorders, and the presence of psychotic symptoms.

The onset of a depressive disorder between approximately the ages of 45 and 65 often suggests a prominent medical cause or comorbidity. In adults aged 65 or older, the prevalence of depressive disorders increases. As people age, there may be age-related psychosocial stressors that contribute to depressive symptoms, including role changes due to retirement (e.g., transition from actively working for several hours a day to being unemployed and primarily engaging in domestic activities) and disability associated with chronic illnesses (e.g., reduced mobility). However, depressive disorders among older adults are often misdiagnosed and undertreated. Relatives and carers may mistake an older adult's symptoms of depression as a reaction to life changes that occur with age or as being due to comorbid medical conditions. Cognitive changes due to depression are frequently attributed to age-associated cognitive decline or to a neurocognitive disorder and not investigated further.

ASSESSMENT

Assessment and treatment planning for individuals with a depressive disorder needs to consider factors beyond the diagnostic requirements for their disorder because these are not homogeneous entities (Maj, 2018). A complete evaluation should include (a) symptom profile and severity, (b) clinical staging, (c) neurocognition, (d) functioning and quality of life, (e) personality traits, (f) a history of present and past syndromes and disorders including previous treatments and response, (g) physical comorbidities and general medical history, (h) family history, (i) protective and risk factors, and (j) previous and current environmental exposures (Maj et al., 2020). This should be considered as only the first phase of a continuous process of evaluation of an individual with depression.

It is important to highlight that the symptoms included in the diagnostic requirements for *ICD-11* may not cover the entire spectrum of depressive symptoms because many of them, although they are frequent among individuals with depressive disorders, do not adequately distinguish between depressive disorders and other mental disorders or medical conditions. Broader, personalized assessment of individuals with depression will enhance personalized management and treatment, increasing the likelihood of successful treatment outcomes (Reynolds, 2020). The evaluation process can be facilitated by integrating clinician- and/or self-administered rating scales, which tend to assess a broader range of depressive symptoms (Fried, 2017), in the initial evaluation and ongoing phases of treatment. The most commonly used rating scales are the clinician-administered Hamilton Rating Scale for Depression (Hamilton, 1960) and Montgomery–Asberg Depression Rating Scale (Montgomery &

Asberg, 1979), as well as the self-administered Patient Health Questionnaire (PHQ-9; Kroenke et al., 2001), Beck Depression Inventory (Beck et al., 1961), and the Center for Epidemiological Studies Depression scale (Radloff, 1977).

Additionally, depending on the psychological intervention approach, evaluation of additional specific psychological and behavioral domains may be important to assist with individual treatment planning and monitoring. For example, if cognitive behavioral therapy is being used as an intervention, it may be important to continuously assess the individual's automatic thoughts and experience of enjoyable or achievement activities. The main tool used to identify personal negative thoughts is the automatic thought record, which includes a column specifying the situation in which specific negative emotions were experienced. These negative emotions are registered and rated for intensity in a 0 to 100 scale in a second column. Then, a third includes related behaviors and physical reactions, and in the last column, all automatic thoughts or images should be recorded. During treatment, additional columns may be added, such as evidence for automatic thoughts, evidence against automatic thoughts, balanced thoughts and type and rate of current emotions. In the case of behavioral interventions, the use of self-recordings is also common. For example, a record of each activity in a person's day may be kept hour by hour, rating each from 0 to 10 for pleasure (indicating how enjoyable the activity was) and mastery (indicating how much of an achievement the activity was; Gautam et al., 2020). There are also valid and reliable measures of cognitive components of depression that could be useful for evaluation purposes. For example, the depression subscale of the Cognition Checklist (Beck et al., 1987) rates the presence of negative views of depressed individuals about themselves, the world, and the future, as well as level of hopelessness.

Comorbidity of Depressive Disorders and Medical Conditions

Depressive disorders are highly comorbid with medical illnesses, particularly chronic and systemic diseases. For example, studies have observed that diagnosable depressive episodes are present in 15% to 25% of individuals with cancer, 15% to 23% of those with coronary heart disease, 25% to 60% of those with chronic pain, and 31% to 80% of those with multiple sclerosis (Thom et al., 2019). Although not completely understood, the relationship between depression and medical illnesses is clearly bidirectional given the direct effects on depression on many physiological parameters, which can have effects on organ systems through a variety of mechanisms (e.g., increased inflammation, disruption of endocrine function). Research across multiple medical conditions has demonstrated that comorbid depressive disorders result in poorer health outcomes and increased mortality among medical populations and therefore require swift detection and treatment. On the basis of their review, Thom et al. (2019) concluded that the diagnostic requirements for depressive episodes should not be altered in medical and surgical populations, despite the acknowledged overlap between symptoms of many medical illnesses and the neurovegetative symptoms of depressive episode. Among hospitalized medical patients, the differential diagnosis of depressive disorders with delirium is particularly important and commonly made incorrectly by nonspecialists (Farrell & Ganzini, 1995).

Cultural Considerations in Depressive Disorders

There appears to be considerable cultural variation in the reporting of depressive symptoms that is partly related to variations in their cultural salience. For example, in some cultures, psychological symptoms (e.g., sadness, emotional numbness, rumination, decreased pleasure) are less important, whereas moral or relational issues (e.g., guilt, worthlessness, lack of productivity, failure in responsibilities to others) or somatic aspects may be emphasized. In particular, a focus on bodily symptoms (e.g., pain, fatigue, weakness) in the experience and reporting of depression has been observed in a variety of cultural contexts (e.g., Muñoz et al., 2005). Symptoms attributed to cultural concepts of distress may also complicate the assessment of depression. The *CDDR* cite cultural concepts including pain in the heart and aching heart, soul loss, complaints related to "nerves," and heat inside the body that different cultural groups use as a framework for understanding and reporting depressive symptoms that will be missed if the clinician does not understand their cultural significance.

Gender Considerations in Depressive Disorders

Epidemiological studies worldwide suggest that there are considerable differences in the prevalence and presentation of depression by gender. Women are more than twice as likely to be diagnosed with depression than men (Albert, 2015), which suggests that gender-related psychosocial and biological features may increase women's susceptibility. Women's prescribed social roles in many cultures may lead to stress, disadvantaged social status, and victimization (Albert, 2015). Moreover, women's hormonal fluctuations may impact neurological systems that mediate depressive states, especially around key reproductive events such as puberty, pregnancy, postpartum, and menopause (Lombardo et al., 2021). Other gender-specific differences reported for depression include the tendency of males to present with irritability rather than sadness (Pollack, 1998), and the higher frequency of women reporting anxiety and less common symptoms, such as mood reactivity, increased sleep or hypersomnia, increased appetite or hyperphagia, and weight gain (Posternak & Zimmerman, 2001).

Additionally, it has been suggested that depression in women is more severe (Cavanagh et al., 2017) and associated with a greater functional impairment (Lopez Molina et al., 2014). However, depressive symptoms may be underreported by men due to psychosocial barriers common in many cultures that discourage help-seeking (e.g., the belief that a man should not cry or complain). Depression among males may also present behaviorally rather than verbally, through risk-taking behaviors and substance use that may exacerbate their symptoms and further jeopardize their health. Co-occurring disorders due to substance use are twice as common among men than among women with depressive disorders (Cavanagh et al., 2017).

Gender differences have also been reported in the response to antidepressant treatments, in terms of both efficacy and safety (i.e., risk for adverse effects; Keers & Aitchison, 2010). In addition, the presence of estrogen in women of childbearing age may interfere with the mechanism of action of several antidepressants, and the potential effects of antidepressant exposure in utero and in breast milk further complicate pharmacological treatment options for women with perinatal depression.

KEY POINTS

- The *ICD-11* provides four main diagnoses of depressive disorders: single episode depressive disorder, recurrent depressive disorder, dysthymic disorder, and mixed depressive and anxiety disorder, representing the continuum of psychopathological manifestations of depressive symptoms. In addition, the category of premenstrual dysphoric disorder, which has important depressive features, is cross-listed from the *ICD-11* chapter on diseases of the genitourinary system.

- The *ICD-11* includes seven possible specifiers to better describe clinical presentations in single episode and recurrent depressive disorders. Specifiers include the severity of the current depressive episode (mild, moderate, or severe), whether the current episode is persistent (i.e., has been continuously present for 2 or years), as well as the presence of psychotic symptoms, melancholia, panic attacks, other significant anxiety symptoms, and a seasonal pattern of onset and remission. An additional code is used to indicate that depressive episodes occur during pregnancy or perinatally. If the depressive episode is not current but rather has occurred in the recent past, another specifier indicating partial or total remission at time of the evaluation may be applied.

- Clinical presentation of depressive disorders varies according to developmental stage, particularly the manifestations of depressed mood, suicidality, and cognitive symptoms. In all cases, symptoms must represent a change from the individual's previous functioning.

- Depressive disorders are more frequent and more often atypical in presentation among women than men. Hormonal fluctuations associated with the menstrual cycle, pregnancy, childbirth, and menopause may mark periods of increased risk of a depressive episode and should be taken into account when planning clinical interventions.

REFERENCES

Albert, P. R. (2015). Why is depression more prevalent in women? *Journal of Psychiatry & Neuroscience, 40*(4), 219–221. https://doi.org/10.1503/jpn.150205

Beck, A. T., Brown, G., Steer, R. A., Eidelson, J. I., & Riskind, J. H. (1987). Differentiating anxiety and depression: A test of the cognitive content-specificity hypothesis. *Journal of Abnormal Psychology*, *96*(3), 179–183. https://doi.org/10.1037/0021-843X.96.3.179

Beck, A. T., Rush, A. J., Shaw, B. E., & Emery, G. (1979). *Cognitive therapy of depression*. Guilford Press.

Beck, A. T., Ward, C. H., Mendelson, M., Mock, J., & Erbaugh, J. (1961). An inventory for measuring depression. *Archives of General Psychiatry*, *4*(6), 561–571. https://doi.org/10.1001/archpsyc.1961.01710120031004

Berenzon, S., Lara, M. A., Robles, R., & Medina-Mora, M. E. (2013). Depresión: Estado del conocimiento y la necesidad de políticas públicas y planes de acción en México [Depression: State of the art and the need for public policy and action plans in Mexico]. *Salud Pública de México*, *55*(1), 74–80. https://doi.org/10.1590/S0036-36342013000100011

Burcusa, S. L., & Iacono, W. G. (2007). Risk for recurrence in depression. *Clinical Psychology Review*, *27*(8), 959–985. https://doi.org/10.1016/j.cpr.2007.02.005

Cavanagh, A., Wilson, C. J., Kavanagh, D. J., & Caputi, P. (2017). Differences in the expression of symptoms in men versus women with depression: A systematic review and meta-analysis. *Harvard Review of Psychiatry*, *25*(1), 29–38. https://doi.org/10.1097/HRP.0000000000000128

Cuijpers, P., Quero, S., Dowrick, C., & Arroll, B. (2019). Psychological treatment of depression in primary care: Recent developments. *Current Psychiatry Reports*, *21*(12), 129. https://doi.org/10.1007/s11920-019-1117-x

Das-Munshi, J., Goldberg, D., Bebbington, P. E., Bhugra, D. K., Brugha, T. S., Dewey, M. E., Jenkins, R., Stewart, R., & Prince, M. (2008). Public health significance of mixed anxiety and depression: Beyond current classification. *The British Journal of Psychiatry*, *192*(3), 171–177. https://doi.org/10.1192/bjp.bp.107.036707

Dubovsky, S. L., Ghosh, B. M., Serotte, J. C., & Cranwell, V. (2021). Psychotic depression: Diagnosis, differential diagnosis, and treatment. *Psychotherapy and Psychosomatics*, *90*(3), 160–177. https://doi.org/10.1159/000511348

Farrell, K. R., & Ganzini, L. (1995). Misdiagnosing delirium as depression in medically ill elderly patients. *Archives of Internal Medicine*, *155*(22), 2459–2464. https://doi.org/10.1001/archinte.1995.00430220119013

Fried, E. I. (2017). The 52 symptoms of major depression: Lack of content overlap among seven common depression scales [erratum at *Journal of Affective Disorders*, *260*, 744]. *Journal of Affective Disorders*, *208*, 191–197. https://doi.org/10.1016/j.jad.2016.10.019

Gautam, M., Tripathi, A., Deshmukh, D., & Gaur, M. (2020). Cognitive behavioral therapy for depression. *Indian Journal of Psychiatry*, *62*(8, Suppl. 2), S223–S229. https://doi.org/10.4103/psychiatry.IndianJPsychiatry_772_19

Goldberg, D. P., Reed, G. M., Robles, R., Bobes, J., Iglesias, C., Fortes, S., de Jesus Mari, J., Lam, T.-P., Minhas, F., Razzaque, B., García, J. A., Rosendal, M., Dowell, C. A., Gask, L., Mbatia, J. K., & Saxena, S. (2016). Multiple somatic symptoms in primary care: A field study for *ICD-11* PHC, WHO's revised classification of mental disorders in primary care settings. *Journal of Psychosomatic Research*, *91*, 48–54. https://doi.org/10.1016/j.jpsychores.2016.10.002

Hamilton, M. (1960). A rating scale for depression. *Journal of Neurology, Neurosurgery, and Psychiatry*, *23*(1), 56–62. https://doi.org/10.1136/jnnp.23.1.56

Joiner, T. E., Jr., Cook, J. M., Hersen, M., & Gordon, K. H. (2007). Double depression in older adult psychiatric outpatients: Hopelessness as a defining feature. *Journal of Affective Disorders*, *101*(1–3), 235–238. https://doi.org/10.1016/j.jad.2005.03.019

Keers, R., & Aitchison, K. J. (2010). Gender differences in antidepressant drug response. *International Review of Psychiatry*, *22*(5), 485–500. https://doi.org/10.3109/09540261.2010.496448

Klein, D. N., Schwartz, J. E., Rose, S., & Leader, J. B. (2000). Five-year course and out-come of dysthymic disorder: A prospective, naturalistic follow-up study. *The American Journal of Psychiatry, 157*(6), 931–939. https://doi.org/10.1176/appi.ajp.157.6.931

Kroenke, K., Spitzer, R. L., & Williams, J. B. (2001). The PHQ-9: Validity of a brief depression severity measure. *Journal of General Internal Medicine, 16*, 606–613. https://doi.org/10.1046/j.1525-1497.2001.016009606.x

Lombardo, G., Mondelli, V., Dazzan, P., & Pariante, C. M. (2021). Sex hormones and immune system: A possible interplay in affective disorders? A systematic review. *Journal of Affective Disorders, 290*, 1–14. https://doi.org/10.1016/j.jad.2021.04.035

Lopez Molina, M. A., Jansen, K., Drews, C., Pinheiro, R., Silva, R., & Souza, L. (2014). Major depressive disorder symptoms in male and female young adults. *Psychology Health and Medicine, 19*(2), 136–145. https://doi.org/10.1080/13548506.2013.793369

Maj, M. (2018). Why the clinical utility of diagnostic categories in psychiatry is intrin-sically limited and how we can use new approaches to complement them. *World Psychiatry, 17*(2), 121–122. https://doi.org/10.1002/wps.20512

Maj, M., Stein, D. J., Parker, G., Zimmerman, M., Fava, G. A., De Hert, M., Demyttenaere, K., McIntyre, R. S., Widiger, T., & Wittchen, H.-U. (2020). The clinical characterization of the adult patient with depression aimed at personalization of management. *World Psychiatry, 19*(3), 269–293. https://doi.org/10.1002/wps.20771

McGlinchey, J. B., Zimmerman, M., Young, D., & Chelminski, I. (2006). Diagnosing major depressive disorder VIII: Are some symptoms better than others? *Journal of Nervous and Mental Disease, 194*(10), 785–790. https://doi.org/10.1097/01.nmd.0000240222.75201.aa

Montgomery, S. A., & Asberg, M. (1979). A new depression scale designed to be sen-sitive to change. *The British Journal of Psychiatry, 134*(4), 382–389. https://doi.org/10.1192/bjp.134.4.382

Muñoz, R. A., McBride, M. E., Brnabic, A. J., López, C. J., Hetem, L. A. B., Secin, R., & Dueñas, H. J. (2005). Major depressive disorder in Latin America: The relationship between depression severity, painful somatic symptoms, and quality of life. *Journal of Affective Disorders, 86*(1), 93–98. https://doi.org/10.1016/j.jad.2004.12.012

National Institute for Health and Care Excellence. (2020, February 11). *Antenatal and postnatal mental health: Clinical management and service guidance* (CG192). https://www.nice.org.uk/guidance/cg192

National Institute of Mental Health. (2022, January). *Major depression.* https://www.nimh.nih.gov/health/statistics/major-depression

Pearlstein, T., Yonkers, K. A., Fayyad, R., & Gillespie, J. A. (2005). Pretreatment pattern of symptom expression in premenstrual dysphoric disorder. *Journal of Affective Disorders, 85*(3), 275–282. https://doi.org/10.1016/j.jad.2004.10.004

Perini, G., Cotta Ramusino, M., Sinforiani, E., Bernini, S., Petrachi, R., & Costa, A. (2019). Cognitive impairment in depression: Recent advances and novel treatments. *Neuropsychiatric Disease and Treatment, 15*, 1249–1258. https://doi.org/10.2147/NDT.S199746

Pollack, W. S. (1998). Mourning, melancholia, and masculinity: Recognizing and treat-ing depression in men. In W. S. Pollack & R. F. Levant (Eds.), *New psychotherapy for men* (pp. 147–166). John Wiley & Sons Inc.

Posternak, M. A., & Zimmerman, M. (2001). Symptoms of atypical depression. *Psychiatry Research, 104*(2), 175–181. https://doi.org/10.1016/S0165-1781(01)00301-8

Radloff, L. S. (1977). The CES-D scale: A self-report depression scale for research in the general population. *Applied Psychological Measurement, 1*(3), 385–401. https://doi.org/10.1177/014662167700100306

Reynolds, C. F. (2020). Optimizing personalized management of depression: The impor-tance of real-world contexts and the need for a new convergence paradigm in mental health. *World Psychiatry, 19*(3), 266–268. https://doi.org/10.1002/wps.20770

Stein, A. T., Carl, E., Cuijpers, P., Karyotaki, E., & Smits, J. A. J. (2021). Looking beyond depression: A meta-analysis of the effect of behavioral activation on depression, anxiety, and activation [addendum at https://doi.org/10.1017/S0033291720003050]. *Psychological Medicine, 51*(9), 1491–1504. https://doi.org/10.1017/S0033291720000239

Thom, R., Silbersweig, D. A., & Boland, R. J. (2019). Major depressive disorder in medical illness: A review of assessment, prevalence, and treatment options. *Psychosomatic Medicine, 81*(3), 246–255. https://doi.org/10.1097/PSY.0000000000000678

Uphoff, E., Ekers, D., Robertson, L., Dawson, S., Sanger, E., South, E., Samaan, Z., Richards, D., Meader, N., & Churchill, R. (2020). Behavioural activation therapy for depression in adults. *Cochrane Database of Systematic Reviews, 7*(7), CD013305. 10.1002/14651858

Wakefield, J. C., & First, M. B. (2012). Validity of the bereavement exclusion to major depression: Does the empirical evidence support the proposal to eliminate the exclusion in *DSM-5? World Psychiatry, 11*(1), 3–10. https://doi.org/10.1016/j.wpsyc.2012.01.002

World Health Organization. (2001). *The international classification of functioning, disability and health.* https://www.who.int/classifications/icf/en/

World Health Organization. (2023a, March 31). *Depressive disorder (depression).* https://www.who.int/news-room/fact-sheets/detail/depression

World Health Organization. (2023b). *ICD-11 for mortality and morbidity statistics* (Version: 01/2023). https://icd.who.int/browse11/l-m/en#/

World Health Organization. (2024). *Clinical descriptions and diagnostic requirements for ICD-11 mental, behavioural and neurodevelopmental disorders.* https://www.who.int/publications/i/item/9789240077263

Young, A. S., Klap, R., Shoai, R., & Wells, K. B. (2008). Persistent depression and anxiety in the United States: Prevalence and quality of care. *Psychiatric Services, 59*(12), 1391–1398. https://doi.org/10.1176/ps.2008.59.12.1391

7

Bipolar and Related Disorders

Thomas D. Meyer, Tania Perich, Steven H. Jones, and Tatia M. C. Lee

OVERARCHING LOGIC

In the 11th revision of the *International Classification of Diseases* (*ICD-11*; World Health Organization [WHO], 2023), bipolar and related disorders (i.e., bipolar type I disorder, bipolar type II disorder, and cyclothymic disorder) are grouped together with depressive disorders in an overarching grouping of mood disorders. The *ICD-11* emphasizes that individual mood episodes—depressive, manic, hypomanic, and mixed episodes—represent specific clinical phenomena that can be present in the context of a variety of disorders but are not independently diagnosable entities. For example, a depressive episode can occur in the context of a depressive disorder, a bipolar type I or type II disorder, or a schizoaffective disorder. All four types of mood episode can occur in bipolar disorders. By combining depressive disorders and bipolar and related disorders in an overarching grouping of mood disorders, the *ICD-11* draws attention to the commonalities among them.

It is essential to view bipolar disorders from a longitudinal perspective that takes into account the pattern of mood episodes over time. Because depressive episodes are addressed in Chapter 6 of this volume, this chapter focuses more on manic, hypomanic, and mixed episodes. We sometimes refer to mania and hypomania collectively as "(hypo)mania," despite their differences in impairment and severity, because there is substantial overlap in their symptoms and the processes underlying both are similar from a biopsychosocial

https://doi.org/10.1037/0000392-007
A Psychological Approach to Diagnosis: Using the ICD-11 as a Framework, G. M. Reed, P. L.-J. Ritchie, and A. Maercker (Editors)

perspective. This is also true of mixed episodes, which have both (hypo)manic and depressive features. However, each of these three types of mood episodes has unique correlates and treatment implications.

The diagnosis of bipolar type I disorder is based on the presence or history of at least one manic or mixed episode and the diagnosis of bipolar type II disorder requires the presence or history of at least one hypomanic disorder and at least one depressive episode (WHO, 2024). Bipolar disorders are substantially less common than depressive disorders; global lifetime prevalence is estimated be between 0.6% and 1.5% (Ferrari et al., 2016; Merikangas et al., 2011). At the same time, bipolar disorders are substantially disabling due to their severity and chronicity and the infrequency of their complete remission. Among mental and substance use disorders they are the fifth leading cause of disability (Ferrari et al., 2016). They are associated with a loss of approximately 10 to 20 potential years of life, partly because people with bipolar disorders die by suicide more frequently than people with any other mental disorder (McIntyre et al., 2020).

Although bipolar disorders are defined based on the presence of (hypo)mania, it is important to keep in mind that in most clinical cases of bipolar disorder, depressive episodes are actually the predominant aspect of the individual's experience. Individuals with bipolar type I and type II disorder can spend up to 50% and 32% of their time, respectively, in a depressive episode (Goodwin & Jamison, 2007). For this reason, depression has a significant effect on many aspects of the lives of people with bipolar disorder, such as their interpersonal relationships, employment, and overall quality of life. Only about 20% of individuals with bipolar type I disorder have no history of clinically relevant depressive episodes at the time of diagnosis, and the great majority of these will experience depressive episodes over time.

This chapter provides an integrative formulation of bipolar and related disorders by focusing on two levels of analysis: (a) the nature of single and recurrent mood episodes in bipolar disorders (i.e., depressive, manic, hypomanic, and mixed episodes) and (b) their longitudinal course.

A PSYCHOLOGICAL APPROACH TO BIPOLAR DISORDERS

It is universally acknowledged that the etiology of bipolar disorders is strongly neurobiological. The heritability of bipolar disorders is estimated at 70%, and first-line treatments are pharmacological (McIntyre et al., 2020). At the same time, pharmacological treatments alone are typically insufficient to achieve complete syndromal recovery and desirable quality of life from the perspective of people living with bipolar disorders (Murray et al., 2017), and there is evidence of superior outcomes when evidence-based psychosocial treatments are integrated into care (National Collaborating Centre for Mental Health, 2014). Areas in which psychosocial treatments can make a specific contribution include cognitive, occupational, and functional remediation (e.g., neurocognitive training, psychoeducation, and problem-solving), health-related behaviors (e.g., smoking, sleep, exercise, diet), adverse and traumatic childhood experiences, treatment of co-occurring disorders (e.g., anxiety or fear-related disorders, disorders due to substance use, personality disorder), suicidality, and internalized stigma (McIntyre et al., 2022).

Psychological models of bipolar disorders are helpful in conceptualizing the emotional and behavioral processes and deficits involved in mood episodes as well as the course of the disorder as a whole. There are two distinct psychological models of bipolar disorders that are relatively well studied. The first is behavioral activation system (BAS) dysregulation theory (e.g., Depue & Iacono, 1989; Urošević et al., 2008), and the second is the integrative cognitive model of bipolar disorders (Mansell et al., 2007).

BAS dysregulation theory predominantly focuses on (hypo)manic episodes in individuals with bipolar disorders. The BAS has its neural substrate in the nucleus accumbens and regulates motivation and goal-directed behavior (Alloy et al., 2015; Johnson et al., 2012). There are individual differences in how easily this system is activated. According to the theory, persons with bipolar disorder are overly sensitive and reactive to goal- and reward-relevant stimuli, which leads to excessive approach-related and reward motivation, which in turn precipitates (hypo)manic symptoms. There is substantial evidence that approach and reward mechanisms play an important role in the development of manic symptoms (Alloy et al., 2015; Ironside et al., 2020; Scott et al., 2017). Several feedback loops make it more likely that the behavioral sequence will escalate and symptoms intensify.

From a psychological perspective, this activation would depend on the external or internal stimuli present, and the types of anticipated rewards that lead to the initiation and maintenance of (hypo)manic behaviors. One class of events that appears especially relevant to bipolar disorders is the achievement of personally meaningful goals (e.g., graduating from college, promotion at work), which have been shown to increases the risk of (hypo)mania in vulnerable individuals (Johnson et al., 2012; Lex et al., 2017). Even when in a normal (euthymic) mood state, individuals with bipolar disorders commonly hold highly ambitious goals and may not disclose these to others for fear of sounding grandiose. Further, risk for bipolar disorders seems to be associated with a strong tendency to react impulsively when positive emotions are experienced.

A criticism of the BAS dysregulation model of bipolar disorders has been that it does a better job of explaining the development and maintenance of (hypo)manic symptoms than recurrent depressive episodes (Koenders et al., 2020). According to the integrative cognitive model (Mansell et al., 2007), both depressive and (hypo)manic mood symptoms can be explained by the extreme negative and positive appraisals of internal affective fluctuations. For example, a person could make an extreme positive appraisal about an activated state (e.g., "I have so much energy, I am the best I have ever been") or an extreme negative appraisal (e.g., "I am losing control of myself, and something terrible is sure to happen"). Behavior is then guided by the content of the appraisal. The person may engage in stimulating activities to "upregulate" the activated state, increasing the risk of developing a hypomanic or manic episode. Or the person may engage in "dampening" behaviors, such as social

withdrawal, to downregulate the activated state, with the possible consequence of increasing depressed mood and triggering a depressive episode.
These different appraisal styles could also apply to more depressive mood fluctuations. Koenders et al. (2020) proposed an integrative bimodal model of
emotion regulation in bipolar disorders, in which some individuals are characterized by the tendency to upregulate positive affect, and others are characterized by the tendency to downregulate both positive and negative affect. The
value of these models is that they can provide a clinically useful framework to
inform and direct assessment as to what factors could increase risk and maintain (hypo)manic and depressive symptoms.

PRESENTATIONS AND SYMPTOM PATTERNS

Bipolar and related disorders are episodic mood disorders defined by the occurrence of manic, mixed or hypomanic episodes or symptoms. These typically
alternate over the course of these disorders with depressive episodes or periods
of depressive symptoms (see Chapter 6), with depressive periods tending to
predominate in the clinical course of the disorder.

Manic Episode

The *Clinical Descriptions and Diagnostic Requirements for ICD-11 Mental, Behavioural
and Neurodevelopmental Disorders* (*CDDR*; WHO, 2024) describe a manic episode as
(a) an extreme mood state characterized by sustained euphoria, expansiveness,
or irritability, together with (b) increased activity or a subjective experience of
increased energy. Mood may also be labile (e.g., alternating euphoria and irritability). The change in mood should represent a significant change from what is
typical for the individual. For example, the individual may laugh substantially
more, have an uncharacteristically optimistic outlook, be surprisingly friendly to
strangers, or react unusually irritably to the comments and feedback of others for
no obvious reason. To assign a diagnosis of bipolar type I disorder, the manic mood
state should be present most of the day, nearly every day and last for at least
1 week. Several other symptoms that are atypical for the person must also be
present in addition to the change in mood and activity level or subjective energy.
Examples include increased self-esteem or grandiosity, increased talkativeness or
pressured speech, flight of ideas, experience of racing thoughts, increased distractibility, a decreased need for sleep, and an increase in impulsive or reckless
behaviors. To diagnose a manic episode, the symptoms must be severe enough to
cause significant impairment in personal, family, social, educational, occupational, or other important areas of functioning or to require intensive treatment
(e.g., hospitalization) to prevent harm to self or others. If the individual requires
urgent treatment (e.g., medication, hospitalization), the change in mood and
activity or feeling of increased energy does not need to last a whole week for
it to be considered a manic episode. The presence of delusions or hallucinations is assumed to be an indicator of an urgent need for treatment.

In a manic episode, the individual's self-esteem may be inflated to the extent that it constitutes a grandiose delusion (e.g., in which the individual believes they are a famous singer, politician, or religious figure). The person may over-estimate their own skills and abilities—for example, believing they have the potential to achieve overly ambitious goals or underestimating how long certain tasks will take them to complete. This could be manifested in delusional form in the belief that they have special abilities or magical powers. Another common symptom is talking much more than usual and feeling unable to stop, talking much faster or louder than usual, or interrupting others frequently or not giving them a chance to speak. The individual may report that their thoughts are racing or jump from topic to topic, making connections between thoughts that may appear logical to them but make little sense to others ("flight of ideas"). The individual may be easily and unusually distractible such that external or irrelevant stimuli can quickly capture their attention, following which the individual may have difficulty returning to a previous task or abandon it for something new. All of these should be atypical of the individual's usual functioning to be counted as symptoms of a manic episode. A person experiencing a manic episode may appraise their symptoms positively (e.g., reports feeling more creative, intelligent, or powerful) or negatively (e.g., reports feeling distressed because they cannot "hold onto their thoughts").

A decreased need for sleep is also often reported as a symptom of a manic episode. For example, individuals may subjectively feel fully rested, despite only getting a few hours of sleep (sometimes as few as 2–3 hours per night) or not sleeping at all for extended periods of time. This decreased need for sleep is different from the symptom of insomnia, such as may occur during a depressive episode (waking up too early, being unable to fall asleep, or having difficulty sleeping through the night). During a manic episode, sleep is often considered a "waste of time" rather than a psychobiological need. Impulsive behaviors or engaging in momentarily pleasurable activities without considering the potential negative consequences can also be symptoms of a manic episode. For example, people experiencing a manic episode may make highly risky financial or business decisions, engage in spontaneous unprotected sex, or follow their "gut feelings" (e.g., quitting their job, making a large purchase). Individuals in a manic state may also show an increase in social contacts (e.g., calling friends more frequently) and goal-directed activities (e.g., scheduling more meetings, taking on more job-related tasks or projects, engaging in more leisure activities and hobbies). These examples highlight that a manic episode is more than just a short-lived extreme change in mood but rather consists of a pattern of changes in mood, behavior, and cognition.

Hypomanic Episode

A hypomanic episode can be viewed as a minor form of a manic episode. Accordingly, the diagnostic requirements for a hypomanic episode in the *CDDR* are similar to those of a manic episode but in attenuated or subthreshold form. The primary differences between a hypomanic and manic episode are the requirements for symptom severity and duration. In a hypomanic episode, the symptoms represent a significant change from the individual's usual behavior or subjective state that would be obvious to someone who knows the person well. However, the symptoms are not sufficiently severe as to cause marked impairment in occupational functioning or in usual social activities or relationships with others. The symptoms must be present most of the day, nearly every day, as in a manic episode, but in a hypomanic episode, they only need to last for "several days." The required duration of symptoms for diagnosing a hypomanic episode is intentionally lower to reduce the risk of misdiagnosing an individual who has a bipolar disorder as having a depressive disorder. When asking about an individual's mood state during a hypomanic episode, it is important that the clinician take the individual's context into account. A change in mood or behavior that represents a normal response to event or situations experienced by the person (e.g., elated mood after having a successful job interview, increased irritability after losing business to a competitor, increased activity due to unusual work demands) should not be considered sufficient to meet the mood or activity requirements for a hypomanic episode.

Other symptoms of a hypomanic episode are often attenuated versions of manic symptoms. For example, an individual with hypomania may only report an elated mood, whereas an individual with mania may report a euphoric mood; an individual with hypomania may make more plans than usual, but these will be more feasible and more closely related to their actual capabilities compared with a person in a manic episode. An individual with hypomania may be more talkative and gregarious than usual, but they can still be stopped or interrupted by others. They may experience increased self-esteem but not to the point of this constituting a grandiose delusion. In fact, if delusions or other psychotic symptoms are present, a manic or mixed episode should be diagnosed rather than a hypomanic episode.

Mixed Episode

In a mixed episode, the individual experiences several prominent manic and several prominent depressive symptoms, consistent with the symptoms of manic episodes and depressive episodes, which either occur simultaneously or alternate rapidly from day to day or sometimes even within the same day. Symptoms must include an altered mood state consistent with a manic and/or depressive episode (i.e., depressed, dysphoric, euphoric, or expansive mood). In mixed episodes where depressive symptoms are predominant, the manic (i.e., "contrapolar") symptoms most likely to be present simultaneously or alternate with depressive symptoms are irritability, talkativeness, psychomotor agitation, and racing thoughts. Conversely, in mixed episodes where manic symptoms are predominant, the most common depressive symptoms are dysphoric mood, feelings of worthlessness, hopelessness, and suicidality.

The symptoms of a mixed episode must last at least 2 weeks and be present most of the day, nearly every day. If the individual requires urgent treatment (e.g., medication, hospitalization), the symptoms do not need to last for the full 2 weeks to meet the diagnostic requirements for a mixed episode. The symptoms must be severe enough to cause significant impairment in personal, family, social, educational, occupational, or other important areas of functioning or to require intensive treatment (e.g., hospitalization) to prevent harm to self or others. This requirement is assumed to be met if delusions or hallucinations are present.

Hallucinations can occur during manic or mixed episodes but are less frequent than would be expected among people diagnosed with schizophrenia. Auditory hallucinations are most common. In terms of delusions, grandiose delusions are the most commonly reported by individuals experiencing a manic episode; however, delusions of a paranoid or self-referential character may also be reported (e.g., believing they are being observed because of their special powers; believing that people have deliberately put obstacles in their way to prevent their success). If there are psychotic symptoms during a mixed episode, they are most often more congruent with those seen among individuals experiencing a depressive episode.

For all types of mood episodes relevant to bipolar disorders, the clinician will need to determine whether the individual's reported symptoms could be the result of a medical condition (e.g., thyroid dysfunctions, epilepsy, brain tumor), or the use of psychoactive substances or medications, including withdrawal. It is especially important to be alert for (hypo)manic symptoms that emerge in response to biological forms of treatment for depressive disorders (e.g., antidepressant medications, electroconvulsive therapy, light therapy, transcranial magnetic stimulation, deep brain stimulation). If a manic, hypomanic, or mixed syndrome arises under such circumstances and persists after the treatment is discontinued and the physiological effects of the treatment are likely to have receded, the corresponding episode should be diagnosed. Thus, establishing a timeline of when the individual's treatments start or change alongside the course of the individual's reported symptoms is essential.

Bipolar Type I and Type II Disorders

Bipolar type I disorder requires a history or presence of at least one manic or mixed episode. In most cases, multiple depressive and manic or mixed episodes typically occur over the course of the disorder, with depressive periods tending to predominate. Manic and mixed episodes are treated as functionally equivalent in the diagnosis of bipolar type I disorder. Either is treated in the *ICD-11* as grounds for a presumptive diagnosis of bipolar type I disorder, even though there is a small proportion of people who experience only manic or mixed episodes without diagnosable depressive episodes, particularly early in the course of the disorder (Angst et al., 2019). It is also important to recognize that individuals with bipolar disorder type I may also have episodes that meet the diagnostic requirements for a hypomanic episode; however, the diagnosis of bipolar disorder type I will still be appropriate as long as the individual has previously had at least one manic or mixed episode.

Bipolar type II disorder requires at least one current or lifetime hypomanic episode and at least one current or lifetime depressive episode, with no history of manic or mixed episodes. One or more hypomanic episodes are not sufficient to diagnose an individual with bipolar type II disorder, and hypomanic episode is not an independently diagnosable disorder in the *ICD-11*. If the individual endorses psychotic symptoms, a diagnosis of bipolar type II disorder can only be made if these psychotic symptoms occur exclusively during a depressive episode. This is because the presence of psychotic symptoms during an otherwise hypomanic episode would automatically meet the diagnostic requirements for manic episode, making the appropriate diagnosis bipolar type I disorder. For some individuals, a diagnosis of bipolar type II disorder is a temporary diagnosis until they later experience a mood episode that meets the diagnostic requirements for a manic or mixed episode.

The *ICD-11* provides mechanisms for coding the current presentation of an individual diagnosed with bipolar type I or II disorder (i.e., current manic, depressive, mixed, hypomanic, partial remission, full remission), episode severity for current depressive episodes, and the presence or absence of psychotic symptoms. When coding "partial remission," it is important to keep in mind that so-called residual symptoms can be attenuated symptoms of the same or the opposite polarity as the most recent mood episode (e.g., being elated, overly confident, or activated after a depressive episode without fulfilling the diagnostic requirements for a hypomanic episode). Additional specifiers may be added to a diagnosis of bipolar type I or bipolar type II disorder to indicate the presence of panic attacks, other significant anxiety symptoms, melancholia in depressive episodes, whether a current depressive episode is persistent (i.e., has been continuously present for 2 or more years), and a seasonal pattern of onset and remission.

There is also a specifier for "rapid cycling," which, in the context of bipolar type I or II, indicates a high frequency of mood episodes (at least four) over the past 12 months. These episodes may involve an immediate switch from one polarity of mood to the other, or the mood episodes may be separated by a period of remission. In individuals with a high frequency of mood episodes, some may have a shorter duration than those usually observed in bipolar type I or type II (e.g., depressive periods that only last for several days). If depressive and manic symptoms alternate rapidly (i.e., from day to day or within the same day), this should be considered a mixed episode rather than rapid cycling.

Cyclothymic Disorder

Cyclothymic disorder is diagnosed based on mood instability over an extended period of time (2 years or more) characterized by numerous periods of hypomanic and depressive symptoms. Mood disturbance has been present on more days than not for at least 2 years, and there has never been a symptom-free period exceeding 2 months during that time. Hypomanic symptoms may or may not meet the diagnostic requirements for hypomanic episode. During the first 2 years of this disorder, the depressive symptoms should never be sufficient in number or duration to meet the diagnostic requirements for a depressive episode. Subsequently, depressive episodes may be superimposed on cyclothymic disorder, with an additional diagnosis of single episode depressive disorder or recurrent depressive disorder assigned as appropriate. A diagnosis of cyclothymic disorder cannot be assigned if the individual has ever experienced a manic or mixed episode. The symptoms must cause subjective distress to the individual and/or cause impairment in personal, family, social, educational, occupational, or other important areas of functioning.

DIFFERENTIAL DIAGNOSIS

It is important to recognize that elated, irritable, and depressive moods are normal human experiences. To differentiate between clinically relevant mood episodes and normal mood, it is helpful to establish (a) whether the mood change is related to specific situational triggers, (b) whether it is transient and not associated with other symptoms (e.g., changes in sleep or appetite), and (c) whether significant functional impairment occurs as a result of the mood changes and not only subjective distress.

Among people with bipolar disorders, there are substantial delays in help-seeking, accurate diagnosis, and appropriate treatment. Available data, primarily from high-income countries, show average durations of untreated bipolar disorder of approximately 6 years (Scott et al., 2022), and up to 10 to 15 years (Lublóy et al., 2020). Delays in correctly diagnosing bipolar disorders contribute to inadequate and ineffective treatment, greater disease progression, and accumulating consequences of impairments in psychosocial functioning (e.g., social, educational, occupational). These factors highlight the importance of differential diagnosis in bipolar disorders.

The main principles for differentiating bipolar disorders from depressive disorders and other conditions with overlapping symptomatology are the following:

1. In bipolar and related disorders, there is an obvious episodic course with recurrence of mood episodes that are not solely of a depressive nature.

2. In bipolar and related disorders, psychotic symptoms occur only occur during mood episodes and are, to some extent, markers of the severity of those episodes.

3. Rapid changes in affect may be observed in other mental disorders, often in response to external or internal triggers. Mood episodes in bipolar and related disorders are characterized by relatively lasting changes in mood and activity levels.

4. In bipolar and related disorders, the change in mood is accompanied by additional symptoms such as changes in energy level, sleep, speech, and social behavior.

5. Symptoms such as emotional instability, distractibility, irritability, or impulsivity that occur during mood episodes are not part of the individual's habitual pattern of behavior, or, if they are, there must be a significant worsening of these symptoms during the episodes.

6. In bipolar and related disorders, there may be a full return to normal functioning between mood episodes, particularly during the early phases of the disorder.

The most common error in the diagnosis of both bipolar type I and type II disorders is mistaking them for single episode or recurrent depressive disorder. This may be especially challenging for bipolar type II disorder because of the relative subtlety of hypomanic compared with manic symptoms. Several factors likely contribute to misdiagnosis: (a) depressive episodes or symptoms are the most common initial presentation of bipolar disorder (McIntyre et al., 2022), which suggests that people are more likely to seek care during these periods; (b) individuals seeking treatment for a depressive episode may not report their experience of manic or hypomanic episodes; and (c) clinicians may be subject to confirmatory bias, relying heavily on typical symptoms or placing insufficient emphasis on evaluating symptoms that do not match their prototypical ideas (e.g., Meyer & Meyer, 2009). In the context of a presenting depressive episode, certain symptoms suggest a greater possibility of bipolar disorder, including consumption of a higher than normal quantity of food, hypersomnia, psychotic features, a higher frequency of mood episodes, and co-occurring disorders due to substance use, anxiety or fear-related disorders, binge eating disorder, and migraines (McIntyre et al., 2020).

Other important differential diagnoses in bipolar disorders include attention deficit hyperactivity disorder (ADHD), personality disorder, anxiety or fear-related disorders, disorders due to substance use, and schizophrenia. The *CDDR* contain more information about making these distinctions. It is important to keep in mind, however, that bipolar disorders can co-occur with any of these disorders, so differential diagnosis is often a matter of determining whether the requirements for both disorders are met rather than one or the other. In the case of ADHD, co-occurrence may be related to shared brain mechanisms. Similarly, bipolar disorder is genetically correlated with schizophrenia (McIntyre et al., 2020). When an individual simultaneously meets the diagnostic requirements for both bipolar type I disorder and schizophrenia, schizoaffective disorder is the appropriate diagnosis (see Chapter 5).

Among children and adolescents, there has been substantial concern about the overdiagnosis of bipolar disorder and consequent overmedication, which appears in part to be related to the idea promulgated by the fourth edition of the *Diagnostic and Statistical Manual of Mental Disorders* that, among young people, irritability could satisfy the mood requirement for a manic episode (Lochman et al., 2015). In the *ICD-11*, a more appropriate diagnosis for many of these cases would be oppositional defiant disorder, often with a specifier for "chronic irritability-anger" (Evans et al., 2017; see Chapter 14). In oppositional defiant disorder, behavior problems of noncompliance and chronic irritability or anger are observed outside of mood episodes.

Psychoactive substances and certain medications, as well as certain medical conditions or injuries (e.g., Cushing syndrome, epilepsy, stroke, tumors, Huntington disease, lesions to the frontal, temporal, and subcortical limbic brain structures) can also cause a manic or hypomanic state. These conditions should be diagnosed as substance-induced mood disorder or secondary mood syndrome, depending on the etiology, with additional coding for depressive, manic, or mixed symptoms as appropriate.

DEVELOPMENTAL COURSE OF BIPOLAR AND RELATED DISORDERS

The developmental course of bipolar and related disorders varies substantially from person to person. Factors that may influence their course include the presence of co-occurring mental disorders and other medical conditions, maltreatment during childhood, trauma, and substance use (McIntyre et al., 2022). Average age of onset for bipolar disorder is most commonly late adolescence to early adulthood (Ferrari et al., 2016), with earlier ages of onset indicative of poorer outcomes and a more severe developmental course (McIntyre et al., 2020). Factors such as having family members with a history of bipolar disorder and early life trauma are associated with earlier onset; a combination of the two seems to contribute to the earliest onset of the disorder (Post et al., 2016).

Although (hypo)mania is rare during childhood and early adolescence, when it does occur, all the characteristic features can be observed (National Collaborating Centre for Mental Health, 2014). The *CDDR* provide additional information about child and adolescent forms of (hypo)manic symptoms. A diagnosis of a manic episode should only be considered when the symptoms are episodic and recurrent (or characterized by rapid onset if a first episode), inappropriate for the context in which they arise, in excess of what might be expected given the person's age or developmental level, represent a distinct change from previous functioning, and are associated with significant impairment in personal, family, social, educational, or other important areas of functioning. Hypomanic episodes may be difficult to distinguish from developmentally normative behaviors in children and adolescents. Factors to consider include an episodic course and marked, co-occurring changes in cognitions (e.g., racing thoughts), or behaviors (e.g., increased activity level). There is limited research on mixed episodes in children and adolescents; however, there is some evidence to suggest that adolescents with bipolar disorders may be more likely than adults with bipolar disorders to experience mixed episodes.

First onset of (hypo)mania in older adults (age 60 years and above) is associated with higher rates of first hospital admission, lower rates of a family history of bipolar disorder, and medical comorbidity, in which case a diagnosis of secondary mood syndrome may be appropriate (Dols & Beekman, 2018).

Stage models of bipolar disorder have been proposed in which each stage is characterized by features that may inform specific treatment approaches (Berk et al., 2017; Kupka et al., 2021). Stage models typically define Stage 0 as characterized by increased risk but no symptoms, Stage 1 as the prodrome, Stage 2 as the first mood episode, Stage 3 as relapse or recurrence, and Stage 4 as chronic or unremitting symptoms. Although stage models capture the general, aggregate characteristics of bipolar disorder, they may obscure substantial levels of individual variation indicating that a linear and stepwise course is not applicable to everyone (McIntyre et al., 2022). Stage models can be clinically useful for conceptualizing targeted interventions for symptom reduction and quality of life that correspond to the characteristics of each stage (Murray et al., 2017), but the clinician should take care not to convey a sense of inevitability about disease progression. What is well established is the need for timely interventions early in the course of the disorder to have a positive influence on its progression (McIntyre et al., 2022).

ASSESSMENT

As noted earlier, delays in correctly diagnosing bipolar disorders can last for years and have serious and cumulative consequences. When the presenting complaint or referral is a co-occurring or related clinical problem, such as depression, anxiety, or alcohol use, it is more likely that the clinician will fail to identify the presence of a bipolar disorder. It is therefore essential to ask every patient directly whether they have experienced periods of elated or irritable mood and increased activity or energy and whether others would have considered these periods unusual for them (National Collaborating Centre for Mental Health, 2014). If one-on-one time is limited, one of the existing screening measures for mania and hypomania can be used. The two most widely used and cross-culturally validated self-administered screening measures are the Mood Disorder Questionnaire for bipolar disorder (Hirschfeld et al., 2000) and the Hypomania Checklist (Angst et al., 2005). Such screening measures do not produce a diagnosis; however, scores above the culturally validated cutoff point should prompt the clinician to conduct a more thorough assessment, typically a detailed clinical interview, to verify or rule out a diagnosis of bipolar disorder.

Several clinician-administered rating scales are available to assess the severity of (hypo)mania, such as the Young Mania Rating Scale (Young et al., 1978) and the Bech Rafaelsen Mania Scale (Bech, 2002). These instruments require training and clinical experience to administer because the clinician must rate different aspects of the individual's presentation (e.g., rate and amount of speech, thought content). There are also self-administered measures that assess the symptoms and severity of (hypo)mania, such as the Altman Self Rating Scale, the Self Rating Mania Inventory, and the Internal State Scale (for a review of all, see Meyer et al., 2020). Despite empirical validation of these scales, some clinicians may still question the validity of an individual's self-ratings during a manic state. Concerns may include deliberate deception and lack of insight. Thus, comparing the clinician's assessment with the individual's self-ratings can help open a discussion about the discrepancies between the clinician's and the patient's perception of their own mood experiences. Reports of family members should also be sought and considered during assessments if they are available.

There is widespread agreement about the benefits of securing self-reports based on daily mood monitoring. A mood diary can have several functions, such as reviewing changes in mood (and other variables) between assessments, monitoring the client's progress, and fostering self-awareness and self-management. A personalized mood diary can be developed jointly with the patient around core emotions, behaviors, cognitions, and life events relevant to the individual. An individualized and context-based approach that integrates the individual's biography can support more sustained use of the daily mood diary, as well as help to develop a sense of collaboration and co-creation in assessment and treatment. A systematic mapping of the course of the disorder conducted in collaboration with the patient can also be of great value in ordinary clinical practice, using flexible and easily usable standardized processes such as the National Institute of Mental Health's Life Chart Method (Post et al., 2003; Roy-Byrne et al., 1985).

Finally, given the substantially elevated risk of suicide among patients with bipolar disorders, it is critical to assess and discuss suicidal thoughts and behaviors at the time of the initial evaluation and throughout treatment. Widely used measures that may be helpful in the evaluation of suicidality include the Scale for Suicide Ideation (Beck et al., 1988) and the Columbia-Suicide Severity Rating Scale (Posner et al., 2011).

CO-OCCURRING DISORDERS

In adults with bipolar disorder, the most commonly co-occurring mental disorders are anxiety and fear-related disorders; a very high proportion meet the diagnostic requirements for generalized anxiety disorder, social anxiety disorder, or panic disorder (Yapici Eser et al., 2018). Between 30% and 50% have a disorder due to substance use, most commonly alcohol (Messer et al., 2017). ADHD, personality disorder, and binge eating disorder (McElroy et al., 2018) are also common. These co-occurring disorders are underdiagnosed among people with bipolar disorder. In addition to requiring specific additional treatments, they can contribute to the severity of mood episodes and exacerbate the course of bipolar disorder (McIntyre et al., 2022). Careful screening for co-occurring mental disorders is therefore critical.

The presentation of co-occurring conditions may also differ depending on the mood state. For example, during (hypo)mania, alcohol or other substance use may be initiated or escalate, which then can contribute to impulsivity. Or some anxiety symptoms may be prominent during depressive episodes but absent during manic or hypomanic episodes. For example, a person with significant social anxiety may find their symptoms disappear during a hypomanic episode, which would feel pleasant and rewarding.

The risk for a number of medical conditions is elevated among people with bipolar disorders (Krishnan, 2005; McIntyre et al., 2022). These include metabolic syndrome, cardiovascular disease, obesity, type 2 diabetes mellitus, thyroid dysfunction, and inflammatory bowel disease. Some of this is due to risk factor clustering in this population. People living with bipolar disorders are less likely to have access to high-quality preventive and primary care health services; are more likely to report economic, housing, and food insecurity; and have high rates of adverse childhood experiences. Unhealthy behaviors (e.g., cigarette smoking, lack of exercise, alcohol and substance use) are additional risk factors that are common among people with bipolar disorders. Exposure to psychotropic medications commonly used to treat bipolar disorder is also a risk factor for several health conditions including obesity, type 2 diabetes mellitus, and dyslipidemia. Beyond that, bipolar disorder is an independent risk factor for cardiovascular disease, which is the most common cause of premature mortality and decreased life expectancy in persons with bipolar disorder, as well as for other noncommunicable and communicable diseases (McIntyre et al., 2022).

CULTURAL AND CONTEXTUAL ISSUES IN BIPOLAR DISORDERS

Although the core symptoms of bipolar disorder are similar across cultures, there are significant cultural variations in the way in which people express and interpret their symptoms and how they respond to treatment. Failure to be aware of and consider these influences may lead to misdiagnosis or inappropriate treatment. For example, Western societies have a strong emphasis on individualism and autonomy, whereas some East Asian cultures focus more on modesty through self-criticism, avoidance of interpersonal conflict, inhibition of emotional expression, preserving group harmony, and overriding personal interests. Although family is an important source of support to individuals with mental health conditions, some families may stigmatize the diagnosis and find it shameful. This may lead to efforts on behalf of the family to convince the individual with bipolar disorder to curb emotional displays and also may impede access to care (Lan et al., 2018). It is essential for clinicians to be mindful of these specific cultural and family values and attitudes to develop and implement a treatment approach that takes into account these factors and anticipates potential barriers. A related issue is the phenomenon of "somatization"—the preferential reporting and experience of somatic over psychological symptoms (Ryder & Chentsova-Dutton, 2012).

Culturally rooted religious beliefs also influence symptom manifestation. For example, in a study conducted in India, more than a third of religious individuals with bipolar disorder conceptualized their psychopathology in a religious context (Grover et al., 2016). Many of these individuals attributed the etiology of their disorder to religious phenomena, and thus sought help from religious figures. Similarly, in a New Zealand study, most remitted religious individuals with bipolar disorder adopted religious coping and had a lower rate of adherence to treatment regimens from medical professionals (Mitchell & Romans, 2003). Cultural factors can also affect clinical judgments, as clinicians from different countries may show marked disparity in identifying manic symptoms (Mackin et al., 2006). Linguistic barriers may also hinder accuracy in diagnostic assessment.

GENDER CONSIDERATIONS IN BIPOLAR DISORDERS

Although there is evidence that women are more likely to be diagnosed with bipolar disorder than men (Dell'Osso et al., 2021), rates of bipolar disorders among men and women are more similar than is the case for depressive disorders. The Global Burden of Disease Study (Ferrari et al., 2016) found that the male-to-female prevalence ratio for combined bipolar disorders was 0.8. The World Mental Health Survey (Merikangas et al., 2011) reported higher lifetime rate of bipolar type I disorder and subthreshold (hypo)manic symptoms among males, but higher rates of bipolar type II disorder among females. In addition, there are some key gender differences in symptoms, course, and co-occurring conditions. For example, rapid cycling is more frequent in women, and suicide rates are higher for men (Goodwin & Jamison, 2007). Late age of onset of bipolar disorders is also more common for women, with approximately 70% of those diagnosed after the age of 50 being women (Depp & Jeste, 2004).

The menstrual period, childbirth, and perimenopause can also affect the presentation and course of bipolar disorders in women. Menstrual periods may be associated with increased mood disturbance and depression. Women with bipolar disorder are also more likely to experience co-occurring premenstrual dysphoric disorder (see Chapter 6). Childbirth, pregnancy, and menopause may also precipitate mood disturbances among women with bipolar disorder (e.g., Diflorio & Jones, 2010; Perich et al., 2017). In cases where the onset of a mood episode occurs during pregnancy or within about 6 weeks after delivery, a diagnosis of mental or behavioral disorders associated with pregnancy, childbirth, or the puerperium should be assigned in addition to the applicable bipolar disorder diagnosis, using a specifier to indicate the presence of psychotic symptoms.

KEY POINTS

- Bipolar and related disorders include bipolar type I disorder, bipolar type II disorder, and cyclothymia. Among mental and substance use disorders, they are the fifth leading cause of disability. They are associated with a loss of approximately 10 to 20 potential years of life, partly because people with bipolar disorders die by suicide more frequently than people with any other mental disorder.

- Bipolar type I disorder is defined based on the presence or history of at least one manic or mixed episode. Bipolar type II disorder requires the presence or history of at least one hypomanic disorder and at least one depressive episode. Cyclothymic disorder is diagnosed based on mood instability over an extended period of time (2 years or more) characterized by numerous periods of hypomanic and subthreshold depressive symptoms.

- A manic episode is defined as (a) an extreme mood state characterized by sustained euphoria, expansiveness, or irritability, together with (b) increased activity or a subjective experience of increased energy. The mood and activity/energy should represent a significant change from what is typical for the individual; be present most of the day, nearly every day, and last for at least 1 week; and cause significant impairment in personal, family, social, educational, occupational, or other important areas of functioning or to require intensive treatment (e.g., hospitalization) to prevent harm to self or others.

- The diagnostic requirements for a hypomanic episode are similar to those of a manic episode but in attenuated or subthreshold form. The symptoms represent an identifiable change in the person's functioning and last for at least several days but are not sufficiently severe to cause marked impairment in occupational functioning or in usual social activities or relationships with others.

- In a mixed episode, the individual experiences several prominent manic and several prominent depressive symptoms, which either occur simultaneously or alternate rapidly from day to day or sometimes even within the same day.

- In bipolar type I and type II disorders, manic, mixed, or hypomanic episodes usually alternate with depressive episodes. Depression is typically the dominant aspect of the experience of most people living with bipolar and related disorders.

- The most common error in the diagnosis of both bipolar disorders is mistaking them for depressive disorders. This may be especially challenging for bipolar type II disorder because of the relative subtlety of hypomanic compared with manic symptoms.

- Pharmacologic treatments alone are typically insufficient to achieve complete syndromal recovery and desirable quality of life from the perspective of people living with bipolar disorders, and there is evidence of superior outcomes when evidence-based psychosocial treatments are integrated into care. Areas in which psychosocial treatments can make a specific contribution include cognitive, occupational, and functional remediation, health-related behaviors, adverse and traumatic childhood experiences, treatment of co-occurring disorders, suicidality, and internalized stigma.

REFERENCES

Alloy, L. B., Nusslock, R., & Boland, E. M. (2015). The development and course of bipolar spectrum disorders: An integrated reward and circadian rhythm dysregulation model. *Annual Review of Clinical Psychology, 11*(1), 213–250. https://doi.org/10.1146/annurev-clinpsy-032814-112902

Angst, J., Adolfsson, R., Benazzi, F., Gamma, A., Hantouche, E., Meyer, T. D., Skeppar, P., Vieta, E., & Scott, J. (2005). The HCL-32: Towards a self-assessment tool for hypomanic symptoms in outpatients. *Journal of Affective Disorders, 88*(2), 217–233. https://doi.org/10.1016/j.jad.2005.05.011

Angst, J., Rössler, W., Ajdacic-Gross, V., Angst, F., Wittchen, H. U., Lieb, R., Beesdo-Baum, K., Asselmann, E., Merikangas, K. R., Cui, L., Andrade, L. H., Viana, M. C., Lamers, F., Penninx, B. W., de Azevedo Cardoso, T., Jansen, K., Dias de Mattos Souza, L., Azevedo da Silva, R., Kapczinski, F., . . . Vandeleur, C. L. (2019). Differences between unipolar mania and bipolar-I disorder: Evidence from nine epidemiological studies. *Bipolar Disorders, 21*(5), 437–448. https://doi.org/10.1111/bdi.12732

Bech, P. (2002). The Bech–Rafaelsen Mania Scale in clinical trials of therapies for bipolar disorder: A 20-year review of its use as an outcome measure. *CNS Drugs, 16*(1), 47–63. https://doi.org/10.2165/00023210-200216010-00004

Beck, A. T., Steer, R. A., & Ranieri, W. F. (1988). Scale for Suicide Ideation: Psychometric properties of a self-report version. *Journal of Clinical Psychology, 44*(4), 499–505. https://doi.org/10.1002/1097-4679(198807)44:4<499::AID-JCLP2270440404>3.0.CO;2-6

Berk, M., Post, R., Ratheesh, A., Gliddon, E., Singh, A., Vieta, E., Carvalho, A. F., Ashton, M. M., Berk, L., Cotton, S. M., McGorry, P. D., Fernandes, B. S., Yatham, L. N., & Dodd, S. (2017). Staging in bipolar disorder: From theoretical framework to clinical utility. *World Psychiatry, 16*(3), 236–244. https://doi.org/10.1002/wps.20441

Dell'Osso, B., Cafaro, R., & Ketter, T. A. (2021). Has bipolar disorder become a predominantly female gender related condition? Analysis of recently published large sample studies. *International Journal of Bipolar Disorders, 9*(1), 3. https://doi.org/10.1186/s40345-020-00207-z

Depp, C. A., & Jeste, D. V. (2004). Bipolar disorder in older adults: A critical review. *Bipolar Disorders, 6*(5), 343–367. https://doi.org/10.1111/j.1399-5618.2004.00139.x

Depue, R. A., & Iacono, W. G. (1989). Neurobehavioral aspects of affective disorders. *Annual Review of Psychology, 40*(1), 457–492. https://doi.org/10.1146/annurev.ps.40.020189.002325

Diflorio, A., & Jones, I. (2010). Is sex important? Gender differences in bipolar disorder. *International Review of Psychiatry, 22*(5), 437–452. https://doi.org/10.3109/09540261.2010.514601

Dols, A., & Beekman, A. (2018). Older age bipolar disorder. *The Psychiatric Clinics of North America, 41*(1), 95–110. https://doi.org/10.1016/j.psc.2017.10.008

Evans, S. C., Burke, J. D., Roberts, M. C., Fite, P. J., Lochman, J. E., de la Peña, F. R., & Reed, G. M. (2017). Irritability in child and adolescent psychopathology: An integrative review for *ICD-11*. *Clinical Psychology Review, 53*, 29–45. https://doi.org/10.1016/j.cpr.2017.01.004

Ferrari, A. J., Stockings, E., Khoo, J. P., Erskine, H. E., Degenhardt, L., Vos, T., & Whiteford, H. A. (2016). The prevalence and burden of bipolar disorder: Findings from the Global Burden of Disease Study 2013. *Bipolar Disorders, 18*(5), 440–450. https://doi.org/10.1111/bdi.12423

Goodwin, F. K., & Jamison, K. R. (2007). *Manic-depressive illness: Bipolar disorders and recurrent depression* (2nd ed.). Oxford University Press.

Grover, S., Hazari, N., Aneja, J., Chakrabarti, S., & Avasthi, A. (2016). Influence of religion and supernatural beliefs on clinical manifestation and treatment practices in patients with bipolar disorder. *Nordic Journal of Psychiatry, 70*(6), 442–449. https://doi.org/10.3109/08039488.2016.1151930

Hirschfeld, R. M. A., Williams, J. B. W., Spitzer, R. L., Calabrese, J. R., Flynn, L., Keck, P. E., Jr., Lewis, L., McElroy, S. L., Post, R. M., Rapport, D. J., Russell, J. M., Sachs, G. S., & Zajecka, J. (2000). Development and validation of a screening instrument for bipolar spectrum disorder: The Mood Disorder Questionnaire. *The American Journal of Psychiatry, 157*(11), 1873–1875. https://doi.org/10.1176/appi.ajp.157.11.1873

Ironside, M. L., Johnson, S. L., & Carver, C. S. (2020). Identity in bipolar disorder: Self-worth and achievement. *Journal of Personality, 88*(1), 45–58. https://doi.org/10.1111/jopy.12461

Johnson, S. L., Edge, M. D., Holmes, M. K., & Carver, C. S. (2012). The behavioral activation system and mania. *Annual Review of Clinical Psychology, 8*(1), 243–267. https://doi.org/10.1146/annurev-clinpsy-032511-143148

Koenders, M. A., Dodd, A. L., Karl, A., Green, M. J., Elzinga, B. M., & Wright, K. (2020). Understanding bipolar disorder within a biopsychosocial emotion dysregulation framework. *Journal of Affective Disorders Reports, 2*, Article 100031. https://doi.org/10.1016/j.jadr.2020.100031

Krishnan, K. R. R. (2005). Psychiatric and medical comorbidities of bipolar disorder. *Psychosomatic Medicine, 67*(1), 1–8. https://doi.org/10.1097/01.psy.0000151489.36347.18

Kupka, R., Duffy, A., Scott, J., Almeida, J., Balanzá-Martínez, V., Birmaher, B., Bond, D. J., Brietzke, E., Chendo, I., Frey, B. N., Grande, I., Hafeman, D., Hajek, T., Hillegers, M., Kauer-Sant'Anna, M., Mansur, R. B., van der Markt, A., Post, R., Tohen, M., . . . Kapczinski, F. (2021). Consensus on nomenclature for clinical staging models in bipolar disorder: A narrative review from the International Society for Bipolar Disorders (ISBD) Staging Task Force. *Bipolar Disorders, 23*(7), 659–678. https://doi.org/10.1111/bdi.13105

Lan, Y. C., Zelman, D. C., & Chao, W. T. (2018). Angry characters and frightened souls: Patients and family explanatory models of bipolar disorder in Taiwan. *Transcultural Psychiatry, 55*(3), 317–338. https://doi.org/10.1177/1363461518761924

Lex, C., Bäzner, E., & Meyer, T. D. (2017). Does stress play a significant role in bipolar disorder? A meta-analysis. *Journal of Affective Disorders, 208*, 298–308. https://doi.org/10.1016/j.jad.2016.08.057

Lochman, J. E., Evans, S. C., Burke, J. D., Roberts, M. C., Fite, P. J., Reed, G. M., de la Peña, F. R., Matthys, W., Ezpeleta, L., Siddiqui, S., & Garralda, M. E. (2015). An empirically based alternative to *DSM-5*'s disruptive mood dysregulation disorder for *ICD-11*. *World Psychiatry, 14*(1), 30–33. https://doi.org/10.1002/wps.20176

Lublóy, Á., Keresztúri, J. L., Németh, A., & Mihalicza, P. (2020). Exploring factors of diagnostic delay for patients with bipolar disorder: A population-based cohort study. *BMC Psychiatry, 20*(1), 75. https://doi.org/10.1186/s12888-020-2483-y

Mackin, P., Targum, S. D., Kalali, A., Rom, D., & Young, A. H. (2006). Culture and assessment of manic symptoms. *The British Journal of Psychiatry, 189*(4), 379–380. https://doi.org/10.1192/bjp.bp.105.013920

Mansell, W., Morrison, A. P., Reid, G., Lowens, I., & Tai, S. (2007). The interpretation of, and responses to, changes in internal states: An integrative cognitive model of mood swings and bipolar disorders. *Behavioural and Cognitive Psychotherapy, 35*(5), 515–539. https://doi.org/10.1017/S1352465807003827

McElroy, S. L., Winham, S. J., Cuellar-Barboza, A. B., Colby, C. L., Ho, A. M., Sicotte, H., Larrabee, B. R., Crow, S., Frye, M. A., & Biernacka, J. M. (2018). Bipolar disorder with binge eating behavior: A genome-wide association study implicates PRR5-ARHGAP8. *Translational Psychiatry, 8*(1), 40. https://doi.org/10.1038/s41398-017-0085-3

McIntyre, R. S., Alda, M., Baldessarini, R. J., Bauer, M., Berk, M., Correll, C. U., Fagiolini, A., Fountoulakis, K., Frye, M. A., Grunze, H., Kessing, L. V., Miklowitz, D. J.,

Parker, G., Post, R. M., Swann, A. C., Suppes, T., Vieta, E., Young, A., & Maj, M. (2022). The clinical characterization of the adult patient with bipolar disorder aimed at personalization of management. *World Psychiatry, 21*(3), 364–387. https://doi.org/10.1002/wps.20997

McIntyre, R. S., Berk, M., Brietzke, E., Goldstein, B. I., López-Jaramillo, C., Kessing, L. V., Malhi, G. S., Nierenberg, A. A., Rosenblat, J. D., Majeed, A., Vieta, E., Vinberg, M., Young, A. H., & Mansur, R. B. (2020). Bipolar disorders. *The Lancet, 396*(10265), 1841–1856. https://doi.org/10.1016/S0140-6736(20)31544-0

Merikangas, K. R., Jin, R., He, J. P., Kessler, R. C., Lee, S., Sampson, N. A., Viana, M. C., Andrade, L. H., Hu, C., Karam, E. G., Ladea, M., Medina-Mora, M. E., Ono, Y., Posada-Villa, J., Sagar, R., Wells, J. E., & Zarkov, Z. (2011). Prevalence and correlates of bipolar spectrum disorder in the world mental health survey initiative. *Archives of General Psychiatry, 68*(3), 241–251. https://doi.org/10.1001/archgenpsychiatry.2011.12

Messer, T., Lammers, G., Müller-Siecheneder, F., Schmidt, R. F., & Latifi, S. (2017). Substance abuse in patients with bipolar disorder: A systematic review and meta-analysis. *Psychiatry Research, 253*, 338–350. https://doi.org/10.1016/j.psychres.2017.02.067

Meyer, F., & Meyer, T. D. (2009). The misdiagnosis of bipolar disorder as a psychotic disorder: Some of its causes and their influence on therapy. *Journal of Affective Disorders, 112*(1–3), 174–183. https://doi.org/10.1016/j.jad.2008.04.022

Meyer, T. D., Crist, N., La Rosa, N., Ye, B., Soares, J. C., & Bauer, I. E. (2020). Are existing self-ratings of acute manic symptoms in adults reliable and valid?—A systematic review. *Bipolar Disorders, 22*(6), 558–568. https://doi.org/10.1111/bdi.12906

Mitchell, L., & Romans, S. (2003). Spiritual beliefs in bipolar affective disorder: Their relevance for illness management. *Journal of Affective Disorders, 75*(3), 247–257. https://doi.org/10.1016/S0165-0327(02)00055-1

Murray, G., Leitan, N. D., Thomas, N., Michalak, E. E., Johnson, S. L., Jones, S., Perich, T., Berk, L., & Berk, M. (2017). Towards recovery-oriented psychosocial interventions for bipolar disorder: Quality of life outcomes, stage-sensitive treatments, and mindfulness mechanisms. *Clinical Psychology Review, 52*, 148–163. https://doi.org/10.1016/j.cpr.2017.01.002

National Collaborating Centre for Mental Health. (2014). Bipolar disorder: The NICE guideline on the assessment and management of bipolar disorder in adults, children and young people in primary and secondary care (2022 update). The British Psychological Society and The Royal College of Psychiatrists. https://www.nice.org.uk/guidance/cg185/evidence/full-guideline-pdf-4840895629

Perich, T., Ussher, J., & Meade, T. (2017). Menopause and illness course in bipolar disorder: A systematic review. *Bipolar Disorders, 19*(6), 434–443. https://doi.org/10.1111/bdi.12530

Posner, K., Brown, G. K., Stanley, B., Brent, D. A., Yershova, K. V., Oquendo, M. A., Currier, G. W., Melvin, G. A., Greenhill, L., Shen, S., & Mann, J. J. (2011). The Columbia-Suicide Severity Rating Scale: Initial validity and internal consistency findings from three multisite studies with adolescents and adults. *The American Journal of Psychiatry, 168*(12), 1266–1277. https://doi.org/10.1176/appi.ajp.2011.10111704

Post, R. M., Altshuler, L. L., Kupka, R., McElroy, S. L., Frye, M. A., Rowe, M., Grunze, H., Suppes, T., Keck, P. E., Jr., Leverich, G. S., & Nolen, W. A. (2016). Age of onset of bipolar disorder: Combined effect of childhood adversity and familial loading of psychiatric disorders. *Journal of Psychiatric Research, 81*, 63–70. https://doi.org/10.1016/j.jpsychires.2016.06.008

Post, R. M., Denicoff, K. D., Leverich, G. S., Altshuler, L. L., Frye, M. A., Suppes, T. M., Rush, A. J., Keck, P. E., Jr., McElroy, S. L., Luckenbaugh, D. A., Pollio, C., Kupka, R., & Nolen, W. A. (2003). Morbidity in 258 bipolar outpatients followed for 1 year with daily prospective ratings on the NIMH life chart method. *The Journal of Clinical Psychiatry, 64*(6), 680–690. https://doi.org/10.4088/JCP.v64n0610

Roy-Byrne, P., Post, R. M., Uhde, T. W., Porcu, T., & Davis, D. (1985). The longitudinal course of recurrent affective illness: Life chart data from research patients at the NIMH. *Acta Psychiatrica Scandinavica. Supplementum, 317*(s317), 1–34. https://doi.org/10.1111/j.1600-0447.1985.tb10510.x

Ryder, A. G., & Chentsova-Dutton, Y. E. (2012). Depression in cultural context: "Chinese somatization," revisited. *The Psychiatric Clinics of North America, 35*(1), 15–36. https://doi.org/10.1016/j.psc.2011.11.006

Scott, J., Graham, A., Yung, A., Morgan, C., Bellivier, F., & Etain, B. (2022). A systematic review and meta-analysis of delayed help-seeking, delayed diagnosis and duration of untreated illness in bipolar disorders. *Acta Psychiatrica Scandinavica, 146*(5), 389–405. https://doi.org/10.1111/acps.13490

Scott, J., Murray, G., Henry, C., Morken, G., Scott, E., Angst, J., Merikangas, K. R., & Hickie, I. B. (2017). Activation in bipolar disorders: A systematic review. *JAMA Psychiatry, 74*(2), 189–196. https://doi.org/10.1001/jamapsychiatry.2016.3459

Urošević, S., Abramson, L. Y., Harmon-Jones, E., & Alloy, L. B. (2008). Dysregulation of the behavioral approach system (BAS) in bipolar spectrum disorders: Review of theory and evidence. *Clinical Psychology Review, 28*(7), 1188–1205. https://doi.org/10.1016/j.cpr.2008.04.004

World Health Organization. (2023). *ICD-11 for mortality and morbidity statistics* (Version: 01/2023). https://icd.who.int/browse11/l-m/en#/

World Health Organization. (2024). *Clinical descriptions and diagnostic requirements for ICD-11 mental, behavioural and neurodevelopmental disorder*s. https://www.who.int/publications/i/item/9789240077263

Yapici Eser, H., Kacar, A. S., Kilciksiz, C. M., Yalçinay-Inan, M., & Ongur, D. (2018). Prevalence and associated features of anxiety disorder comorbidity in bipolar disorder: A meta-analysis and meta-regression study. *Frontiers in Psychiatry, 9*, 229. https://doi.org/10.3389/fpsyt.2018.00229

Young, R. C., Biggs, J. T., Ziegler, V. E., & Meyer, D. A. (1978). A rating scale for mania: Reliability, validity and sensitivity. *The British Journal of Psychiatry, 133*(5), 429–435. https://doi.org/10.1192/bjp.133.5.429

8

Anxiety and Fear-Related Disorders

Cary S. Kogan, Chee-Wing Wong, and Paul M. G. Emmelkamp

OVERARCHING LOGIC

The grouping of anxiety and fear-related disorders (AFRDs) in the 11th revision of the *International Classification of Diseases* (*ICD-11*; World Health Organization [WHO], 2023) brings together disorders characterized by anxiety or fear as their primary clinical feature. Many other mental disorders (e.g., mood disorders, obsessive-compulsive and related disorders, disorders specifically associated with stress) can have anxiety as an aspect of their clinical presentation, but in these other disorders, anxiety occurs alongside other symptoms that are considered more central to the disorder. Anxiety refers to future-oriented perceptions of anticipated threat. Fear refers to present-state psychophysiological reactions to perceived immediate threat. A variety of internal and external stimuli or situations can be the source of anxiety and fear. *ICD-11* AFRDs occur across the life span and include generalized anxiety disorder (GAD), panic disorder, agoraphobia, specific phobia, social anxiety disorder, separation anxiety disorder, and selective mutism. The *Clinical Descriptions and Diagnostic Requirements for ICD-11 Mental, Behavioural and Neurodevelopmental Disorders* (*CDDR*; WHO, 2024) conceptualize AFRDs in terms of their prominent physiological, cognitive, and behavioral features, which are clinically useful as a basis for identification and treatment planning.

https://doi.org/10.1037/0000392-008
A Psychological Approach to Diagnosis: Using the ICD-11 as a Framework, G. M. Reed, P. L.-J. Ritchie, and A. Maercker (Editors)

A PSYCHOLOGICAL APPROACH TO AFRDs

A psychological perspective on AFRDs focuses on aspects that are common across all these disorders. These key areas inform diagnosis, case conceptualization, and treatment planning (Kogan et al., 2016). The *ICD-11 CDDR* present these aspects of AFRDs systematically in the essential features section for each disorder, making it easy for clinicians to compare how each disorder differs from other AFRDs in terms of these features.

While all AFRDs have the experience of fear or anxiety as the primary clinical feature, the best means of differentiating among them is the *focus of apprehension*, which refers to cognitions related to the specific stimuli or contexts that are associated with anxiety or fear. The essential features section for each AFRD begins with a description of the defining focus of apprehension, which can be highly circumscribed as in specific phobia or relate to a broader class of situations as in GAD. Because anxiety and fear are normal reactions and can have protective functions, the essential features also focus on the frequency, persistence, and intensity of symptoms and the level of associated distress or functional impairment that demarcate the boundary between normal reactions and those that warrant clinical attention.

Specifically, following a description of the focus of apprehension, the essential features describe behavioral manifestations of each AFRD, which are typically forms of avoidance, or recurrent escape from, the stimuli that represent the focus of apprehension. Alternatively, confrontation with the focus of apprehension may be endured with intense fear or anxiety. The essential features then specify the required duration of symptoms, typically several months, to help differentiate the disorder from more transitory or temporary reactions. The *ICD-11* essential features also require significant distress about the experience of anxiety symptoms or significant impairment in functioning to assign a diagnosis.

Symptoms associated with AFRDs often vary in severity across time and contexts depending on several factors such as previous experiences with the focus of apprehension, degree of avoidance, or use of safety behaviors, and co-occurring mental disorders. Anxiety may become so severe as to culminate in a panic attack, which in addition to being a cardinal feature of panic disorder can also occur in other AFRDs when an individual is confronted with or anticipates confronting the relevant focus of apprehension. It is important to distinguish between such "cued" attacks that may be a part of the clinical picture of a given AFRDs and the "uncued" panic attacks that occur in panic disorder. The presence of severe anxiety or panic attacks in AFRDs suggests greater likelihood of co-occurring disorder, higher risk of suicidality, and possible need for specific interventions such as interoceptive exposure.

GENERAL PRINCIPLES FOR ASSESSING AFRDs

This chapter provides information for each of the AFRDs to assist clinicians in planning a comprehensive assessment. We recommend a sequential, multimodal approach—that is, an assessment that integrates information from a clinical interview, self-report measures, behavioral observation, and interviews with collateral informants. Such an approach serves several objectives, including differential diagnosis; establishing baseline severity, frequency, and duration of symptoms; developing a case formulation; selecting treatments; evaluating treatment efficacy; and monitoring for treatment relapse (Antony & Rowa, 2005; Shear et al., 2008).

Clinical interviews should be conducted to elicit a history of the symptoms including onset and contextual factors (e.g., stressors) as well as information about current symptom frequency, intensity, and duration, including the presence of "cued" or "uncued" panic attacks. It is important to ask specifically about what the person is concerned about when confronting or anticipating the situation or stimulus that provokes anxiety. Treatment selection and planning are also informed by the pervasiveness and degree of avoidance behaviors, presence of unhelpful coping strategies, content of anxious cognitions, treatment history, motivation for treatment, suitability and preference for therapies, and identification of skills deficits (Antony & Rowa, 2005). Generally, higher levels of severity, longer duration, and higher levels of behavioral avoidance, as well as co-occurrence with other mental disorders, predict a more difficult course (Asselmann & Beesdo-Baum, 2015).

In settings where it is not feasible to conduct lengthy interviews due to time constraints, psychometrically sound self-report screening measures such as the GAD-7 (Spitzer et al., 2006), which assesses the most common symptoms of anxiety, or the DASS (Lovibond & Lovibond, 1995), which provides a broader assessment of depressive, stress, and anxiety symptoms, can assist in identifying areas in greatest need of intervention for adolescents and adults. These screening tools are available in the public domain and have been translated into multiple languages. Self-report and caregiver/parent report measures for specific AFRDs can be useful in treatment planning and can also be administered throughout treatment to assess response to intervention. Psychometric properties of measures should be considered as well as whether the norms available for a particular test are representative of the individual being tested.

GENERALIZED ANXIETY DISORDER

Presentations and Symptom Patterns

GAD is characterized by excessive, intense, pervasive, and generalized anticipatory apprehension of multiple events or situations that result in significant subjective distress or impairment of daily functioning. The focus of apprehension shifts across a range of everyday life concerns or may be articulated as "free-floating" apprehension, discomfort, or dread related to unspecified negative outcomes. Some individuals with GAD have difficulty specifying the cognitive content of their worries and instead report chronic generalized somatic symptoms. Despite significant associated distress or impairment, many individuals with GAD believe that their worry has a positive functional value, such as helping them to be better prepared for future threats. Avoidance behaviors are not as prominent as those found in other AFRDs; if present, they often take the form of social isolation, procrastination, and refraining from participating in day-to-day activities (Hendriks et al., 2014).

Differential Diagnosis

GAD shares a number of symptoms with depressive disorders, such as poor concentration, dread, sleep disturbance, and pessimistic thoughts. However, unlike depression, GAD lacks prominent signs of depressed mood, anhedonia, vegetative symptoms of decreased appetite and weight loss, periodic crying, suicidal ideation, early morning awakening, and desperate feelings of hopelessness and worthlessness. GAD and depression can be diagnosed together if symptoms of GAD have been present before the onset or following complete remission of a depressive episode.

Developmental Course

The clinical course of GAD is insidious and chronic. Median age of onset tends to be later than for other AFRDs. GAD is rarely diagnosed in young children and more often diagnosed during or after late adolescence with the development of cognitive capacities related to worry. In general, females have an earlier symptom onset than males as well as twice the prevalence (Copeland et al., 2014). Earlier onset of GAD is associated with greater co-occurrence with other mental disorders. Across the life span, worry content changes in developmentally expected ways such that children are usually more concerned about school, sports, family, and safety, whereas adolescents are more concerned about performance, perfectionism, and meeting expectations. Among older adults, the focus of worry shifts to that of health status, illnesses, and personal safety, such as falling. Untreated, worry and anxiety in GAD wax and wane but usually persist across the life span, with gradual reduction after middle age, including spontaneous remission.

Assessment

It is common for individuals seeking help to report worry. Often these worries are associated with acute life stressors and need to be differentiated from the chronic worry or apprehension characteristic of GAD. Eliciting information about the duration of symptoms of worry/apprehension, the amount of time spent worrying each day, and whether symptoms occur outside periods of low mood or anhedonia is important for establishing a diagnosis. Individuals with GAD often report that they have a long-standing history of worrying regardless of what the topic might be. Establishing the impact of worry/apprehension on functioning, such as sleep duration and quality, behavioral rigidity (e.g., taking the same route home), and avoidance is useful for planning targeted interventions.

PANIC DISORDER

Presentations and Symptom Patterns

Panic disorder is characterized by recurrent and unexpected panic attacks that are not restricted to particular stimuli or situations. A panic attack is an episode of intense fear that reaches a peak within minutes, during which a number of physical and cognitive symptoms occur. The sudden onset and intense severity of panic attacks differentiate them from normal situation-bound anxiety. Panic disorder is also differentiated from normal fear reactions by recurrence of panic attacks, persistent concern about future panic attacks or their meaning (e.g., impending heart attack), or changes in behavior. These symptoms are sufficiently severe to result in significant impairment in important areas of functioning.

An isolated panic attack is a common experience in the general population and often associated with periods of extreme stress or life changes and is typically not associated with concerns about the meaning of bodily symptoms of anxiety or with changes in behavior. Panic-related apprehension may be a key factor in the subsequent development of panic disorder and usually consists of three aspects: (a) perceived likelihood of panic occurrence, (b) the perceived negative consequences, and (c) the perceived efficacy in panic coping.

Panic attacks can also occur in the context of other AFRDs when they are specifically "cued" by exposure or anticipation of exposure to the focus of apprehension in the particular disorder (e.g., anticipating giving a speech in social anxiety disorder). If panic attacks occur specifically in response to anticipation or confrontation with the focus of apprehension in another AFRD or are entirely explained by the phenomenology of another disorder, a "with panic attacks" specifier can be added to the main diagnosis to indicate the presence of such "cued" panic attacks; a separate diagnosis of panic disorder should not be given.

Panic disorder is also characterized by frequent worries about having panic attacks and their possible consequences, including (a) the presence of a life-threatening illness (e.g., a heart attack); (b) social concerns, such as embarrassment or fear of being judged negatively by others because of visible panic symptoms; and (c) concerns about mental functioning, such as "going crazy" or losing control. The frequency and severity of panic attacks can vary widely depending on individual coping style and avoidance behavior. Often maladaptive behaviors are employed to minimize occurrence of panic attacks. Examples include avoiding physical exertion, reorganizing daily life to ensure help is available in the event of a panic attack, restricting usual daily activities, and avoiding situations (e.g., public transportation). If intense fear of multiple situations is present, a separate diagnosis of agoraphobia can be assigned.

Panic attacks in panic disorder should not be explained by another medical condition (e.g., adrenal gland tumor), although panic disorder can be comorbid with medical conditions (e.g., asthma). Panic attacks in panic disorder should also be differentiated from the effects of substances (e.g., stimulants), as well as the withdrawal effects of various medications (e.g., sedatives) and alcohol.

Differential Diagnosis

Symptoms of panic/anxiety are common during substance use or withdrawal, which should be distinguished from primary AFRDs. Although a substantial number of individuals with panic disorder also eventually develop agoraphobia as a result of experiencing multiple "uncued" panic attacks in various situations, agoraphobia in *ICD-11* is classified as a distinct disorder, based on evidence that agoraphobia exists in individuals who never experienced panic attacks or panic-like symptoms (Wittchen et al., 2010). Severity of initial panic attacks may be predictive of the development of co-occurring agoraphobia (Pané-Farré et al., 2014).

Developmental Course

Mean onset of panic disorder is between 21 and 35 years, and prevalence gradually reduces with age (Olaya et al., 2018). Panic disorder is rarely diagnosed in young children because attributions about the meaning of bodily symptoms is not yet developed at this stage. Significant life events often precede the onset of panic disorder, including interpersonal and work-related stressors or threats to physical well-being.

Assessment

Interviews should include detailed questions about panic symptoms, onset (typically within 10 to 15 minutes), as well as recurrence and frequency of panic attacks. Assessment of the context in which symptoms have their onset can assist in differentiating "uncued" panic attacks in panic disorder from those that occur in other AFRDs. The focus of apprehension in panic disorder is elicited by asking what the individual was afraid of during the panic attack. It may be necessary to ask the patient to monitor their symptoms, the context in which they occur, and the associated thoughts that arise to confirm the diagnosis as well as obtain useful information for treatment planning (e.g., distorted cognitions about the danger of bodily symptoms). It is common for individuals with panic disorder to begin avoiding situations in which they have experienced panic attacks. Therefore, behavioral changes related to panic symptoms such as avoidance, adoption of safety behaviors, and escape, which all serve to reinforce the mistaken notion that panic attacks are dangerous, should be assessed. Suicide risk should be evaluated; individuals with panic disorder, particularly those with co-occurring depressive disorders, are at higher risk (Teismann et al., 2018).

AGORAPHOBIA

Presentations and Symptom Patterns

Agoraphobia is characterized by marked and excessive fear or anxiety that occurs in response to exposure or anticipation of a wide range of situations where escape might be difficult or help might not be available, such as using public transportation, being in crowds, being outside the home alone, in shops, in theatres, or standing in line. The focus of apprehension in these situations is the fear of specific negative outcomes such as panic attacks or other incapacitating (e.g., falling) or embarrassing physical symptoms (e.g., incontinence). These situations are actively avoided or are entered only when accompanied by a trusted person, or else they are endured with intense fear or anxiety. Other avoidance strategies may include going to certain places only at particular times of day or carrying specific materials (e.g., medication) in case of the feared negative outcome.

Differential Diagnosis

Fear or anxiety is evoked nearly every time the individual comes into contact with the feared situations. An individual who becomes anxious occasionally in one agoraphobic situation is not diagnosed with agoraphobia (Emmelkamp & Meyerbröker, 2019); in this case, diagnosis of specific phobia may be more appropriate. Avoidance of multiple situations can occur in a variety of mental disorders including other AFRDs. Eliciting the focus of apprehension assists in determining whether the avoidance relates to a fear of a negative outcome in situations in which escape is difficult or help is unavailable. For example, individuals with separation anxiety disorder avoid situations but do so to prevent or limit being away from an attachment figure for fear of losing them. Individuals with psychotic disorders may avoid situations because of persecutory or paranoid delusions.

Panic attacks associated with agoraphobia occur exclusively in or in anticipation of entering feared situations rather than "uncued" as in panic disorder. The "with panic attacks" specifier can be included in the diagnosis to indicate presence of "cued" panic attacks. It is unclear why some individuals with panic attacks start avoiding situations while others do not. Both disorders may be diagnosed if both "cued" and "uncued" panic attacks are present.

Developmental Course

Initial onset of agoraphobia is typically before age 35, with a chronic course and low remission rate if untreated (de Lijster et al., 2017). The clinical features of agoraphobia are relatively consistent across the life span, although situations that trigger fear and avoidance as well as the type of cognitions may change. For example, for children being outside their home alone is the most frequently feared situation, whereas in adults standing in line in a shop and being in open spaces are most often feared, and in older adults fear of falling is common (Emmelkamp & Meyerbröker, 2019). Most individuals with agoraphobia experience some panic attacks or show some signs of anxiety before the onset of agoraphobia or panic disorder. Severity is predictive of chronicity and lower remission rates in treated individuals.

Assessment

A key issue is correctly ascertaining the focus of apprehension. Individuals with agoraphobia often report specific scenarios that they anticipate will occur upon entering situations where they fear no one will be there to assist them or it will be impossible to escape. Obtaining a list of feared situations as well as the degree of avoidance of those situations helps with making the diagnosis as well as planning exposure exercises. Similarly, eliciting the specific cognitions that arise during or in anticipation of entering feared situations informs targets for cognitive restructuring and behavioral experiments.

SPECIFIC PHOBIA

Presentations and Symptom Patterns

Specific phobia is characterized by marked and excessive fear/anxiety that consistently occurs upon exposure or in anticipation of exposure to one or more objects or situations. The fear is out of proportion to the actual danger posed by the specific object or situation. The focus of apprehension in specific phobia is directly connected to the feared stimulus. Deciding whether fears are out of proportion to the actual danger can sometimes be difficult (e.g., snake phobia where poisonous species are common) and further complicated by the person's subjective cognitive appraisal of danger. Determination of whether fears are excessive should be made with developmentally and culturally normative fears in mind. To qualify for a diagnosis of specific phobia, a person must experience intense fear nearly every time they are exposed to the feared object or situation. Feared objects or situations are clearly circumscribed and most often external to the person.

Feared stimuli are either actively avoided or tolerated with distress. Functioning can also be significantly affected by specific phobia. In other cases, however, fears of specific situations or objects do not engender functional impairment. For example, a person with flying phobia may not experience any impairment until there is a sudden and unavoidable need for air travel. The diagnosis should only be made if the symptoms result in significant distress or significant impairment in functioning.

When confronted with the feared object or situation, individuals with specific phobia exhibit immediate and intense autonomic nervous system arousal giving rise to a sudden surge of concurrent physiological symptoms such as palpitations, flushing, trembling, shortness of breath, and dizziness. Anxiety may become so intense that it results in panic attacks, which can be indicated using the "with panic attacks" specifier. Alternatively, an individual may exhibit a startle response with overwhelming fear resulting in either freezing or escape behavior. Fear of blood, injection, or injury may also include reactions of disgust or a vasovagal crisis, which can cause fainting spells.

Differential Diagnosis

Specific phobia shares symptoms with panic disorder, agoraphobia, and social anxiety disorder. A diagnosis of specific phobias is often made after considering the focus of apprehension and through a process of elimination.

Developmental Course

Because specific phobia usually precedes the onset of other mental disorders, it has sometimes been considered a possible early-life indicator of vulnerability (Wardenaar et al., 2017). The etiology of specific phobia may be attributable to real-life experiences with the feared object or situation, learned vicariously, or through information transmission. Active avoidance of contact of the feared stimulus serves as a maintaining factor through negative reinforcement whereby individuals do not have the opportunity to learn that the stimulus or situation is not dangerous.

Specific phobia can occur in children as young as 3 but must be distinguished from developmentally normative fears (e.g., fear of the dark). Children usually fear tangible objects or situations, and fear is often manifested by freezing, tantrums, or crying rather than verbal expression of fears. In adolescence and adulthood, cognitively mediated fear responses such as perceived proximity to the feared stimuli, or expectations of encountering the feared stimuli, are sometimes sufficient to trigger a full-blown fear response or panic attack.

Assessment

Interviews should focus on eliciting a description of the focus of apprehension, intensity of symptoms, and degree of avoidance. To determine whether fear is excessive, patients can be queried as to whether they believe they are more fearful of the stimulus or situation than other people or than they believe they ought to be. The determination of excessiveness must consider what is developmentally and culturally normative.

SOCIAL ANXIETY DISORDER

Presentations and Symptom Patterns

Social anxiety disorder is characterized by marked and excessive fear or anxiety that occurs consistently in one or more social situations such as social interactions, doing something while feeling observed, or performing in front of others. The focus of apprehension is the concern that the individual will act in a way that will be negatively evaluated by others or show symptoms of anxiety that will be humiliating, embarrassing, lead to rejection, or be offensive to others. These social situations are consistently avoided or endured with intense fear or anxiety.

The social situations that represent the focus of apprehension may be limited or may be generalized to all social situations, which is a marker of greater severity. Common features include physical symptoms of blushing, sweating, trembling, and fears of negative evaluation. Fear in social situations may be so intense as to result in panic attacks in which case the "with panic attacks" specifier can be assigned. People with social anxiety disorder often have difficulty functioning in work settings that require interaction with others, tend to have fewer social supports, and have elevated rates of suicide attempts.

Differential Diagnosis

The diagnosis of social anxiety disorder should not be diagnosed to describe shyness, a normal temperamental variant, or developmentally appropriate stranger anxiety or behavioral inhibition in children. Other AFRDs may also manifest in social situations but the respective foci of apprehension differ from the fear of negative evaluation that characterizes social anxiety disorder. Many individuals with social anxiety disorder also experience panic attacks that are cued by social situations or in anticipation of social situations and individuals with panic disorder may report a fear of social situations because of their concern that others will judge them negatively if their panic symptoms are observable. Both disorders can co-occur, and it is important to ask about both recurrent "cued" and "uncued" panic attacks.

Assessment

Interviews should query the individual's focus of apprehension in a variety of social settings that can be roughly grouped into those that are performance related and interactional. Generally, severity increases with the number of social situations that trigger anxiety. Self-monitoring of symptoms by patients can be useful in determining social situations that are most feared, which informs treatment sequencing as well as reveals fearful cognitions that are targets of treatment themselves.

SEPARATION ANXIETY DISORDER

Presentations and Symptom Patterns

Separation anxiety disorder is characterized by marked and excessive fear or anxiety about being separated from attachment figures, defined as those to whom an individual has a deep emotional bond (Kogan et al., 2016). Separation anxiety disorder can be diagnosed across the life span, although the symptoms vary based on developmental stage. Separation anxiety disorder is the most frequently diagnosed AFRDs of childhood (Cartwright-Hatton et al., 2006) and is more common among adults than once thought (Silove et al., 2015). The focus of apprehension typically involves imagined scenarios of prolonged separation or harm befalling an attachment figure or to the individual themselves. Childhood fears of separation can continue into adulthood; even when it is not persistent, its presence increases risk of developing a variety of disorders. However, a substantial proportion of adults with separation anxiety disorder experience adult onset without a childhood history of the disorder (Silove et al., 2015).

Level of impairment is relevant for determining current treatment needs. School refusal among children is common and impairing for both the affected individual and parents/caregivers and other family members. School refusal also reduces opportunities for peer interactions, serving as a risk factor for future social skills deficits and isolation (Shear et al., 2006). Most adults with separation anxiety disorder report one or more social role impairments, and half of those individuals experience severe impairment (Shear et al., 2006). Some individuals with separation anxiety disorder may have such intense anxiety cued by separation or anticipated separation from attachment figures that they may experience panic attacks, which can be documented using the "with panic attacks" specifier. The presence of panic attacks is often a marker of severity.

Differential Diagnosis

Separation anxiety disorder often co-occurs with other mental disorders, particularly other AFRDs (Shear et al., 2006). Possible differential diagnoses vary according to age. Oppositional behaviors (e.g., school refusal) are more likely to be observed in children and adolescents and may be related to fears of separation rather than evidence of oppositional defiant disorder. Childhood adversity and lifetime trauma have also been associated with separation anxiety disorder across the life span (Silove et al., 2015), highlighting the need to assess for the presence of disorders specifically associated with stress, which may co-occur with or better explain symptoms. Among adults, it is important to consider the possibility that fear of separation may be consistent with personality disorders, particularly among those individuals exhibiting dependency or a borderline pattern.

Developmental Course

Although separation anxiety disorder is the most common AFRD during childhood, in the majority of individuals, it does not persist into adulthood (Copeland et al., 2014; Kessler et al., 2012). Family adversity and exposure to trauma are often antecedents, although not predictive of disorder persistence (Silove et al., 2015). In contrast, severity of symptoms (rather than impairment) appears to be predictive of a longer course (Foley et al., 2008). Separation anxiety disorder is a waxing and waning disorder with periods of exacerbation often coinciding with life transitions associated with separation.

Symptoms vary across the life span. Young children are more likely to experience nightmares and distress in anticipation of separation. They are less likely to articulate specific concerns but rather manifest their symptoms behaviorally by refusing to sleep alone, throwing tantrums, or becoming excessively clingy. Adolescents are more likely to present with physical symptoms with accompanying specific worries of separation. Among adults, the focus of apprehension typically shifts to their own children and romantic partners. Although physical symptoms may be reported, more elaborate worries of separation and catastrophic outcomes are likely to be endorsed (Allen et al., 2010).

Assessment

Concerns about separation from attachment figures is common among children (Muris et al., 2002), particularly at developmental milestones. Interview questions and measures should distinguish developmentally normative reactions from problematic behaviors warranting clinical attention. The degree of severity of symptoms, impact on functioning, environmental factors, and co-occurring disorders provide valuable information for case conceptualization and treatment planning. Attribution of problematic behaviors such as tantrums and school refusal are more difficult to assess in younger children, for whom assessment relies more heavily on parental interviews and reports, behavioral observations, and functional behavioral analysis (Krajniak et al., 2016). Observations of parent–child interactions are useful, including assessment of parental intrusiveness and overprotectiveness, which may inadvertently undermine acquisition of autonomy skills (Wood, 2006). For adults, it is usually possible to elicit the focus of apprehension and distinguish fears of separation from fears characteristic of other AFRDs.

SELECTIVE MUTISM

Presentations and Symptom Patterns

Selective mutism, a relatively rare disorder, has an early age of onset. Clinical features include a consistent pattern of restricted or absent speech in specific settings where speech is expected with normal speech in other settings (most typically at school vs. home). Symptoms are expected to be present for at least 1 month and not during the first month of beginning school when many children are reluctant to speak until they adjust to the novel environment and social demands. Selective mutism is classified as an AFRD based on evidence that the primary characteristic of the disorder is fear/anxiety (e.g., Sharp et al., 2007). A focus of apprehension is not included as an essential feature because the preponderance of those affected are young children who are often not able to verbalize reasons for their fears.

Selective mutism often co-occurs with other AFRDs, particularly social anxiety disorder (Vecchio & Kearney, 2005; Yeganeh et al., 2003). However, most children with selective mutism also exhibit distinct characteristics in addition to anxiety—in particular, mild speech and language problems or oppositional behaviors not typically observed in children with social anxiety disorder. Impairment ranges in severity and is usually defined by the number of individuals and contexts in which a child is able to speak as well as the extent of communication observed in those contexts. Paucity of speech can interfere with the development of social and academic skills leading to further isolation and reinforcement of selectivity of speech.

Differential Diagnosis

Although commonly co-occurring, selective mutism and social anxiety disorder can often be differentiated based on typical age of onset (between 3 and 5 years for selective mutism compared with 11 to 13 years for social anxiety disorder; Kristensen, 2001). Children with selective mutism often enjoy social interactions where there is no expectation of speech, whereas those with social anxiety disorder typically avoid all social interactions (Kotrba, 2015). Many children who are reluctant to speak may be temperamentally shy rather than have selective mutism. Shy children are usually slower to connect with others but, with time, will engage in conversation.

Communication difficulties in selective mutism are typically mild and may not meet the diagnostic threshold for a developmental speech or language disorder. Unlike those with selective mutism, individuals with developmental speech or language disorder exhibit the same difficulties across situations and people. When oppositional behaviors are present in children with selective mutism, they typically occur in response to anxiety-provoking situations— namely, when speech is required (Cohan et al., 2008). Speech may be limited for some individuals with autism spectrum disorder, but unlike those with selective mutism, paucity of speech and impairment in social communication is generalized across contexts. Measures of intellectual ability focusing less on verbal performance can assist in differentiating selective mutism from disorders of intellectual development. Panic attacks are not a feature of selective mutism and would suggest the presence of another disorder.

Developmental Course

The natural course of selective mutism is not well established. However, absence of speech in selective contexts tends to remit with increasing age (Remschmidt et al., 2001). Many individuals with selective mutism go on to develop another disorder, most often social anxiety disorder. Follow-up after treatment with CBT suggests increasing remission rates over time from 50% at 1 year to 70% at 5 years (Oerbeck et al., 2014, 2015). Selective mutism in adulthood is exceedingly rare, and selectivity of speech is typically consistent with clinical features of social anxiety disorder.

Assessment

Direct assessment of the child may be difficult because of refusal to speak. Gradual building of rapport and emphasizing alternative means of interacting often results in engagement on the part of the child. Asking about parental/ caregiver responses to children's restricted speech informs whether parental behavior should also be a target of treatment. As described in the *CDDR*, it is important to establish whether restricted speech may be related to language proficiency in a second language or other environmental factors that may better explain the lack of speech in particular contexts. Evaluation of speech, language, and academic functioning should be conducted, emphasizing receptive language tests and parent/caregiver reports.

CO-OCCURRING DISORDERS FOR AFRDs

More than half of patients with AFRDs report symptoms consistent with more than one of the included disorders (Kessler et al., 2005). As such, *ICD-11* permits diagnosis of multiple AFRDs if the diagnostic requirements for each disorder are met. Co-occurrence of AFRDs and anxiety symptoms more generally with other mental disorders is common, including depressive disorders and disorders of substance use, as well as, among children, externalizing disorders (e.g., oppositional defiant disorder; Essau, 2003). AFRDs often precede the onset of co-occurring disorders. However, comprehensive assessments should attempt to attribute symptoms to the minimum number of disorder entities necessary to account for the symptoms. If, after this process, co-occurrence is still present, it will influence the sequence and content of treatment.

AFRDs should be also differentiated from medical conditions. The *CDDR* note that various medical conditions (e.g., respiratory diseases) can present with somatic symptoms that are akin to or exacerbate those observed in AFRDs. Collaboration with a patient's primary care physician or other health professional as well as eliciting information about medical history in a clinical interview will help determine whether medical conditions may better explain or be exacerbating an existing AFRDs.

CULTURAL AND CONTEXTUAL CONSIDERATIONS IN AFRDs

In some cultures, anxiety and associated distress are more likely to be reported as somatic complaints rather than in emotional and cognitive terms. Furthermore, psychological attributions of anxiety may be perceived as socially stigmatizing, leading to an underreporting of anxiety. Therefore, it may be more difficult to elicit the focus of apprehension and consequently differentiate among the AFRDs. An evaluation of behavior can be used to infer a focus of apprehension. In the case of GAD, the *CDDR* specify that general apprehensiveness, which may be manifested as somatic symptoms rather than worry, is sufficient to meet one of the core diagnostic requirements.

The *ICD-11 CDDR* rely on clinical judgment to assess the presence of certain required features. For example, in specific phobia, it is expected that the fear of a specific stimulus must be excessive. Therefore, determinations of what is normative should be made based on comparisons with an individual's stated cultural identity. For example, people from collectivistic cultures are more accepting of socially reticent and withdrawn behaviors, whereas those from individualistic cultures see such behaviors as socially inadequate. Self-report measures of anxiety are also influenced by culture. The validity of translations of measures as well as adequate cross-cultural testing to establish comparable norms should be established before administration and interpretation.

KEY POINTS

- In the *ICD-11*, all disorders with anxiety or fear as the primary clinical feature are classified in the grouping of anxiety and fear-related disorders (AFRDs). Most AFRDs occur across the life span, although with developmentally distinct presentations.

- AFRDs are the most prevalent type of mental disorder. Untreated, they are associated with a chronic course, often resulting in significant impairment.

- AFRDs are distinguished from one another by their focus of apprehension. The focus of apprehension is the specific stimulus or situation that the individual reports as triggering their fear or anxiety.

- In the *ICD-11*, panic attacks can occur in the context of panic disorder, as well as another AFRD or mental or behavioral disorder. For panic disorder to be diagnosed, the individuals must have recurrent "uncued" attacks. For other AFRDs (except selective mutism), "cued" panic attacks may occur in response to exposure or anticipation of the focus of apprehension. A "with panic attacks" specifier can be applied in such cases, and a separate diagnosis of panic disorder should not be assigned.

- Severity is reflected in the degree of generalization of the anxiety or fear to multiple contexts, the frequency, intensity, and duration of anxiety symptoms, as well as co-occurrence with other AFRDs and other mental disorders.

- Behavioral manifestations of AFRDs include various avoidance, escape, and safety behaviors. For treatment planning, it is critical to understand behaviors specific to the individual through clinical interview and ongoing monitoring. The use of validated measures can also be helpful.

- AFRDs often co-occur and can be diagnosed together if the diagnostic requirements for multiple disorders are met. AFRDs also co-occur frequently with other mental disorders, particularly depressive disorders and disorders due to substance use. Co-occurring conditions are an indicator of greater severity and suggest a higher risk of suicidality.

- Multiple sources are used to conduct a differential diagnosis; establish the baseline severity, frequency, and duration of symptoms; develop a case formulation; select treatments; evaluate treatment efficacy; and monitor for relapse.

REFERENCES

Allen, J. L., Lavallee, K. L., Herren, C., Ruhe, K., & Schneider, S. (2010). *DSM-IV* criteria for childhood separation anxiety disorder: Informant, age, and sex differences. *Journal of Anxiety Disorders*, *24*(8), 946–952. https://doi.org/10.1016/j.janxdis.2010.06.022

Antony, M. M., & Rowa, K. (2005). Evidence-based assessment of anxiety disorders in adults. *Psychological Assessment, 17*(3), 256–266. https://doi.org/10.1037/1040-3590. 17.3.256

Asselmann, E., & Beesdo-Baum, K. (2015). Predictors of the course of anxiety disorders in adolescents and young adults. *Current Psychiatry Reports, 17*(2), Article 7. https://doi.org/10.1007/s11920-014-0543-z

Cartwright-Hatton, S., McNicol, K., & Doubleday, E. (2006). Anxiety in a neglected population: Prevalence of anxiety disorders in pre-adolescent children. *Clinical Psychology Review, 26*(7), 817–833. https://doi.org/10.1016/j.cpr.2005.12.002

Cohan, S. L., Chavira, D. A., Shipon-Blum, E., Hitchcock, C., Roesch, S. C., & Stein, M. B. (2008). Refining the classification of children with selective mutism: A latent profile analysis. *Journal of Clinical Child and Adolescent Psychology, 37*(4), 770–784. https://doi.org/10.1080/15374410802359759

Copeland, W. E., Wolke, D., Lereya, S. T., Shanahan, L., Worthman, C., & Costello, E. J. (2014). Childhood bullying involvement predicts low-grade systemic inflammation into adulthood. *Proceedings of the National Academy of Sciences of the United States of America, 111*(21), 7570–7575. https://doi.org/10.1073/pnas.1323641111

de Lijster, J. M., Dierckx, B., Utens, E. M. W. J., Verhulst, F. C., Zieldorff, C., Dieleman, G. C., & Legerstee, J. S. (2017). The age of onset of anxiety disorders. *Canadian Journal of Psychiatry, 62*(4), 237–246. https://doi.org/10.1177/0706743716640757

Emmelkamp, P. M. G., & Meyerbröker, K. (2019). *Personality disorders* (2nd ed.). Routledge. https://doi.org/10.4324/9781351055901

Essau, C. A. (2003). Comorbidity of anxiety disorders in adolescents. *Depression and Anxiety, 18*(1), 1–6. https://doi.org/10.1002/da.10107

Foley, D. L., Rowe, R., Maes, H., Silberg, J., Eaves, L., & Pickles, A. (2008). The relationship between separation anxiety and impairment. *Journal of Anxiety Disorders, 22*(4), 635–641. https://doi.org/10.1016/j.janxdis.2007.06.002

Hendriks, S. M., Licht, C. M., Spijker, J., Beekman, A. T., Hardeveld, F., de Graaf, R., & Penninx, B. W. (2014). Disorder-specific cognitive profiles in major depressive disorder and generalized anxiety disorder. *BMC Psychiatry, 14*(1), Article 96. https://doi.org/10.1186/1471-244X-14-96

Kessler, R. C., Berglund, P., Demler, O., Jin, R., Merikangas, K. R., & Walters, E. E. (2005). Lifetime prevalence and age-of-onset distributions of *DSM-IV* disorders in the National Comorbidity Survey Replication [see correction at *Archives of General Psychiatry, 62*(7), 768]. *Archives of General Psychiatry, 62*(6), 593–602. https://doi.org/10.1001/archpsyc.62.6.593

Kessler, R. C., Petukhova, M., Sampson, N. A., Zaslavsky, A. M., & Wittchen, H.-U. (2012). Twelve-month and lifetime prevalence and lifetime morbid risk of anxiety and mood disorders in the United States. *International Journal of Methods in Psychiatric Research, 21*(3), 169–184. https://doi.org/10.1002/mpr.1359

Kogan, C. S., Stein, D. J., Maj, M., First, M. B., Emmelkamp, P. M. G., & Reed, G. M. (2016). The classification of anxiety and fear-related disorders in the *ICD-11*. *Depression and Anxiety, 33*(12), 1141–1154. https://doi.org/10.1002/da.22530

Kotrba, A. (2015). *Selective mutism: A guide for therapists, educators, and parents*. PESI Publishing and Media.

Krajniak, M. I., Anderson, K., & Eisen, A. R. (2016). Separation anxiety. In *Encyclopedia of mental health* (2nd ed., pp. 128–132). Elsevier. https://doi.org/10.1016/B978-0-12-397045-9.00251-2

Kristensen, H. (2001). Multiple informants' report of emotional and behavioural problems in a nation-wide sample of selective mute children and controls. *European Child & Adolescent Psychiatry, 10*(2), 135–142. https://doi.org/10.1007/s007870170037

Lovibond, P. F., & Lovibond, S. H. (1995). The structure of negative emotional states: Comparison of the Depression Anxiety Stress Scales (DASS) with the Beck Depression and Anxiety Inventories. *Behaviour Research and Therapy, 33*(3), 335–343. https://doi.org/10.1016/0005-7967(94)00075-U

Muris, P., Merckelbach, H., Ollendick, T., King, N., & Bogie, N. (2002). Three traditional and three new childhood anxiety questionnaires: Their reliability and validity in a normal adolescent sample. *Behaviour Research and Therapy, 40*(7), 753–772. https://doi.org/10.1016/S0005-7967(01)00056-0

Oerbeck, B., Stein, M. B., Pripp, A. H., & Kristensen, H. (2015). Selective mutism: Follow-up study 1 year after end of treatment. *European Child & Adolescent Psychiatry, 24*(7), 757–766. https://doi.org/10.1007/s00787-014-0620-1

Oerbeck, B., Stein, M. B., Wentzel-Larsen, T., Langsrud, Ø., & Kristensen, H. (2014). A randomized controlled trial of a home and school-based intervention for selective mutism—Defocused communication and behavioural techniques. *Child and Adolescent Mental Health, 19*(3), 192–198. https://doi.org/10.1111/camh.12045

Olaya, B., Moneta, M. V., Miret, M., Ayuso-Mateos, J. L., & Haro, J. M. (2018). Epidemiology of panic attacks, panic disorder and the moderating role of age: Results from a population-based study. *Journal of Affective Disorders, 241*, 627–633. https://doi.org/10.1016/j.jad.2018.08.069

Pané-Farré, C. A., Stender, J. P., Fenske, K., Deckert, J., Reif, A., John, U., Schmidt, C. O., Schulz, A., Lang, T., Alpers, G. W., Kircher, T., Vossbeck-Elsebusch, A. N., Grabe, H. J., & Hamm, A. O. (2014). The phenomenology of the first panic attack in clinical and community-based samples. *Journal of Anxiety Disorders, 28*(6), 522–529. https://doi.org/10.1016/j.janxdis.2014.05.009

Remschmidt, H., Poller, M., Herpertz-Dahlmann, B., Hennighausen, K., & Gutenbrunner, C. (2001). A follow-up study of 45 patients with elective mutism. *European Archives of Psychiatry and Clinical Neuroscience, 251*(6), 284–296. https://doi.org/10.1007/PL00007547

Sharp, W. G., Sherman, C., & Gross, A.M. (2007). Selective mutism and anxiety: A review of the current conceptualization of the disorder. *Journal of Anxiety Disorders, 21*(4), 568–579. https://doi.org/10.1016/j.janxdis.2006.07.002

Shear, K., Jin, R., Ruscio, A. M., Walters, E. E., & Kessler, R. C. (2006). Prevalence and correlates of estimated *DSM-IV* child and adult separation anxiety disorder in the National Comorbidity Survey Replication. *The American Journal of Psychiatry, 163*(6), 1074–1083. https://doi.org/10.1176/ajp.2006.163.6.1074

Shear, M. K., Brown, C., & Clark, D. B. (2008). Anxiety disorders measures. In A. J. Rush, M. B. First, & D. Blacker (Eds.), *Handbook of psychiatric measures* (2nd ed., pp. 529–558). American Psychiatric Publishing.

Silove, D., Alonso, J., Bromet, E., Gruber, M., Sampson, N., Scott, K., Andrade, L., Benjet, C., Caldas de Almeida, J. M., De Girolamo, G., de Jonge, P., Demyttenaere, K., Fiestas, F., Florescu, S., Gureje, O., He, Y., Karam, E., Lepine, J. P., Murphy, S., . . . Kessler, R. C. (2015). Pediatric-onset and adult-onset separation anxiety disorder across countries in the World Mental Health Survey. *The American Journal of Psychiatry, 172*(7), 647–656. https://doi.org/10.1176/appi.ajp.2015.14091185

Spitzer, R. L., Kroenke, K., Williams, J. B., & Löwe, B. (2006). A brief measure for assessing generalized anxiety disorder: The GAD-7. *Archives of Internal Medicine, 166*(10), 1092–1097. https://doi.org/10.1001/archinte.166.10.1092

Teismann, T., Brailovskaia, J., Siegmann, P., Nyhuis, P., Wolter, M., & Willutzki, U. (2018). Dual factor model of mental health: Co-occurrence of positive mental health and suicide ideation in inpatients and outpatients. *Psychiatry Research, 260*, 343–345. https://doi.org/10.1016/j.psychres.2017.11.085

Vecchio, J. L., & Kearney, C. A. (2005). Selective mutism in children: Comparison to youths with and without anxiety disorders. *Journal of Psychopathology and Behavioral Assessment, 27*(1), 31–37. https://doi.org/10.1007/s10862-005-3263-1

Wardenaar, K. J., Lim, C. C. W., Al-Hamzawi, A. O., Alonso, J., Andrade, L. H., Benjet, C., Bunting, B., de Girolamo, G., Demyttenaere, K., Florescu, S. E., Gureje, O., Hisateru, T.,

Hu, C., Huang, Y., Karam, E., Kiejna, A., Lepine, J. P., Navarro-Mateu, F., Oakley Browne, M., . . . de Jonge, P. (2017). The cross-national epidemiology of specific phobia in the World Mental Health Surveys. *Psychological Medicine*, *47*(10), 1744–1760. https://doi.org/10.1017/S0033291717000174

Wittchen, H.-U., Gloster, A. T., Beesdo-Baum, K., Fava, G. A., & Craske, M. G. (2010). Agoraphobia: A review of the diagnostic classificatory position and criteria. *Depression and Anxiety*, *27*(2), 113–133. https://doi.org/10.1002/da.20646

Wood, J. J. (2006). Parental intrusiveness and children's separation anxiety in a clinical sample. *Child Psychiatry and Human Development*, *37*(1), 73–87. https://doi.org/10.1007/s10578-006-0021-x

World Health Organization. (2023). *ICD-11 for mortality and morbidity statistics* (Version: 01/2023). https://icd.who.int/browse11/l-m/en#/

World Health Organization. (2024). *Clinical descriptions and diagnostic requirements for ICD-11 mental, behavioural and neurodevelopmental disorders*. https://www.who.int/publications/i/item/9789240077263

Yeganeh, R., Beidel, D. C., Turner, S. M., Pina, A. A., & Silverman, W. K. (2003). Clinical distinctions between selective mutism and social phobia: An investigation of childhood psychopathology. *Journal of the American Academy of Child & Adolescent Psychiatry*, *42*(9), 1069–1075. https://doi.org/10.1097/01.CHI.0000070262.24125.23

Obsessive-Compulsive and Related Disorders

Christine Lochner, Paulomi M. Sudhir, and Dan J. Stein

OVERARCHING LOGIC

The grouping of obsessive-compulsive and related disorders (OCRDs) in the 11th revision of the *International Classification of Diseases* (*ICD-11*; World Health Organization [WHO], 2023) includes obsessive-compulsive disorder (OCD), body dysmorphic disorder, olfactory reference disorder, hypochondriasis (health anxiety disorder), and hoarding disorder. It also includes the subgrouping of body-focused repetitive behavior disorders, which comprise trichotillomania (hair-pulling disorder) and excoriation (skin-picking) disorder. Because hypochondriasis, also referred to as health anxiety disorder, is associated with anxiety about illness, this disorder is cross-listed in the *ICD-11* grouping of anxiety and fear-related disorders. Tourette syndrome, which is classified as a tic disorder in the section on movement disorders in the *ICD-11* chapter on diseases of the nervous system, is also cross-listed in the OCRD grouping as well as in the neurodevelopmental disorders grouping because of frequent co-occurrence and familiality with other disorders in these sections.

OCRDs are characterized by persistent intrusive thoughts and/or repetitive behaviors. OCRD symptoms are egodystonic (i.e., inconsistent with one's fundamental beliefs and self-image), time-consuming, and result in significant distress and/or functional impairment. Emerging evidence suggests that parallel clinical features seen in different OCRDs are based in part on overlapping neuroanatomical, neurochemical, and genetic features of these conditions, as well as

https://doi.org/10.1037/0000392-009
A Psychological Approach to Diagnosis: Using the ICD-11 as a Framework, G. M. Reed, P. L.-J. Ritchie, and A. Maercker (Editors)

155

cognitive and affective similarities (Stein et al., 2016). This helps explain why the conditions in the OCRD grouping frequently co-occur, why similar approaches to assessment and evaluation are useful across the grouping, and why some OCRDs also share similar responses to specific pharmacological and psychological interventions (Fineberg et al., 2014). By establishing a grouping of OCRDs, the *ICD-11* emphasizes the clinical importance of repetitive thoughts and behaviors in assessment and treatment. The grouping is also intended to increase awareness of often-overlooked conditions such as excoriation disorder as well as often misdiagnosed conditions such as olfactory reference disorder, therefore facilitating the use of evidence-based treatments. So, for example, even though people with body dysmorphic disorder often present to cosmetic surgeons with thoughts or beliefs that appear to be delusional, the OCRD grouping signals the appropriate treatment is likely to have more in common with OCD than with delusional disorder.

The different OCRDs are distinguished by the fact that the focus of preoccupation and the nature of the repetitive behaviors are distinct for each (World Health Organization, 2024). In body dysmorphic disorder, symptoms are focused on appearance concerns and related behaviors, in olfactory reference disorder, symptoms are centered on body odor concerns and related behaviors, and in hypochondriasis, symptoms focus on illness concerns and related behaviors. A description of the specific presentations of each of the OCRDs is provided in subsequent sections of this chapter.

A PSYCHOLOGICAL APPROACH TO OCRDs

Cognitive behavioral models of OCRDs emphasize the role of faulty appraisals and dysfunctional beliefs in the development and maintenance of these disorders (Calkins et al., 2013). Misappraisals of the significance of intrusive thoughts—particularly those that interpret them as informative, important, dangerous, or predictive of harm—are at the core of OCRDs such as OCD, body dysmorphic disorder, olfactory reference disorder, hypochondriasis, and hoarding disorder. These misappraisals lead to increased anxiety and distress, and performance of behaviors aimed at reducing these emotions or the perceived likelihood of the catastrophic consequence occurring, thus preserving the symptoms through negative reinforcement.

In turn, dysfunctional beliefs may underlie vulnerability to develop misappraisals in response to intrusive thoughts. For example, an inflated sense of responsibility and overestimation of threat, based in a belief that harm can happen if one is not careful, are implicated in the development and maintenance of OCD and other OCRDs that involve the enactment of rituals (e.g., "If I do not pray correctly, I will be responsible for my child's death"). Beliefs related to perfectionism may also play a role—for example, through their contribution to a sense of "just right" experiences in OCD, or the need to complete repetitive behaviors in "just the right way" in body-focused repetitive behavior disorders. Other beliefs that can play a role in the development and maintenance of OCRDs are the beliefs that absolute certainty is necessary, all thoughts are meaningful and should be controlled, and thoughts are equivalent to actions (sometime referred to as *thought–action fusion*).

It is notable, however, that some individuals with OCRDs do not seem to have dysfunctional cognitions. An alternative psychological model is that compulsions in OCRDs are derived from excessive habit formation and deficits in the ability to inhibit behaviors and typical OCRD cognitions may, therefore, be post hoc rationalizations of the compulsive behavior (Gillan & Robbins, 2014). This is consistent with some OCRDs having been historically termed *habit disorders* and with the observation that the repetitive behaviors characteristic of OCRDs are often characterized by automaticity and reduced awareness. Precipitants of behaviors such as hair-pulling and skin-picking in trichotillomania and excoriation disorder, respectively, may include negative emotional states such as low mood or boredom. Learning theories also describe the maintenance of these body-focused repetitive behaviors through a cycle of negative reinforcement as a result of tension release and positive reinforcement in the form of relief or pleasure (Roberts et al., 2013).

Experiential avoidance, which refers to an avoidance of or reluctance to be in contact with unpleasant emotional states or experiences (Hayes et al., 1996), is another core aspect of OCRDs. Experiential avoidance occurs in response to distress and anxiety and has a maladaptive regulatory function because it ultimately maintains distress through inadequate emotional processing. In OCD, for example, it manifests as the avoidance of discomfort when negative affect is diminished by the enactment of compulsions. Experiential avoidance is a transdiagnostic phenomenon, present in OCRDs but also in other disorders (e.g., the anxiety or fear-related disorders), where anxiety is central.

There is a growing integration of cognitive-behavioral models of OCRDs with work on neuropsychology and neuroimaging. Cortical–striatal–thalamo–cortical (CSTC) circuitry, for example, is involved in response inhibition, reversal learning and set-shifting, cognitive flexibility, planning, and goal-directed behavior, which are impaired in various OCRDs (Abramovitch et al., 2013; Robbins et al., 2019). Furthermore, cognitive-behavioral models have provided a key foundation for intervention in OCRDs; cognitive-behavioral techniques including cognitive restructuring, exposure and response prevention, awareness training, emotion regulation, and habit reversal training are first-line approaches to the treatment of these conditions.

OBSESSIVE-COMPULSIVE DISORDER

Presentations and Symptom Patterns

OCD is the prototypic exemplar of the OCRDs in the *ICD-11*, with intrusive, repetitive, and persistent thoughts, images and impulses/urges, and repetitive behaviors (including mental acts) at its core. The explicit content of these intrusive thoughts and compulsions most commonly fall on a few well-described dimensions: contamination fears with washing and cleaning compulsions; concerns about harm to self or others with checking compulsions; forbidden or taboo aggressive, sexual, or religious thoughts with related mental rituals or other compulsions; and symmetry obsessions with repeating, ordering, and counting compulsions. These thoughts, images, urges, or impulses are distressing and commonly associated with anxiety, disgust, or shame. Compulsions are typically performed in response to an obsession, to reduce the associated anxiety or distress, according to rigid rules, or to achieve a sense of "completeness." As noted, several belief domains are central in OCD: an inflated sense of responsibility; overestimation of threat; perfectionism; intolerance of uncertainty; and overvaluation of the power of thoughts. Symptoms involving a sense of incompleteness may be associated with tics and anankastic personality traits (see Chapter 17, this volume, on personality disorder).

Differential Diagnosis

Subclinical obsessions and compulsions are relatively common in the general population. However, OCD is diagnosed only when these symptoms are time-consuming (e.g., take more than 1 hour per day) and cause functional impairment or significant distress. OCD should also be differentiated from feeding and eating disorders, which may involve intrusive thoughts and repetitive behaviors that are mainly related to body weight or shape. There may also be strong similarities between repetitive behavior patterns associated with OCD and those observed in people with autism spectrum disorder. Unlike in OCD, people with autism spectrum disorder generally experience their repetitive interests or behaviors as egosyntonic and consistent with their identity and self-image. OCRDs and anxiety and fear-related disorders share recurrent thoughts, avoidance behaviors, anxiety, and requests for reassurance. However, in OCD, recurrent thoughts are more likely to involve odd or irrational content (e.g., intrusive images of harming a friend) and are typically accompanied by compulsions. Panic attacks may also be seen in OCD; when these are entirely explained by OCD (e.g., when an individual is prevented from enacting a compulsion), an additional diagnosis of panic disorder is not warranted. The *Clinical Descriptions and Diagnostic Requirements for ICD-11 Mental, Behavioural and Neurodevelopmental Disorders* (*CDDR*; WHO, 2024) for OCD describe its differentiation from a range of other disorders.

Developmental Course

Onset of OCD is usually gradual, typically in late adolescence or the early 20s. Childhood-onset OCD is more common in boys, whereas the gender ratio reverses during or after puberty. Earlier age of onset is associated with poorer outcomes due to interference of symptoms with achieving developmental milestones (e.g., forming peer relationships or acquiring academic skills). Diagnostic requirements for OCD are the same for all ages. However, children with OCD are more likely than adults to have tic-like compulsions, which may constitute simple, repetitive movements (e.g., tapping and touching). Young children often lack insight into the irrationality of their actions, with almost half of them denying that their compulsions are driven by obsessions. Co-occurrence of attention deficit hyperactivity disorder (ADHD) and tics is associated with childhood-onset OCD, whereas co-occurring depressive and anxiety symptoms are more common when the onset of OCD is during or after puberty.

BODY DYSMORPHIC DISORDER

Presentations and Symptom Patterns

In body dysmorphic disorder, the intrusive, repetitive, and persistent thoughts and behaviors characteristic of OCRDs are focused on one or more perceived defects or flaws in appearance or on ugliness and imperfection in general, when these are either unnoticeable or only slightly noticeable to others. The symptoms are usually accompanied by ideas of reference (i.e., the conviction that people are taking special notice of or judging the perceived defect or flaw). Repetitive behaviors (e.g., mirror checking; excessive grooming; elaborate efforts to cover, alter, or camouflage the defect) or mental acts (e.g., comparing one's appearance with that of others) are performed to reduce anxiety. Some individuals with body dysmorphic disorder, more commonly males, present with muscle dysmorphia (Pope et al., 2005), characterized by the belief that one's body is too small or insufficiently muscular. Body dysmorphic disorder is associated with distressing emotions such as shame, disgust, anxiety, and excessive self-consciousness. Avoidance of triggers (i.e., social situations or other stimuli such as reflective surfaces that increase anxiety and distress about the perceived defect) is central. Over time, there may be physical complications such as infections, blood loss, and scarring due to unnecessary or excessive cosmetic surgeries.

Differential Diagnosis

Concerns about appearance are common, especially during adolescence. Subclinical body dissatisfaction or body image concerns are differentiated from body dysmorphic disorder where the symptoms are clearly excessive and significant. Some anxiety or fear-related disorders share features with body dysmorphic disorder. In generalized anxiety disorder, individuals may worry about their appearance; however, these preoccupations occur together with worries about other everyday aspects of life. Individuals with social anxiety disorder are mainly concerned about being negatively evaluated by others due to their anxiety symptoms, not because of a perceived bodily flaw or deformity as in body dysmorphic disorder. When panic attacks are entirely explained by body dysmorphic disorder (e.g., occurring when feeling that others are scrutinizing the perceived flaw in appearance), an additional diagnosis of panic disorder is not warranted. Symptoms of feeding and eating disorders and body dysmorphic

disorder may also overlap; however, body dysmorphic disorder is not characterized by excessive concern about weight per se as is typical of anorexia
nervosa or bulimia nervosa, but rather with dissatisfaction with several other
aspects of their appearance (e.g., skin, face, hair). The *CDDR* for body dysmorphic disorder describe its differentiation from a range of other disorders.

Developmental Course

Subclinical symptoms of body dysmorphic disorder start gradually, during
childhood and early adolescence, several years before individuals meet the full
diagnostic requirements, typically during mid-adolescence. Adolescence constitutes a vulnerable developmental period during which the quest for an unrealistic ideal image may result in a negative body image, fear of negative evaluation,
depression, and anxiety, ultimately contributing to body dysmorphic disorder
(Rautio et al., 2022). Youth with this disorder are at increased risk for school
dropout, potentially having an impact on their academic and social development. The clinical presentation of the disorder is largely similar in children,
adolescents, and adults, with similar lifetime rates of functional impairment
and co-occurring conditions. However, there is evidence suggesting that youth
may have poorer insight into the excessiveness or irrationality of their symptoms,
to the point of presenting with beliefs that appear more frankly delusional, and
a higher rate of suicide attempts than adults (Phillips et al., 2012).

OLFACTORY REFERENCE DISORDER

Presentations and Symptom Patterns

Olfactory reference disorder is a new diagnostic entity in the *ICD-11*. Individuals with olfactory reference disorder present with intrusive, repetitive, and
persistent thoughts about a perceived foul or offensive body odor or halitosis
that is either unnoticeable or only slightly noticeable to others. These patients
typically present with excessive self-consciousness about the perceived odor,
often including ideas of self-reference (i.e., the conviction that people are
taking notice of, or judging the odor). The preoccupation with the perceived
smell may be accompanied by repetitive and excessive behaviors, such as
repeatedly checking for body odor or excessive attempts to camouflage, alter,
or prevent the perceived odor. Individuals with olfactory reference disorder
generally believe that their odor will be offensive to others; consequently,
interpersonal interactions are avoided or endured with distress, shame, and
embarrassment (Veale & Matsunaga, 2014).

Differential Diagnosis

Fear of emitting offensive odors is a concern found in many cultures. Subclinical
symptoms are differentiated from olfactory reference disorder where the degree

of the olfactory preoccupation, the frequency of related recurrent behaviors performed, and the degree of distress or interference the individual experiences are clearly excessive and clinically significant. Olfactory reference disorder should also be differentiated from medical illnesses with objectively verifiable body odors and related complaints (e.g., various dermatological, otolaryngeal, dental, metabolic, or genitourinary conditions). Olfactory reference disorder must be differentiated from social anxiety disorder, OCD, and body dysmorphic disorder, conditions that are also characterized by anxiety and avoidance of social situations and obsessional triggers. In contrast to these other conditions, symptoms of olfactory reference disorder all relate to concerns about body odor specifically. The *CDDR* for olfactory reference disorder describe its differentiation from a range of other disorders.

Developmental Course

Olfactory reference disorder usually has its onset during adolescence or in the mid-20s. Most individuals with ORD report a chronic, and often unremitting, course. Although the literature on this condition in youth is sparse, it is assumed that the symptoms in children and adolescents are reminiscent of those reported by adults. Similar to adults, many younger individuals have strong beliefs about imagined body odor to the point that these may appear to be delusional. Olfactory reference disorder is associated with depression and anxiety, with many individuals becoming increasingly socially isolated from adolescence onwards due to avoidance of interaction with others for fear of embarrassment or fear offending others with their smell.

HYPOCHONDRIASIS (HEALTH ANXIETY DISORDER)

Presentations and Symptom Patterns

Hypochondriasis, also referred to as health anxiety disorder, is characterized by intrusive, repetitive, and persistent preoccupation or anxiety about having one or more serious, progressive, or life-threatening illnesses. The preoccupation or health anxiety is accompanied by repetitive and excessive health-related behaviors such as repeatedly checking of the body for evidence of illness; repeated, unnecessary medical examinations and diagnostic tests; and, more recently, extensively searching the internet for medical information. Alternatively, some individuals with hypochondriasis may present with maladaptive avoidance related to health (e.g., avoiding medical appointments fearing diagnosis of a serious illness or avoiding social interactions due to associated health risks). The experience of anxiety, which may include panic attacks, is a significant presenting feature. For this reason, health anxiety disorder is designated as an alternative name for the disorder, and hypochondriasis is cross-listed in the *ICD-11* grouping of anxiety and fear-related disorders.

Differential Diagnosis

Health anxiety falls along a continuum; subclinical or mild health anxiety may be adaptive in the sense that it leads to medical attention seeking. In hypochondriasis, however, the preoccupation, fear, or avoidance are extreme, not proportional to experienced symptoms or risk, and not related to a circumscribed situation (e.g., awaiting results of testing for a serious illness). In hypochondriasis, the preoccupation and repetitive behaviors or avoidance are all focused on health concerns, whereas in OCD, these rather encompass a variety of obsessions (e.g., of contamination, of causing harm) and compulsions (e.g., excessive washing, counting, checking). Some individuals with depressive disorders may also present with health concerns, but in depression, these are usually an integral part of a range of preoccupations (e.g., related to guilt, nihilism, poverty) and occur alongside other depressive symptoms (e.g., anhedonia, sleep disturbance, weight changes). Individuals with hypochondriasis may present with symptoms that are similar to presentations of anxiety or fear-related disorders. However, people with generalized anxiety disorder may worry about their health in addition to other worries (e.g., work, finances, family). Panic attacks can occur in hypochondriasis, but if exclusively associated with fears of having a life-threatening illness, an additional diagnosis of panic disorder is not warranted.

Developmental Course

There is growing evidence for early onset of health anxiety in children and adolescents (Thorgaard, 2017). Onset of hypochondriasis may be at any age, with the most common age being in early adulthood. Hypochondriasis in youth shares the same cognitive and behavioral features seen in adults (Wright et al., 2017). Early environmental risk factors may contribute to the development and maintenance of hypochondriasis, including illness in self or in significant others and safety-seeking behavior. Exposure to a negative parental style during childhood and adolescence, and exposure to early aversive experiences that may lead to an insecure attachment style, have both been associated with severe health anxiety. In addition, genetic factors may also have a role to play; children in families with a mother with severe health anxiety may be at higher risk of developing such symptoms themselves due to both environmental and genetic risk factors (Taylor et al., 2006).

HOARDING DISORDER

Presentations and Symptom Patterns

Individuals with hoarding disorder accumulate possessions to such an extent that living spaces are cluttered and their use or safety is compromised. Accumulation, which may be passive (e.g., accumulation of mail or newspapers) or active (e.g., excessive acquisition of free items), occurs due to repetitive urges or behaviors related to amassing items. There is significant difficulty discarding possessions due to a perceived need to save items and distress associated with discarding them. Generally, items are hoarded because of their emotional significance (sentimental value), their perceived usefulness, or their intrinsic value (e.g., perceived aesthetic qualities). Symptoms of hoarding disorder may be egosyntonic (i.e., associated with positive feelings of excitement and pleasure). The clutter caused by the hoarding behaviors may be distressing, however, and compromise functioning in several ways, including not being able to find important items (e.g., bills, tax forms), not being able to move easily inside the home, or even being unable to exit the home in the event of an emergency.

Differential Diagnosis

Hoarding must be distinguished from normal collecting. Collectors are more targeted in their acquisitions (e.g., stamp collecting), are more selective (e.g., purchasing only predetermined items), organize their acquisitions, and their collecting does not compromise the use and safety of their living space. OCD patients may also present with compulsive hoarding symptoms, but these are generally in response to unwanted and distressing thoughts; for example, the belief that something bad will happen if something is thrown away. Clutter may also result from decreased energy, lack of initiative, or apathy, typical of depressive episodes. In bipolar disorder, hoarding may be secondary to excessive shopping, and thus restricted to manic episodes. Panic attacks can occur in hoarding disorder, but if they are exclusively associated with having to discard accumulated possessions, an additional diagnosis of panic disorder is not warranted. When hoarding occurs in schizophrenia and other psychotic disorders, accumulation is driven by delusions, generally restricted to a small number of themes (e.g., hoarding of animals or books), and typically not accompanied by pleasure or enjoyment. In individuals with dementia, hoarding usually results from cognitive deficits or severe personality and behavioral changes, with no specific interest in accumulating objects or distress about discarding items.

Developmental Course

The first signs of the disorder usually begin in pre- and mid-adolescence. Treatment seeking begins at a later age, however. It is debatable whether the diagnostic requirements for adults with hoarding symptoms are suitable for younger individuals because hoarding may differ in several respects across different age groups. The requirement of cluttering, for example, may not apply to youth because they generally have limited resources and control over their living spaces (e.g., parents may throw objects away). Hoarding disorder is generally thought to follow a chronic course, with hoarding behaviors generally worsening over each decade of life. Hoarding disorder–specific risk factors and co-occurring mental disorders in children and adolescents are largely unknown.

BODY-FOCUSED REPETITIVE BEHAVIOR DISORDERS

Presentations and Symptom Patterns

Body-focused repetitive behavior disorders is an umbrella term used to describe conditions characterized by repetitive behaviors aimed at the surface of the body such as hair-pulling and skin-picking. These conditions differ from the other OCRDs in that they usually comprise repetitive behaviors without involving the intrusive repetitive persistent thoughts typical of other OCRDs. Body-focused repetitive behavior disorders lead to significant dermatological sequelae (e.g., hair loss, skin lesions), are characterized by unsuccessful attempts to decrease or stop the behavior, and produce significant distress or impairment. Negative feelings regarding the consequences of hair-pulling and skin-picking, such as a sense of loss of control or shame, are typical. In the *ICD-11*, trichotillomania and excoriation disorder constitute specific categories under the subgrouping of body-focused repetitive behavior disorders. Other similar behaviors (e.g., nail-biting or lip-biting) can be diagnosed as other specified body-focused repetitive behavior disorders if they are sufficiently severe and meet the other diagnostic requirements.

Differential Diagnosis

The behaviors in body-focused repetitive behavior disorders are differentiated from normal variants of these behaviors because they are recurrent, can result in extensive consequences to the body (e.g., bald spots, ulcerations), and are associated with significant distress or impairment. Individuals with other OCRDs such as body dysmorphic disorder may also present with pulling or picking as a symmetry ritual that is meant to "balance" appearance. Similarly, in OCD, skin may be picked to remove contamination when there are contamination obsessions. Excoriation disorder is differentiated from self-injurious and self-mutilating behaviors because they are not performed with the express purpose of self-injury, although injury may result.

Developmental Course

The diagnostic requirements for trichotillomania and excoriation disorder are suitable for individuals of all ages. The clinical presentation may vary over the lifetime, however, with some data suggesting that older children with trichotillomania may report more urges and have a more focused type of hair-pulling (Panza et al., 2013). The most common age of trichotillomania and excoriation disorder onset is early to mid-adolescence, typically coinciding with the onset of puberty. Onset of trichotillomania in very early childhood (in children younger than 5 years) may occur, potentially representing a subtype that is less chronic than later onset cases. In excoriation disorder, there is evidence for bimodal onset, with earlier onset often triggered by acne or eczema, and later onset occurring in middle adulthood, with increased rates of co-occurring depression, anxiety, and posttraumatic stress disorder.

Trichotillomania (Hair-Pulling Disorder)

The core feature of trichotillomania is the recurrent pulling of one's hair with a persistent inability to resist or decrease pulling (Lochner, Grant, Odlaug, & Stein, 2012). Hair loss is typically concealed or camouflaged (e.g., by using makeup, scarves, or wigs). Pathological hair-pulling may be associated with numerous additional behaviors such as visually or tactilely examining the hair or orally manipulating it after it has been pulled. Some individuals swallow or eat the hair that has been pulled (trichophagia) and may experience serious and even life-threatening gastrointestinal symptoms warranting medical attention, depending on the volume of hair consumed. Individuals with trichotillomania vary in the degree to which they pull hair in a more automatic or more intentional way.

Excoriation Disorder

Individuals with excoriation disorder pick anywhere and from multiple body sites, with the most picked sites being the face, arms, and hands. Many associated behaviors may be present, including visually or tactilely examining the skin, orally manipulating, and eating the skin or scab after it has been picked. There are numerous unsuccessful attempts to stop or decrease the behavior, which leads to significant distress or functional impairment (Lochner, Grant, Odlaug, Woods, et al., 2012). Skin-picking by individuals with excoriation disorder frequently leads to significant tissue damage and scarring, sometimes warranting antibiotic treatment or even surgery, and, in rare cases, can be life threatening (Odlaug & Grant, 2008).

TOURETTE SYNDROME

Presentations and Symptom Patterns

Tourette syndrome is classified under the grouping of primary tics and tic disorders in the chapter on diseases of the nervous system and is cross-listed with OCRDs for several reasons. There is high co-occurrence and familial association of Tourette syndrome with OCD, a finding that is consistent with a range of neurobiological data indicating overlap between these conditions, including brain imaging studies indicating disruption in CSTC circuits in both (Burton, 2017). Tourette syndrome is characterized by multiple motor and phonic tics that may or may not manifest concurrently or continuously, and that have been present for at least 1 year, with onset typically in childhood. They occur frequently and are associated with distress and impairment. The condition typically begins with transient bouts of simple motor tics, such as eye blinking, head jerks, or head banging, which eventually become more persistent, sometimes resulting in inadvertent self-injury. Phonic tics also tend to be simple in character at the onset (e.g., throat clearing, grunting, or squeaking) but may gradually develop into more complex vocal symptoms.

Differential Diagnosis

Tics are common in childhood but are transient in most cases, which is one reason for the long duration requirement for a diagnosis of Tourette syndrome. Tics in Tourette syndrome are differentiated from the repetitive and stereotyped motor movements that may occur in autism spectrum disorder because the latter last longer than a typical tic, usually emerge at a younger age, are not characterized by premonitory sensory urges, are often experienced by the individual as soothing or rewarding, and can generally be interrupted with distraction. Tourette syndrome and OCD also have features in common; differentiating complex tics and compulsions in OCD may be challenging. In contrast to compulsions of OCD, tics are not aimed at neutralizing unwanted or intrusive thoughts or images (obsessions).

Developmental Course

In Tourette syndrome, the onset of tics most commonly ranges between the ages of 4 and 6 years, peaking in severity between the ages of 10 and 12 years. Tics typically follow a waxing and waning course. The impact of the disorder is particularly pronounced for adolescents during this vulnerable phase of development, especially with regard to their social lives and relationships. The co-occurrence of Tourette syndrome and ADHD is well established, with ADHD occurring in half of children with Tourette syndrome, and predominantly affecting boys. OCD is also present in half of youth with Tourette syndrome (Hirschtritt et al., 2015). With increasing age, many individuals with Tourette syndrome develop the ability to temporarily suppress tics, with some effort.

INSIGHT SPECIFIER FOR OCRDs

An insight specifier is provided for those OCRDs in which cognitive phenomena are a prominent aspect of the clinical phenomenology—namely, OCD, body dysmorphic disorder, olfactory reference disorder, hypochondriasis, and hoarding disorder. The insight specifier describes the extent to which the individual is able to consider that the beliefs and perceptions underlying their symptoms may be untrue or excessive. Level of insight is specified by applying a dichotomous specifier: either "fair to good" or "poor to absent." A dichotomous specifier was chosen based on *ICD-11* field study data indicating that clinicians were not able to reliably distinguish between three proposed levels of insight (Kogan et al., 2020). When an individual expresses fixed and inaccurate beliefs that are restricted to beliefs specifically related to their OCRDs, with no history of other delusions, and the presentation is fully consistent with the other clinical features of the disorder, a diagnosis of an OCRD with poor to absent insight rather than delusional disorder should be assigned, even if the beliefs appear to be delusional in strength or fixity. Individuals with poor or absent insight are less likely to seek or receive mental health treatment. Indeed, a large proportion of patients with body dysmorphic disorder or hypochondriasis present in non–mental health settings (e.g., in body dysmorphic disorder, to dermatology or cosmetic surgery; in hypochondriasis, to emergency or internal medicine). Moreover, poor insight has been associated with several factors contributing to worse clinical outcome, including, for example, increased disorder severity, lower intellectual ability, poorer social functioning and quality of life, greater depressive symptoms, reduced compliance with treatment, and risk for suicidality (Gan et al., 2022). Some treatment interventions such as cognitive behavior therapy may also be less effective for people with low insight, at least initially, given that these techniques in part depend on the ability to challenge one's thoughts and beliefs.

ASSESSMENT

Individuals with OCRDs frequently do not spontaneously disclose their unwanted thoughts or repetitive due to shame, anxiety, or lack of insight, so it is important to ask about these specifically as a part of a psychological assessment. Questions about whether the person has intrusive thoughts that are recurrent, difficult to control, and cause fear or anxiety can assist in establishing the presence of obsessions or the focus of preoccupations. Questions about the presence of repetitive behaviors that are time-consuming, hard to control, and cause distress can yield information on the presence of compulsions typical of these conditions. Additional questions to determine the content of these obsessions and compulsions will assist in the diagnostic formulation. For example, to establish a diagnosis of body dysmorphic disorder, the patient can be asked whether their intrusive thoughts are about the appearance of some part(s) of their body that they consider unattractive and whether their lives and normal routines have been affected by these appearance concerns. Questions about whether there is substantial worry about the possibility of having a serious illness or whether it is hard to believe their doctor when told there is nothing to worry about can assist in establishing a diagnosis of hypochondriasis. To establish presence of olfactory reference disorder, patients can be asked whether their concerns are focused on concerns about body odor and whether there are any actions that they often or repeatedly perform in response to these concerns. The clinician can further assist in this process by providing examples of such thoughts and behaviors to patients. For example, in olfactory reference disorder, examples may include repeated and excessive teeth-brushing, washing or changing clothes very frequently, and repeatedly asking others for reassurance that there is no odor. In those OCRDs with a cognitive component (i.e., OCD, body dysmorphic disorder, olfactory reference disorder, hypochondriasis, and hoarding disorder), the assessment should also include questions aimed at determining level of insight. For example, a patient being interviewed for OCD could be asked whether they consider their concerns about preoccupation to be realistic or whether they sometimes think they are excessive. Presence of panic attacks within the context of obsessions and compulsions (e.g., in situations in which compulsions cannot be performed) should also be determined because this will have treatment implications.

Severity of the core symptoms and related functional impairment should be assessed at baseline and throughout treatment. For patients with OCD, the psychometrically sound clinician-administered Yale-Brown Obsessive-Compulsive Scale (Y-BOCS) is the "gold standard" severity scale (Goodman et al., 1989). The Y-BOCS has been adapted for use in some of the other OCRDs, including body dysmorphic disorder, olfactory reference disorder, hypochondriasis, and excoriation disorder. Severity measures of trichotillomania include the self-report Massachusetts General Hospital Hair-Pulling Scale (Keuthen et al., 1995). The clinician-administered Brown Assessment of Beliefs Scale provides information about level of insight (Eisen et al., 1998). These instruments can assist the clinician in deciding on the type of treatment that would be optimal. For example, patients scoring low on these measures and who are at least sometimes able to entertain the possibility that their disorder-specific beliefs may not be true and to accept an alternative explanation for their experience can typically be treated on an outpatient basis. Other patients with extremely high scores will likely require more intensive form of intervention, possibly including inpatient treatment.

A functional analysis can clarify the relationships between stimuli and responses associated with the disorder and is useful in treatment planning. This would include identifying the antecedent or trigger of the behavior, identifying and operationalizing the problem behaviors themselves, and identifying the maintaining consequences of the behavior. For example, a functional analysis for an individual with a trichotillomania would include collection and logging of information about critical antecedents or triggers of pulling (e.g., studying or watching TV, being bored or anxious), pulling-related behaviors (e.g., twirling or playing with hair, feeling the texture of hair, biting hair, swallowing), and consequences of hair-pulling (e.g., gratification or pleasure, shame, depression, anxiety). A functional analysis would also include information on how the person's cultural context shapes their symptoms. For example, in an individual with OCD, it should address whether aspects of behaviors such as extensive washing can be considered "normal" within their culture (for more discussion on this, see the next section, "Cultural Considerations"). The functional analysis would then guide behavioral treatment strategies (e.g., self-monitoring, replacing the problem behavior with a competing response) targeting the critical causal and maintenance factors.

The process of assessment and diagnosis also represents an important opportunity to provide psychoeducation to patients and their significant others.

People with OCD are often relieved to learn basic facts about their condition, including the fact that OCRDs are relatively common, that many others are also embarrassed or ashamed of their symptoms, and that treatments are effective for many. Myths such as that these conditions are due to bad parenting may be detrimental and should be addressed. Several consumer advocacy organizations such as the International OCD Foundation (https://iocdf.org/) and the TLC Foundation for Body-Focused Repetitive Behaviors (https://www.bfrb.org/) can assist in conveying such information.

CULTURAL CONSIDERATIONS IN OCRDs

OCRDs occur worldwide, with common features and similar pathophysiology across diverse ethnic groups and cultures (Reddy et al., 2018). However, cultural factors may shape the content of symptoms and level of distress that the individual experiences through faulty appraisals. For example, in OCD, there is evidence of increased prevalence of religiously themed obsessions and compulsions in the Middle East, and increased distress related to scrupulosity obsessions among individuals of certain faith groups. Cultural norms regarding beauty also play an important role in shaping the content of preoccupations in individuals with body dysmorphic disorder. For example, concerns about the appearance of eyelids are common in Eastern countries. In Western countries, fears of displeasing others is rare in body dysmorphic disorder, whereas in some cultures, faulty perceptions of abnormal or ugly bodily features or emitting a foul smell are characterized by intense anxiety about offending, embarrassing, or hurting others (e.g., *shubo-kyofu* or *taijin kyofusho* in Japan and related conditions in Korea and other societies). Help-seeking and clinical disclosure are less likely when the obsessions or compulsions are considered by the individual to be culturally taboo, leading to underdiagnosis and undertreatment of OCRDs. Familiarity with the cultural norms of the patient will assist in recognizing irrational cognitions and behavioral excesses that lead to clinically significant distress and functional impairment, in appropriate diagnosis of symptoms, and in selecting culturally appropriate treatment targets and techniques.

GENDER-RELATED FEATURES

The clinical features of OCRDs in men and women have many similarities but also important differences. Cognizance of these gender-related differences may be helpful during assessment and may facilitate rapport building and understanding. For example, women with OCD are more likely than men to report contamination-related symptoms, particularly in the context of perinatal OCD, whereas men are more likely to report sexual and symmetry-related obsessions. In body dysmorphic disorder, men are more likely to be preoccupied by the appearance of their genitals, body build, and thinning hair/balding whereas women with this condition are more likely to present with dissatisfaction with several aspects of their appearance including their shape (not weight per se) and excessive body hair. Patterns of co-occurrence with other mental disorders may also differ between men and women with OCRDs. In OCD, for example, men are more likely to experience co-occurring disorders due to substance use, whereas women more commonly present with co-occurring mood disorders and anxiety and fear-related disorders. In body dysmorphic disorder, women may present with a co-occurring eating disorder, whereas males are more likely to present with muscle dysmorphia and/or genital preoccupation. Women may be more likely to seek treatment than men, but no major differences in treatment responsivity between men and women diagnosed with OCRDs have been identified. Therefore, a treatment plan that involves targeting the inaccurate beliefs, along with exposure exercises and other strategies to address compulsive behaviors and anxiety, specific to each OCRD, would remain the first-line treatment, irrespective of gender.

PREVALENCE

OCD and body dysmorphic disorder are relatively common; for example, a survey in the United States indicated a lifetime prevalence of OCD in adults of 2.3% (Ruscio et al., 2010), and a global study suggested a lifetime prevalence of body dysmorphic disorder in adults in the community of 1.9% (Veale et al., 2016). Prevalence of other OCRDs such as hypochondriasis and olfactory reference disorder appears to be within the same range but is not yet well established. Prevalence of these conditions vary depending on the type of setting. In mental health and medical settings, rates of some OCRDs (such as body dysmorphic disorder and hypochondriasis) may be higher than in community settings. Prevalence rates of many OCRDs in the literature may be an underestimation because individuals may not report all their symptoms due to shame or embarrassment or being culturally taboo.

KEY POINTS

- Obsessive-compulsive and related disorders (OCRDs) are characterized by intrusive thoughts or repetitive behaviors (or both) that are time-consuming, distressing, and impairing.

- OCRDs include obsessive-compulsive disorder (OCD), body dysmorphic disorder, olfactory reference disorder, hypochondriasis (health anxiety disorder), and hoarding disorder. It also comprises the subgrouping of body-focused repetitive behavior disorders, including trichotillomania (hair-pulling disorder) and excoriation (skin-picking) disorder, which are characterized by repetitive behaviors but not obsessions.

- A specifier for level of insight is applied to those OCRDs with a prominent cognitive component, which describes the extent to which the individual is able to consider that the beliefs and perceptions underlying their symptoms may be untrue or excessive. Insight may be specified as "fair to good" or "poor to absent."

- Grouping these conditions has clinical utility because similar assessment and treatment approaches, adapted for each disorder, are helpful for these conditions.

- Cognitive-behavioral theories of OCRD emphasize the misappraisals of the significance of intrusive thoughts, leading to increased anxiety and distress, and performance of behaviors aimed at reducing these emotions and/or the likelihood of the catastrophic consequences occurring. The cognitions that underlie the vulnerability to develop such negative misappraisals in response to intrusive thoughts include inflated sense of responsibility and overestimation of threat, perfectionism, the need for absolute certainty, and the belief that all thoughts are meaningful and should be controlled.

- Individuals with an OCRD frequently do not spontaneously disclose their unwanted or repetitive thoughts due to shame, anxiety, or lack of insight, so it is important to ask about these specifically as a part of a psychological assessment.

- Well-established symptom scales may assist in the assessment process to identify antecedents or triggers and associated emotional and behavioral responses. A functional analysis will guide the cognitive-behavioral treatment strategies (e.g., self-monitoring, replacing the problem behavior with a competing response), so targeting the critical causal and maintenance factors. Assessment and diagnosis should be accompanied by psychoeducation to patients and their significant others.

REFERENCES

Abramovitch, A., Abramowitz, J. S., & Mittelman, A. (2013). The neuropsychology of adult obsessive-compulsive disorder: A meta-analysis. *Clinical Psychology Review, 33*(8), 1163–1171. https://doi.org/10.1016/j.cpr.2013.09.004

Burton, F. H. (2017). Back to the future: Circuit-testing TS & OCD. *Journal of Neuroscience Methods, 292*, 2–11. https://doi.org/10.1016/j.jneumeth.2017.07.025

Calkins, A. W., Berman, N. C., & Wilhelm, S. (2013). Recent advances in research on cognition and emotion in OCD: A review. *Current Psychiatry Reports, 15*(5), 357. https://doi.org/10.1007/s11920-013-0357-4

Eisen, J. L., Phillips, K. A., Baer, L., Beer, D. A., Atala, K. D., & Rasmussen, S. A. (1998). The Brown Assessment of Beliefs Scale: Reliability and validity. *The American Journal of Psychiatry, 155*(1), 102–108. https://doi.org/10.1176/ajp.155.1.102

Fineberg, N. A., Chamberlain, S. R., Goudriaan, A. E., Stein, D. J., Vanderschuren, L. J., Gillan, C. M., Shekar, S., Gorwood, P. A., Voon, V., Morein-Zamir, S., Denys, D., Sahakian, B. J., Moeller, F. G., Robbins, T. W., & Potenza, M. N. (2014). New developments in human neurocognition: Clinical, genetic, and brain imaging correlates of impulsivity and compulsivity. *CNS Spectrums, 19*(1), 69–89. https://doi.org/10.1017/S1092852913000801

Gan, J., He, J., Fu, H., & Zhu, X. (2022). Association between obsession, compulsion, depression and insight in obsessive-compulsive disorder: A meta-analysis. *Nordic Journal of Psychiatry, 76*(7), 489–496. https://doi.org/10.1080/08039488.2021.2013532

Gillan, C. M., & Robbins, T. W. (2014). Goal-directed learning and obsessive-compulsive disorder. *Philosophical Transactions of the Royal Society of London: Series B. Biological Sciences*, *369*(1655), Article 20130475. https://doi.org/10.1098/rstb.2013.0475

Goodman, W. K., Price, L. H., Rasmussen, S. A., Mazure, C., Fleischmann, R. L., Hill, C. L., Heninger, G. R., & Charney, D. S. (1989). The Yale–Brown Obsessive Compulsive Scale. I. Development, use, and reliability. *Archives of General Psychiatry*, *46*(11), 1006–1011. https://doi.org/10.1001/archpsyc.1989.01810110048007

Hayes, S. C., Wilson, K. G., Gifford, E. V., Follette, V. M., & Strosahl, K. (1996). Experimental avoidance and behavioral disorders: A functional dimensional approach to diagnosis and treatment. *Journal of Consulting and Clinical Psychology*, *64*(6), 1152–1168. https://doi.org/10.1037/0022-006X.64.6.1152

Hirschtritt, M. E., Lee, P. C., Pauls, D. L., Dion, Y., Grados, M. A., Illmann, C., King, R. A., Sandor, P., McMahon, W. M., Lyon, G. J., Cath, D. C., Kurlan, R., Robertson, M. M., Osiecki, L., Scharf, J. M., Mathews, C. A., & the Tourette Syndrome Association International Consortium for Genetics. (2015). Lifetime prevalence, age of risk, and genetic relationships of comorbid psychiatric disorders in Tourette syndrome. *JAMA Psychiatry*, *72*(4), 325–333. https://doi.org/10.1001/jamapsychiatry.2014.2650

Keuthen, N. J., O'Sullivan, R. L., Ricciardi, J. N., Shera, D., Savage, C. R., Borgmann, A. S., Jenike, M. A., & Baer, L. (1995). The Massachusetts General Hospital (MGH) Hairpulling Scale: 1. Development and factor analyses. *Psychotherapy and Psychosomatics*, *64*(3-4), 141–145. https://doi.org/10.1159/000289003

Kogan, C. S., Stein, D. J., Rebello, T. J., Keeley, J. W., Chan, K. J., Fineberg, N. A., Fontenelle, L. F., Grant, J. E., Matsunaga, H., Simpson, H. B., Thomsen, P. H., van den Heuvel, O. A., Veale, D., Grenier, J., Kulygina, M., Matsumoto, C., Domínguez-Martínez, T., Stona, A. C., Wang, Z., & Reed, G. M. (2020). Accuracy of diagnostic judgments using *ICD-11* vs. *ICD-10* diagnostic guidelines for obsessive-compulsive and related disorders. *Journal of Affective Disorders*, *273*, 328–340. https://doi.org/10.1016/j.jad.2020.03.103

Lochner, C., Grant, J. E., Odlaug, B. L., & Stein, D. J. (2012). *DSM-5* field survey: Skin picking disorder. *Annals of Clinical Psychiatry*, *24*(4), 300–304.

Lochner, C., Grant, J. E., Odlaug, B. L., Woods, D. W., Keuthen, N. J., & Stein, D. J. (2012). *DSM-5* field survey: Hair-pulling disorder (trichotillomania). *Depression and Anxiety*, *29*(12), 1025–1031. https://doi.org/10.1002/da.22011

Odlaug, B. L., & Grant, J. E. (2008). Clinical characteristics and medical complications of pathologic skin picking. *General Hospital Psychiatry*, *30*(1), 61–66. https://doi.org/10.1016/j.genhosppsych.2007.07.009

Panza, K. E., Pittenger, C., & Bloch, M. H. (2013). Age and gender correlates of pulling in pediatric trichotillomania. *Journal of the American Academy of Child & Adolescent Psychiatry*, *52*(3), 241–249. https://doi.org/10.1016/j.jaac.2012.12.019

Phillips, K. A., Pinto, A., Hart, A. S., Coles, M. E., Eisen, J. L., Menard, W., & Rasmussen, S. A. (2012). A comparison of insight in body dysmorphic disorder and obsessive-compulsive disorder. *Journal of Psychiatric Research*, *46*(10), 1293–1299. https://doi.org/10.1016/j.jpsychires.2012.05.016

Pope, C. G., Pope, H. G., Menard, W., Fay, C., Olivardia, R., & Phillips, K. A. (2005). Clinical features of muscle dysmorphia among males with body dysmorphic disorder. *Body Image*, *2*(4), 395–400. https://doi.org/10.1016/j.bodyim.2005.09.001

Rautio, D., Jassi, A., Krebs, G., Andrén, P., Monzani, B., Gumpert, M., Lewis, A., Peile, L., Sevilla-Cermeño, L., Jansson-Fröjmark, M., Lundgren, T., Hillborg, M., Silverberg-Morse, M., Clark, B., Fernández de la Cruz, L., & Mataix-Cols, D. (2022). Clinical characteristics of 172 children and adolescents with body dysmorphic disorder. *European Child & Adolescent Psychiatry*, *31*(1), 133–144. https://doi.org/10.1007/s00787-020-01677-3

Reddy, Y. J., Simpson, H. B., & Stein, D. J. (2018). Obsessive-compulsive and related disorders in *International Classification of Diseases–11* and its relation to *International*

Classification of Diseases–10 and *Diagnostic and Statistical Manual of Mental Disorders–5*. *Indian Journal of Social Psychiatry*, *34*(5), 34–43. https://doi.org/10.4103/ijsp.ijsp_38_18

Robbins, T. W., Vaghi, M. M., & Banca, P. (2019). Obsessive-compulsive disorder: Puzzles and prospects. *Neuron*, *102*(1), 27–47. https://doi.org/10.1016/j.neuron.2019.01.046

Roberts, S., O'Connor, K., & Bélanger, C. (2013). Emotion regulation and other psychological models for body-focused repetitive behaviors. *Clinical Psychology Review*, *33*(6), 745–762. https://doi.org/10.1016/j.cpr.2013.05.004

Ruscio, A. M., Stein, D. J., Chiu, W. T., & Kessler, R. C. (2010). The epidemiology of obsessive-compulsive disorder in the National Comorbidity Survey Replication. *Molecular Psychiatry*, *15*(1), 53–63. https://doi.org/10.1038/mp.2008.94

Stein, D. J., Kogan, C. S., Atmaca, M., Fineberg, N. A., Fontenelle, L. F., Grant, J. E., Matsunaga, H., Reddy, Y. C. J., Simpson, H. B., Thomsen, P. H., van den Heuvel, O. A., Veale, D., Woods, D. W., & Reed, G. M. (2016). The classification of obsessive-compulsive and related disorders in the *ICD-11*. *Journal of Affective Disorders*, *190*, 663–674. https://doi.org/10.1016/j.jad.2015.10.061

Taylor, S., Thordarson, D. S., Jang, K. L., & Asmundson, G. J. (2006). Genetic and environmental origins of health anxiety: A twin study. *World Psychiatry*, *5*(1), 47–50.

Thorgaard, M. V. (2017). Health anxiety and illness behaviour in children of mothers with severe health anxiety. *Danish Medical Journal*, *64*(5), B5365.

Veale, D., Gledhill, L. J., Christodoulou, P., & Hodsoll, J. (2016). Body dysmorphic disorder in different settings: A systematic review and estimated weighted prevalence. *Body Image*, *18*, 168–186. https://doi.org/10.1016/j.bodyim.2016.07.003

Veale, D., & Matsunaga, H. (2014). Body dysmorphic disorder and olfactory reference disorder: Proposals for *ICD-11*. *Brazilian Journal of Psychiatry*, *36*(Suppl. 1), 14–20. https://doi.org/10.1590/1516-4446-2013-1238

World Health Organization. (2023). *ICD-11 for mortality and morbidity statistics* (Version: 01/2023). https://icd.who.int/browse11/l-m/en#/

World Health Organization. (2024). *Clinical descriptions and diagnostic requirements for ICD-11 mental, behavioural and neurodevelopmental disorders*. https://www.who.int/publications/i/item/9789240077263

Wright, K. D., Reiser, S. J., & Delparte, C. A. (2017). The relationship between childhood health anxiety, parent health anxiety, and associated constructs. *Journal of Health Psychology*, *22*(5), 617–626. https://doi.org/10.1177/1359105315610669

10

Disorders Specifically Associated With Stress

Chris R. Brewin, Marylène Cloitre, Amy Y. M. Chow, and Andreas Maercker

OVERARCHING LOGIC

The grouping of disorders specifically associated with stress in the 11th revision of the *International Classification of Diseases* (*ICD-11*; World Health Organization [WHO], 2023) replaces the *ICD-10* grouping of reaction to severe stress and adjustment disorders. Although the onset and course of many mental disorders can be influenced by past and current stressors, this grouping acknowledges that some disorders are so intimately connected with stressful events that they could not have occurred in their absence. At the same time, most people do not develop a disorder even when faced with a severe stressor, so psychological, social, and biological vulnerabilities also contribute to these disorders. Disorders specifically associated with stress include posttraumatic stress disorder (PTSD), complex PTSD, prolonged grief disorder, and adjustment disorder, which are the focus of this chapter. The *ICD-11* grouping of disorders specifically associated with stress also includes reactive attachment disorder and disinhibited social engagement disorder, which are not discussed in this chapter. Both of these last two disorders are typically diagnosed in young children with a history of grossly inadequate child care (e.g., severe neglect, maltreatment, institutional deprivation) and are not commonly seen in general practice.

The principles of clinical utility and global applicability that underpin the *ICD-11* suggest that, where possible, diagnostic requirements should be simplified, describing disorders with the most parsimonious set of distinctive

https://doi.org/10.1037/0000392-010
A Psychological Approach to Diagnosis: Using the ICD-11 as a Framework, G. M. Reed, P. L.-J. Ritchie, and A. Maercker (Editors)

symptoms. Accordingly, PTSD in the *ICD-11* involves the presence of three core elements that distinguish it from other disorders. Preliminary evidence suggests the application of the *ICD-11* requirements may result in a lower prevalence of PTSD in adult samples while reducing diagnostic co-occurrence with depression (Brewin et al., 2017). Thus, PTSD in *ICD-11* may be considered a more specific disorder than it is in *ICD-10*, and individuals who do not meet the *ICD-11* requirements for PTSD may instead be more appropriately diagnosed as experiencing another disorder (e.g., a depressive disorder, an anxiety or fear-related disorder, an adjustment disorder).

The *ICD-11* development process took account of long-standing arguments for the introduction of a complex PTSD diagnosis that reflects the additional effects of exposure to repeated or chronic traumatic stress (Brewin et al., 2017; Robles et al., 2014). *ICD-11* has introduced this distinction based on specific scientific and clinical evidence. *ICD-11* complex PTSD, in part a reformulation of *ICD-10* diagnosis "enduring personality change after catastrophic experience," focuses on disturbances in self-organization that can result from multiple, chronic, or repeated traumas, typically of an interpersonal nature, from which escape is difficult or impossible (e.g., exposure to childhood abuse, domestic violence, torture, slavery, genocide campaigns). Importantly, however, *ICD-11* complex PTSD differs from all previous formulations of complex responses to trauma in that it is symptom-based rather than requiring a particular form of trauma exposure. Complex PTSD is not a subtype of PTSD but rather a separate and distinct disorder. If a person is diagnosed with complex PTSD, an additional diagnosis of PTSD is not assigned.

Prolonged grief disorder is also a new diagnosis classified in the *ICD-11* grouping of disorders specifically associated with stress. It may be assigned to individuals who have experienced the death of a partner, parent, child, or other person close to them and is characterized by abnormally chronic and pervasive responses to bereavement that interfere with functioning (Killikelly & Maercker, 2017). Like PTSD, diagnostic requirements for prolonged grief disorder were designed to be as parsimonious as possible to enhance clinical utility. In addition, the *ICD-11 Clinical Descriptions and Diagnostic Requirements* (*CDDR*) emphasize known social and cultural influences on the form and intensity of symptoms as well as on the duration of grief to facilitate global applicability.

Adjustment disorder has been a widely used diagnosis (Evans et al., 2013; Reed et al., 2011) but one that is poorly defined, owing to the wide variety of possible presenting symptoms and the relative absence of distinctive features. It has often been used as a residual category for individuals who do not meet the diagnostic requirements for a depressive or anxiety disorder, or as a provisional diagnosis when it is not clear whether a posttraumatic or mood disorder will emerge. By contrast, in the *ICD-11* adjustment disorder is characterized by preoccupation with a stressor and failure to adapt, as shown by a range of symptoms that interfere with everyday functioning. Lack of evidence for the validity of various subtypes specified in the *ICD-10* resulted in their omission from the *ICD-11*.

This chapter mentions several relatively new measures that have been developed to be used in the assessment of disorders specifically associated with stress. Some are available in multiple languages and may be used free of charge.

These measures help describe symptoms and evaluate thresholds, but it is important to keep in mind that a diagnosis cannot be made based on any single measure, and measures used should be culturally and linguistically appropriate for the individual being tested.

A PSYCHOLOGICAL APPROACH TO DISORDERS SPECIFICALLY ASSOCIATED WITH STRESS

The *ICD-11* recognizes a distinction between disorders linked to *traumatic* stress, consisting of extremely threatening or horrific events, and disorders linked to other kinds of stress (such as relationship breakdown or housing and financial problems). There is no assumption here that one kind of stress is more severe than another; rather, the distinction reflects the experience that stressors which elicit intense responses of fear or horror tend to be accompanied by different sorts of symptoms. The symptoms are consistent with a model in which psychopathology arises from events that have exceeded the individual's capacity to adapt, leading to psychological responses not fully integrated with the person's sense of self or knowledge of other people and the world. This is reflected in comments such as "I still cannot believe this has happened," or "I don't want to accept that this has happened." The symptoms vary between disorders but reflect common constructs such as the influence of the memory of the event (e.g., reexperiencing), making sense of the event (e.g., preoccupation), physiological responses (e.g., increased startle reaction), attempts to control reactions (e.g., avoidance), and goal-oriented behavior (e.g., yearning). Symptoms are only relevant if they first appeared after the event, although this may be difficult to establish in the case of long-ago or repeated events.

POSTTRAUMATIC STRESS DISORDER

Presentations and Symptom Patterns

PTSD can follow an event or situation that is experienced by the individual as extremely threatening or horrific. As described in the *Clinical Descriptions and Diagnostic Requirements for ICD-11 Mental, Behavioural and Neurodevelopmental Disorders* (*CDDR*; WHO, 2024), such events include, but are not limited to, directly experiencing combat, disasters, serious accidents, physical and sexual assaults, and acute life-threatening illness; witnessing the threatened or actual injury or death of others in a sudden, unexpected, or violent manner; and learning about the sudden, unexpected, or violent death of a loved one. A series of events, such as being repeatedly stalked, handling or retrieving body parts after people have died violently, or witnessing abuse, may qualify if the result is that the person comes to experience extreme fear or horror. Conditions that alter normal perception (such as experiencing threatening delusions and hallucinations, whether psychotic or drug-induced, and the atypical processing of the social and sensory world associated with conditions such as autism spectrum disorder) may result in other types of experiences qualifying as triggering events because they are subjectively experienced with extreme fear and horror (Brewin et al., 2019).

After a qualifying event, a PTSD diagnosis requires the simultaneous presence of three core elements, which must last for at least several weeks. The first element is evidence that the traumatic event is being reexperienced in the present. That is, the individual has the experience that the traumatic event is happening again in the "here and now." The reexperiencing may occur in the form of nightmares that closely recapitulate the themes of the event (without necessarily reproducing it exactly), intrusive memories, or flashbacks.

The second core element is evidence of deliberate avoidance of the traumatic event, either in the form of internal avoidance of thoughts and memories or of external avoidance of people, conversations, activities, or situations reminiscent of the event. The third core element is evidence of persistent perceptions of heightened current threat—for example, as indicated by hypervigilance or by an enhanced startle reaction to stimuli such as unexpected noises. Again, evidence of the presence of all three core elements is required. Symptoms must also be accompanied by significant impairment in personal, family, social, educational, occupational, or other important areas of functioning. Alternately, if functioning is maintained, it is only through significant additional effort.

In the *ICD-11*, therefore, the diagnosis of PTSD depends only on the presence of these three core elements (WHO, 2024). Many other symptoms (e.g., suicidal thoughts and impaired concentration) will commonly be encountered but are not unique to PTSD; they may indicate a co-occurring condition. Although fear and horror will be present to some degree, other emotions such as anger, shame, sadness, humiliation, and guilt, including survivor guilt, are often more prominent features of the clinical presentation.

Differential Diagnosis

A history of exposure to an event or situation of an extremely threatening or horrific nature does not in itself indicate the presence of PTSD. Most people who experience such stressors do not develop a disorder. Moreover, normal acute reactions to traumatic events can show all the symptoms of PTSD including reexperiencing, but these begin to subside fairly quickly (e.g., within 1 week after the event terminates or removal from the threatening situation, or 1 month in the case of continuing stressors). If clinical intervention is warranted in these situations, assignment of the category acute stress reaction from the chapter on factors influencing health status or contact with health services (i.e., a nondisorder category) is generally more appropriate.

When people do develop a disorder after exposure to a traumatic event, it is most commonly a depressive disorder or an anxiety or fear-related disorder (either the onset of a new disorder or a recurrence of a preexisting disorder). If the event has not produced extreme fear or horror and the diagnostic requirements for these other disorders are not met, a diagnosis of adjustment disorder can be considered. More typical triggering events for adjustment disorder are divorce, loss of a job, or diagnosis of a life-threatening or chronic illness. Adjustment disorder is also often the most appropriate diagnosis after traumatic events characteristic of PTSD (i.e., those that produce extreme fear or horror) when the PTSD symptom requirements are not met; rather, the individual's reaction is characterized by preoccupation with the event or its consequences.

A variety of dissociative symptoms can occur after exposure to an extremely threatening or horrific event, including trance or fugue states as well as somatic symptoms, and a dissociative disorder may be considered as an alternative or co-occurring diagnosis if these symptoms are prominent. Both PTSD and prolonged grief disorder may occur in individuals who experience bereavement as a result of the death of a loved one under traumatic circumstances. Unlike in PTSD, where the individual reexperiences the event or situation associated with the death, in prolonged grief disorder, the person may be preoccupied with memories of the circumstances surrounding the death but does not reexperience them as occurring again in the here and now.

Co-Occurring Conditions

The disorders that most commonly co-occur with PTSD are depressive disorders, anxiety or fear-related disorders, and disorders due to substance use.

Developmental Course

There is considerable evidence that diagnostic requirements developed primarily with adults in mind may not always be suitable for school-age and younger children (Danzi & La Greca, 2016). Younger children are typically unable to describe reexperiencing, for example, but evidence of it is often notable in behavioral manifestations such as trauma-specific reenactments (e.g., repetitive play or drawings with traumatic themes), frightening dreams without clear content, or night terrors. A sense of threat may be manifested by uncharacteristic impulsivity. Children may not appear distressed when talking about or playing out their traumatic recollections, despite substantial impact on psychosocial functioning and development. Other manifestations of PTSD in preschool children may include inhibited behaviors, such as excessive reassurance seeking, or disinhibited behaviors, such as increased frequency and intensity of temper tantrums or acting out.

Adolescents may also deny feelings of fear or horror associated with reexperiencing and instead report either no affect or other types of strong or overwhelming emotions. Reluctance to pursue developmental opportunities (e.g., to gain autonomy from caregivers) may occur as a sign of psychosocial impairment. Self-injurious or risky behaviors (e.g., substance use or unprotected sex) occur at elevated rates among adolescents with PTSD.

Assessment

Reexperiencing of the traumatic event may occur in the form of nightmares, intrusive memories, or flashbacks. The term *flashback* refers to a continuum of reexperiencing phenomena. At the milder end, it is synonymous with intrusive traumatic memories containing sensory elements such as sights, sounds, or physical sensations that are repeatedly experienced, even only briefly, as though they were occurring in the present. Clinicians should be careful to question individuals to distinguish these symptoms from ordinary intrusive memories, which are common in many mental disorders. Ordinary intrusive memories are not experienced as though they were happening again in the here and now but rather as belonging to the past. At the more extreme end, flashbacks are reexperiencing episodes in which people become absorbed, sometimes for a considerable period, in the traumatic memory and lose touch with their current surroundings. If the individual does not have any conscious memory of the traumatic event (e.g., because they were very young when it happened or because they sustained a head injury), the reexperiencing requirement can be met by the presence of a strong emotional or physical response to reminders of the event.

In assessing avoidance of thoughts and feelings, clinicians should note this refers only to *attempts* to avoid; often these attempts are only partially successful. Increased alcohol or substance use after the trauma may represent an attempt at avoidance. Avoidance may not be possible in some work contexts—for example, members of the armed forces or emergency services who are required to attend situations that stimulate reexperiencing as part of their duties.

In assessing a continued sense of threat, the clinicians should be careful to assess whether any objective threat is still occurring. PTSD should not be diagnosed given evidence that the threat (e.g., from an assailant or from a natural hazard such as an earthquake) is realistically still present and thus could account for hypervigilance or exaggerated startle reactions. Impairment is recognized when performance (e.g., at work) has suffered or is maintained only with considerable extra effort. All symptoms, including impairment, should have begun or become markedly worse after the traumatic event.

The International Trauma Questionnaire (Cloitre et al., 2018) is a validated instrument designed to assess *ICD-11* PTSD and complex PTSD, with translations into more than 30 languages available (https://www.traumameasuresglobal.com). Measurement of PTSD involves six symptom items and a further three items that assess impairment in functioning, making the International Trauma Questionnaire useful both as a diagnostic tool and as a brief screening instrument. However, a diagnosis cannot be made solely on the administration of a single instrument. Measures should be culturally appropriate and usually administered in the individual's preferred language. When these conditions are not met, test results should be interpreted with caution.

COMPLEX PTSD

Presentations and Symptom Patterns

Complex PTSD most commonly develops after prolonged or repetitive events from which escape is difficult or impossible (e.g., torture, slavery, genocide campaigns, prolonged domestic violence, repeated childhood sexual or physical abuse). Complex PTSD comprises six symptom clusters, described in the *CDDR*. The first three are identical to those of PTSD—namely, reexperiencing in the present, avoidance, and persistent perceptions of heightened threat. The three additional symptom clusters describe disturbances in self-organization (DSO)—namely, severe and persistent (a) problems in affect regulation; (b) beliefs about oneself as diminished, defeated, or worthless, accompanied by feelings of shame, guilt, or failure related to the traumatic event; and (c) difficulties in sustaining relationships and in feeling close to others. To meet the diagnostic requirements for complex PTSD, the PTSD and DSO symptoms must cause significant impairment in personal, family, social, educational, occupational, or other important areas of functioning.

Chronic trauma is a risk factor, not a requirement, for the diagnosis of complex PTSD. This approach recognizes and allows for the influence of internal or environmental factors on psychological outcome. The presence (or lack thereof) of personal (e.g., optimism, resilience) or environmental resources (e.g., social support) can determine an individual's response to events. For example, an individual with a history of chronic childhood sexual abuse who has positive social support, personal strengths, or other protective factors may not develop complex PTSD but rather PTSD or no disorder. Alternatively, an individual who experiences a single adult trauma (e.g., gang rape, witnessing the murder of their child) whose psychological resources are limited or depleted or who experiences an absence of social support or rejection by their community may develop complex PTSD rather than PTSD.

Problems in affect regulation include hyperreactivity such as difficulty recovering from minor stressors, violent outbursts, or reckless behaviors (e.g., unprotected sex, driving at high speeds), as well as hyporeactivity such as emotional numbing, difficulty experiencing pleasure or positive emotions (anhedonia), and dissociation (e.g., feeling outside of one's body, feeling the world is unreal, gaps in memory). Problems in self-concept include persistent beliefs about oneself as diminished, defeated, or worthless accompanied by deep and pervasive feelings of shame, guilt, or failure. Interpersonal problems are characterized by persistent difficulties in sustaining relationships. Examples of such difficulties include problems feeling close to others, avoidance of relationships, ending relationships when difficulties or conflicts emerge, or deriding the value or importance of relationships.

Associated features are symptoms and problems that may be observed in the individual with complex PTSD but are not necessary to making the diagnosis. In complex PTSD, these include problems such as suicidal ideation or behavior and substance use, which have been related to emotion regulation difficulties, and significant depressive symptoms, possibly including psychotic symptoms. Somatic complaints (e.g., pain) may be present but vary by culture and may also be a more direct result of the trauma (e.g., torture; physical punishment; being deprived of adequate food, clothing, or shelter).

Differential Diagnosis

A history of exposure to an event or situation of an extremely threatening or horrific nature, even those of a prolonged or repetitive nature from which escape is difficult or impossible (e.g., sexual abuse, domestic violence, exposure to genocide) does not in itself indicate the presence of complex PTSD. People can experience such stressors without developing a disorder, or they may develop a depressive disorder or an anxiety or fear-related disorder. To diagnose complex PTSD, the presentation must meet the diagnostic requirements for the disorder.

Complex PTSD shares three symptom clusters with PTSD (reexperiencing in the here and now, avoidance, and sense of current threat). In addition, there must be clinically significant symptoms in each domain of emotion dysregulation, negative self-concept, and relationship difficulties, which must be persistent and pervasive (i.e., occurring across a variety of situations and contexts and not dependent on the presence of trauma-related cues). If these additional symptoms are not present, a diagnosis of PTSD may be made. Disturbances in self-organization may occasionally be seen in PTSD but most commonly occur as an acute response to a recent stressor that tends to resolve relatively quickly, wax and wane over the reported period, or do not present simultaneously in all three areas as is required for complex PTSD.

As with complex PTSD, personality disorders include problems in functioning related to the self (e.g., identify, self-worth) and/or interpersonal dysfunction (ability to develop and maintain close and mutually satisfying relationships) that are of a pervasive nature. Personality disorders differ in that the presence of the symptoms must have persisted over an extended period (generally 2 years or more) and are not specifically tied to a traumatic stressor. Complex PTSD symptoms must emerge after a trauma and the symptoms representing DSO must co-occur with the PTSD symptoms of reexperiencing, avoidance, and sense of current threat. Although all the symptoms of complex PTSD must co-occur for a sustained period, the duration is not specified and can be less than the 2 years specified for a personality disorder. Research to date has not identified a required duration for complex PTSD.

A diagnosis of personality disorder can include a specifier for "borderline pattern." The borderline pattern has similar domains of disturbances as complex PTSD (self-concept, affect dysregulation, and interpersonal difficulties), but the content and character of the problems are quite different. In the borderline pattern, self-concept difficulties reflect an instability in identity with shifting overly positive or overly negative self-appraisals, whereas in complex PTSD, the self-concept is stable but persistently negative. Relational difficulties in the context of the borderline pattern are characterized by volatile patterns of interactions with alternating overidealization or denigration of the other person, whereas in complex PTSD, relational difficulties are characterized by a persistent tendency to avoid relationships and distancing in times of difficulties. Affect dysregulation is the most phenomenologically similar problem in both disorders, typically characterized by lability in emotional reactions and difficulty returning to baseline.

Following an experience of a traumatic event, individuals with complex PTSD may experience a variety of dissociative symptoms including somatic symptoms, trance, or fugue state. These symptoms are also experienced by individuals with PTSD but are more strongly associated with and occur at substantially higher levels of severity among those with complex PTSD (Hyland et al., 2020). The presence of persistent experiences of a fugue or trance state may warrant an additional dissociative disorder diagnosis.

Dysthymic disorder typically includes low self-esteem, which may be expressed as a sense of worthlessness and failure and may be similar to some of symptoms of complex PTSD. A diagnosis of dysthymic disorder can be considered if insufficient PTSD symptoms are present. Dysthymic disorder also requires additional depressive symptoms such as significant problems in sleeping or eating, which are not core symptoms of complex PTSD.

Co-Occurring Conditions

The disorders that most commonly co-occur with complex PTSD are identical to those associated with PTSD but occur at significantly greater rates—namely, depressive disorders, anxiety and fear-related disorders, and disorders due to substance use (Brewin et al., 2017).

Developmental Course

Complex PTSD symptoms related to disturbances in self-organization reflect the developmental stage of the child or adolescent. Among school-age children, affect dysregulation may be expressed by excessive crying and increased irritability, negative self-concept by feeling like a "bad person," and interpersonal difficulties expressed as social withdrawal or increased aggressiveness (Cook et al., 2005). In adolescence, affect dysregulation may be expressed by increased moodiness; increased risky behavior such as unsafe sex, unsafe driving, and substance use; and negative self-concept by feelings of self-hatred, worthlessness, shame, and guilt. Interpersonal problems in adolescence may include aggressive or highly sexualized behaviors or feeling exceptionally distant from peers.

Assessment

To be recognized as part of the complex PTSD symptom profile, disturbances in self-organization specific to complex PTSD must emerge or worsen after the trauma exposure. This may be hard to determine if the trauma began in early childhood. In such cases, problems can be attributed to trauma exposure even if there is no definitive information about timing available. This can include inferences made based on the individual describing feeling changed after the traumatic experience, reports from others who observed the individual during the years surrounding the trauma (e.g., teachers, relatives, friends), or documentation of changes in behavior around the time of the trauma (e.g., school or medical records). The International Trauma Questionnaire (Cloitre et al., 2018), described in the section on PTSD earlier in this chapter, can also be used to assess complex PTSD.

In assessing complex PTSD, it is important to keep in mind that problems in affect regulation can be expressed in symptoms of hyperreactivity (e.g., difficulty calming down), deactivation (e.g., numbing, dissociation), or both. Clinicians should be careful to ask about both types of problems.

Negative self-concept is typically represented by endorsements of feeling worthless or like a failure. This can emerge from a diversity of experiences. A person can feel worthless from either having been a victim of violence or alternatively not having been able to stop violence from being perpetrated against a loved one (e.g., parent or spouse) or perpetrated within their community. The individual may express feelings of shame or guilt, but these are likely to vary according to the nature of the traumatic experience and are not required to meet the negative self-concept requirement.

In diagnosing complex PTSD, the clinician should consider two distinct dimensions of interpersonal difficulties. A sense of distance or not feeling close can arise from feeling "different" from those who have not experienced similar events with an accompanying sense of being stigmatized or not feeling understood. This experience can lead to interpersonal problems, particularly in initiating relationships. Difficulty in maintaining relationships may emerge from emotion dysregulation (e.g., numbing or anger) and a desire to avoid or difficulty in managing conflict or emotionally charged situations. Clinicians should ask about difficulties in initiating as well as maintaining relationships.

PROLONGED GRIEF DISORDER

Presentations and Symptom Patterns

Prolonged grief disorder is a distinct disorder that shares symptoms with other disorders specifically associated with stress as well as with depressive disorders (Boelen et al., 2010). The essential features of prolonged grief disorder include persistent and pervasive longing for the deceased or continuous and uncontrollable preoccupation with the deceased. Additionally, these features are accompanied by intense emotional pain, which can be manifested as sadness, guilt, anger, or blame. This may include experiences such as difficulty accepting the death, feeling one has lost a part of oneself, an inability to experience positive mood, or emotional numbness.

The severity of functional impairment in personal, family, social, educational, occupational, and other important areas of functioning is also taken into consideration when establishing the diagnosis. A postloss duration of at least 6 months is required for the diagnosis, although the duration requirement may be lengthened in light of the individual's social, cultural, and religious norms. Prigerson et al. (2009) found that grief experienced at 6 to 12 months postloss, in contrast to that experienced in the first 6 months, is associated with suicidal ideation and poor quality of life.

Differential Diagnoses

Prolonged grief disorder should be differentiated from uncomplicated bereavement (expected grief responses) after the death of a family member or other loved one. First, this is achieved by the "prolonged" duration of intense reactions in which a diagnosis of prolonged grief disorder requires the symptoms to persist for a minimum of 6 months post-loss. Second, prolonged grief disorder is distinguished from uncomplicated bereavement by the level of impact on the functioning of the bereaved.

Death of a family member can be a traumatic event for the bereaved persons because of the nature of the death or its suddenness. In contrast to avoidance and continuing sense of threat, individuals with prolonged grief disorder have strong yearnings and longings to meet the deceased. Additionally, the content of the intrusive memories should be related to the deceased and not the circumstances related to the death. Prolonged grief disorder and adjustment disorder share the core symptom of preoccupation, but in prolonged grief disorder, preoccupation focuses on the deceased person. Adjustment disorder typically resolves within 6 months of the stressor and should not be applied to normal bereavement. Prolonged grief disorder cannot be diagnosed if the bereavement has occurred less than 6 months earlier. Depressive disorders manifest in symptoms such as sadness and loss of pleasure that significantly affect the functioning of the individual. Prolonged grief disorder shares common symptoms such as the inability to experience positive mood and social withdrawal. However, persistent and pervasive longing and preoccupation with the deceased are characteristic of prolonged grief disorder and not depression.

Developmental Course

Prolonged grief disorder can occur at any age as long as individuals have the cognitive ability to experience longing and preoccupation. The way symptoms are expressed differs according to developmental stage as well as cognitive and coping ability. Some children, who might have limited verbal expression, communicate their grief through behaviors such as waiting for the return of the deceased and continued searching for the deceased. They might have intense pain as reflected through the drastic loss of interest in activities that they enjoyed previously, excessive anger or guilt, avoidance of reminders about the death, and thoughts that a part of themselves has died with the death (Boelen et al., 2019). Bereaved children may also express their grief in their play or dreams or though developmental regression.

Bereaved older adults have similar grief reactions as other age groups (O'Connor et al., 2019). Yearning and longing for the deceased are commonly expressed through strong attachment to possessions of the deceased. Bereaved persons are comforted by touching and smelling the clothing of the deceased. Sometimes, they avoid social contacts to focus on memories with the deceased. Dwelling in the past may lead them to neglect self-care and further affect their functioning.

Assessment

The Inventory of Complicated Grief, developed by Prigerson and colleagues (1995), is the most commonly used measure for assessing disturbed grief through self-report. Persistent and persuasive yearning and longing may also be manifest in a variety of observable behaviors. Despite acknowledging the reality of death, bereaved persons with prolonged grief disorder tend to spend excessive time in searching for or accompanying the deceased, which is associated with impairment in functioning. The bereaved person may visit places where they spent time with the deceased or place phone calls to the deceased. Some spend a long time at the cemetery to be physically close to the deceased. They cry and call the name of the deceased, wishing to have them return. Some spend a lot of time sleeping, hoping to meet the deceased in dreams. Intense emotional pain may also be expressed through somatization (e.g., "my heart is aching," "I feel pain in my heart"). In addition to the core manifestations of grief reactions, assessment of functioning by self-report, report of others, or observation is essential to making the diagnosis. Special attention should be paid to the cultural, social, and religious norms of bereaved persons. In some cultures, for example, maintaining a connection with the deceased by visiting the cemetery frequently, preparing meals for the deceased, or talking to the deceased is perceived as an expression of love rather than as pathological.

ADJUSTMENT DISORDER

Presentations and Symptom Patterns

Adjustment disorder refers to a maladaptive reaction to an important and generally negative psychosocial life event (e.g., breakdown of relationship, loss of job) or to prolonged stressful circumstances (e.g., conflicts in the family or at work, poverty). Precipitating events in adjustment disorder are usually nontraumatic in the sense that they are not extremely threatening or horrific as in PTSD and complex PTSD. It is assumed that adjustment disorder is a relatively transient disorder that remits within 6 months after the acute or chronic stressor and its consequences have ended. Nevertheless, it is associated with significant distress and a risk for chronic or worsening symptoms (Bachem & Casey, 2018). It is one of the most frequently diagnosed mental disorders in mental health settings (Evans et al., 2013; Reed et al., 2011). Several clinical studies have shown that people with adjustment disorder have an increased risk for suicide and self-injurious behavior, which may be substantial (Casey et al., 2015; Nock et al., 2008). In one Indian study, adjustment disorder was the most common mental disorder among suicidal individuals (e.g., Manoranjitham et al., 2010).

The diagnostic requirements for adjustment disorder in *ICD-11* include an identifiable psychological stressor or multiple stressors (e.g., single stressful event, ongoing psychosocial difficulty, or combination of stressful life situations). Common stressors in adjustment disorder include interpersonal events, such as separation, divorce, family conflict, conflicts with work associates or superiors, parenthood, and adoption; occupational or scholastic stressors, such as academic overload or failure, retirement, unemployment, too much or too little work, high pressure on deadlines and time, financial problems; severe illness or medical intervention; being the victim of a crime; or changes in living or social environment (e.g., relocating to another residence, emigration, refugee status).

Adjustment disorder is characterized by preoccupation or mental fixation on the stressor. This may be manifested as excessive worry, recurring and distressing thoughts, or constant rumination about the stressor and its implications. There is a failure to adapt to the stressor, which in turn leads to significant impairments in functioning. Symptoms are not better explained by another mental disorder and resolve within 6 months after the stressor and its consequences have ended. Adjustment disorder may also present with a variety of other symptoms, such as depressive or anxiety symptoms, as well as impulsive or "externalizing" symptoms, including increased use of tobacco, alcohol, or other substance use. However, these symptoms are not required for the diagnosis and are not a sufficient basis for the diagnosis of adjustment disorder if the core features of preoccupation and failure to adapt are not present.

Differential Diagnoses

The *ICD-11 CDDR* mention various disorders that, if present, exclude a diagnosis of adjustment disorder based on overlapping symptoms: separation anxiety disorder in childhood, single episode or recurrent depressive disorder, generalized anxiety disorder, PTSD, prolonged grief disorder, and uncomplicated bereavement. However, adjustment disorder can also be diagnosed together with other disorders, provided there are substantial, nonoverlapping symptoms and a distinct onset and progression of each disorder can be identified. This would be plausible, for example, if specific phobia or panic disorder is already present before the onset of the stressor and is not etiologically related to the symptoms of the adjustment disorder. However, if a critical life event mainly leads to an exacerbation of earlier symptoms (e.g., intensification of depressive symptoms after separation), an additional diagnosis of adjustment disorder should not be made.

A careful differential diagnosis is particularly important in relation to the other disorders specifically associated with stress, such as prolonged grief disorder and PTSD. Both adjustment disorder and prolonged grief disorder have preoccupation as a clinical feature. However, in prolonged grief disorder, the preoccupation is related to feelings of longing and a strong desire to be close to the deceased person. Unlike prolonged grief disorder, avoidance behavior can often be observed in relation to the relevant preoccupation in adjustment disorder. If an individual exhibits significant symptoms after a traumatic experience that do not meet the diagnostic requirements for PTSD, the diagnosis of adjustment disorder should be considered. A key differentiating feature is that PTSD involves intrusive reexperiencing of events in the here and now, whereas preoccupation in the context of the adjustment disorder involves a mental reminiscence; the events are perceived by the person as situated in the past.

Developmental Course

Although adjustment disorder is conceptualized as a transient disorder that is expected to remit within 6 months after the termination of the stressor and its consequences, initial longitudinal studies suggest there is a serious risk of chronicity or intensification of symptoms. For example, in adjustment disorder following involuntary job loss, a majority of individuals reported symptomatology that persisted after 6 months, and a subset of individuals reported a high severity of symptoms that continued to increase beyond 6 months (Lorenz et al., 2018). The *CDDR* indicate that if the disorder persists beyond 6 months, a different diagnosis should be considered.

Assessment

The core *ICD-11* symptoms of adjustment disorder can be measured by two relatively new assessment methods: the Adjustment Disorder–New Module (ADNM; Glaesmer et al., 2015) and the International Adjustment Disorder Questionnaire (IADQ; Shevlin et al., 2020). The ADNM is based on the *ICD-11* and is available as a structured clinical interview or a self-report questionnaire, the latter being more widely used. It contains a list of potential stressors, as well as 20 items in Likert format on preoccupations and failure to adapt symptoms together with various accessory symptoms and has satisfactory reliability and validity (Lorenz et al., 2016). The ADNM-8 is a short version with eight items for the screening of the core symptoms, which also shows sufficient reliability (Kazlauskas et al., 2018).

The IADQ is also based on the *ICD-11* and measures the core diagnostic requirements of adjustment disorder—stressor exposure, preoccupation with and failure to adapt to the stressor, and timing of symptom onset—and includes a psychosocial stressor checklist. The assessment of psychosocial and functional impairment consists of three separate items and is thus formulated more concisely than in the ADNM.

CULTURAL CONSIDERATIONS

Research thus far on disorders specifically related to stress suggests that the interpretations of symptoms and traumatic events are likely subject to wide cultural variations (Hinton & Lewis-Fernández, 2011; Humayun & Somasundaram, 2018). Descriptions of symptoms differ with regard to attention to somatic symptoms and in the use of metaphors related to the body or to the environment (Maercker & Heim, 2016). For example, *ataque de nervios* (an attack of the nerves) is an expression that appears in Latino populations in the Americas and is associated with a sense of instability of the entire person (Migliore, 1993). In some Asian cultures, such as the Tamil culture in India, manifestations of traumatic stress include *perumuchu* (deep, sighing breathing).

The *CDDR* include descriptions of cultural differences in the ramifications of traumatic events on a family, community, and social level in the context of disorders specifically associated with stress to the extent they are known. The *CDDR* also acknowledge phenomena such as cultural bereavement and collective trauma (Humayun & Somasundaram, 2018). In collectivistic or sociocentric cultures, the impact of traumatic events may be experienced not so much through changes in individual self-concept but rather through changes in family and community relationships including collective distrust, loss of values and norms, and antisocial behavior (Abramowitz, 2005; Bhugra & Becker, 2005).

GENDER-RELATED FEATURES

Previous studies suggest women have a higher risk of PTSD than men despite less overall trauma exposure (McGinty et al., 2021). Gender differences in prevalence of complex PTSD are less clear (McGinty et al., 2021), although some research suggests that complex PTSD symptoms tend to be more severe among women (Giarratano et al., 2020). This may be related to their experience of more interpersonal violence, particularly of a sexual nature, their younger age at the time of trauma exposure, and their stronger perceptions of threat and loss of control during traumatic events. Consistent differences to date have not been found in the prevalence of prolonged grief disorder or adjustment disorder among men and women.

KEY POINTS

- The grouping of disorders specifically associated with stress comprises four disorders, two of which are new: complex posttraumatic stress disorder and prolonged grief disorder. The remaining two, PTSD and adjustment disorder, have been reorganized, in part by including more specific and focused symptom requirements.

- The formulation of all disorders in this grouping, whether new or refined, was empirically guided by evidence from studies of symptom profiles and were later evaluated in field studies to confirm their consistency of application by clinicians and their clinical utility (e.g., ease of use and goodness of fit to observed clinical phenomena; Keeley, Reed, Roberts, Evans, Medina-Mora, et al., 2016; Keeley, Reed, Roberts, Evans, Robles, et al., 2016).

- The inclusion of the new diagnosis of complex PTSD was in response to clinical and research evidence of the greater complexity and impairment associated with sustained and repeated exposure to trauma.

- The introduction of prolonged grief disorder was in response to a perceived clinical need and substantial evidence of impairment associated with prolonged grief.

- The revised adjustment disorder diagnosis places greater emphasis on positive symptoms and impairment and has eliminated subtypes, which were not widely used and undermined clinical utility.

REFERENCES

Abramowitz, S. A. (2005). The poor have become rich, and the rich have become poor: Collective trauma in the Guinean Languette. *Social Science & Medicine, 61*(10), 2106–2118. https://doi.org/10.1016/j.socscimed.2005.03.023

Bachem, R., & Casey, P. (2018). Adjustment disorder: A diagnosis whose time has come. *Journal of Affective Disorders, 227,* 243–253. https://doi.org/10.1016/j.jad.2017.10.034

Bhugra, D., & Becker, M. A. (2005). Migration, cultural bereavement and cultural identity. *World Psychiatry, 4*(1), 18–24.

Boelen, P. A., Spuij, M., & Lenferink, L. I. M. (2019). Comparison of *DSM-5* criteria for persistent complex bereavement disorder and *ICD-11* criteria for prolonged grief disorder in help-seeking bereaved children. *Journal of Affective Disorders, 250,* 71–78. https://doi.org/10.1016/j.jad.2019.02.046

Boelen, P. A., van de Schoot, R., van den Hout, M. A., de Keijser, J., & van den Bout, J. (2010). Prolonged grief disorder, depression, and posttraumatic stress disorder are distinguishable syndromes. *Journal of Affective Disorders, 125*(1–3), 374–378. https://doi.org/10.1016/j.jad.2010.01.076

Brewin, C. R., Cloitre, M., Hyland, P., Shevlin, M., Maercker, A., Bryant, R. A., Humayun, A., Jones, L. M., Kagee, A., Rousseau, C., Somasundaram, D., Suzuki, Y., Wessely, S., van Ommeren, M., & Reed, G. M. (2017). A review of current evidence regarding the *ICD-11* proposals for diagnosing PTSD and complex PTSD. *Clinical Psychology Review, 58,* 1–15. https://doi.org/10.1016/j.cpr.2017.09.001

Brewin, C. R., Rumball, F., & Happé, F. (2019). Neglected causes of post-traumatic stress disorder. *BMJ, 365,* Article l2372. https://doi.org/10.1136/bmj.l2372

Casey, P., Jabbar, F., O'Leary, E., & Doherty, A. M. (2015). Suicidal behaviours in adjustment disorder and depressive episode. *Journal of Affective Disorders, 174,* 441–446. https://doi.org/10.1016/j.jad.2014.12.003

Cloitre, M., Shevlin, M., Brewin, C. R., Bisson, J. I., Roberts, N. P., Maercker, A., Karatzias, T., & Hyland, P. (2018). The International Trauma Questionnaire: Development of a self-report measure of *ICD-11* PTSD and complex PTSD. *Acta Psychiatrica Scandinavica, 138*(6), 536–546. https://doi.org/10.1111/acps.12956

Cook, A., Spinazzola, J., Ford, J., Lanktree, C., Blaustein, M., Cloitre, M., DeRosa, R., Hubbard, R., Kagan, R., Liautaud, J., Mallah, K., Olafson, E., & van der Kolk, B. (2005). Complex trauma in children and adolescents. *Psychiatric Annals, 35*(5), 390–398. https://doi.org/10.3928/00485713-20050501-05

Danzi, B. A., & La Greca, A. M. (2016). *DSM-IV, DSM-5,* and *ICD-11*: Identifying children with posttraumatic stress disorder after disasters. *Journal of Child Psychology and Psychiatry, and Allied Disciplines, 57*(12), 1444–1452. https://doi.org/10.1111/jcpp.12631

Evans, S. C., Reed, G. M., Roberts, M. C., Esparza, P., Watts, A. D., Correia, J. M., Ritchie, P., Maj, M., & Saxena, S. (2013). Psychologists' perspectives on the diagnostic classification of mental disorders: Results from the WHO-IUPsyS Global Survey. *International Journal of Psychology, 48*(3), 177–193. https://doi.org/10.1080/00207594.2013.804189

Giarratano, P., Ford, J. D., & Nochajski, T. H. (2020). Gender differences in complex posttraumatic stress symptoms, and their relationship to mental health and substance abuse outcomes in incarcerated adults. *Journal of Interpersonal Violence, 35,* 1133–1157. https://doi.org/10.1177/0886260517692995

Glaesmer, H., Romppel, M., Brähler, E., Hinz, A., & Maercker, A. (2015). Adjustment disorder as proposed for *ICD-11*: Dimensionality and symptom differentiation. *Psychiatry Research, 229*(3), 940–948. https://doi.org/10.1016/j.psychres.2015.07.010

Hinton, D. E., & Lewis-Fernández, R. (2011). The cross-cultural validity of posttraumatic stress disorder: Implications for *DSM-5. Depression and Anxiety, 28*(9), 783–801. https://doi.org/10.1002/da.20753

Humayun, A., & Somasundaram, D. (2018). Using *International Classification of Diseases 11* "mental disorders specifically associated with stress" in developing countries. *Indian Journal of Social Psychiatry, 34*(Suppl. 5), S23–S28. https://doi.org/10.4103/ijsp.ijsp_25_18

Hyland, P., Shevlin, M., Fyvie, C., Cloitre, M., & Karatzias, T. (2020). The relationship between *ICD-11* PTSD, complex PTSD and dissociative experiences. *Journal of Trauma & Dissociation, 21*(1), 62–72. https://doi.org/10.1080/15299732.2019.1675113

Kazlauskas, E., Gegieckaite, G., Eimontas, J., Zelviene, P., & Maercker, A. (2018). A brief measure of the *International Classification of Diseases–11* adjustment disorder: Investigation of psychometric properties in an adult help-seeking sample. *Psychopathology, 51*(1), 10–15. https://doi.org/10.1159/000484415

Keeley, J. W., Reed, G. M., Roberts, M. C., Evans, S. C., Medina-Mora, M. E., Robles, R., Rebello, T., Sharan, P., Gureje, O., First, M. B., Andrews, H. F., Ayuso-Mateos, J. L., Gaebel, W., Zielasek, J., & Saxena, S. (2016). Developing a science of clinical utility in diagnostic classification systems field study strategies for *ICD-11* mental and behavioral disorders. *American Psychologist, 71*(1), 3–16. https://doi.org/10.1037/a0039972

Keeley, J. W., Reed, G. M., Roberts, M. C., Evans, S. C., Robles, R., Matsumoto, C., Brewin, C. R., Cloitre, M., Perkonigg, A., Rousseau, C., Gureje, O., Lovell, A. M., Sharan, P., & Maercker, A. (2016). Disorders specifically associated with stress: A case-controlled field study for *ICD-11* mental and behavioural disorders. *International Journal of Clinical and Health Psychology, 16*(2), 109–127. https://doi.org/10.1016/j.ijchp.2015.09.002

Killikelly, C., & Maercker, A. (2017). Prolonged grief disorder for *ICD-11*: The primacy of clinical utility and international applicability. *European Journal of Psychotraumatology, 8*(Suppl. 6), Article 1476441. https://doi.org/10.1080/20008198.2018.1476441

Lorenz, L., Bachem, R. C., & Maercker, A. (2016). The Adjustment Disorder–New Module 20 as a screening instrument: Cluster analysis and cut-off values. *The International Journal of Occupational and Environmental Medicine, 7*(4), 215–220. https://doi.org/10.15171/ijoem.2016.775

Lorenz, L., Perkonigg, A., & Maercker, A. (2018). The course of adjustment disorder following involuntary job loss and its predictors of latent change. *Clinical Psychological Science, 6*(5), 647–657. https://doi.org/10.1177/2167702618766290

Maercker, A., & Heim, E. (2016). A new approach to culturally sensitive PTSD research in Zurich: Inspired by contributions from Carl Gustav Jung. *International Psychology Bulletin, 20*, 67–71.

Manoranjitham, S. D., Rajkumar, A. P., Thangadurai, P., Prasad, J., Jayakaran, R., & Jacob, K. S. (2010). Risk factors for suicide in rural south India. *The British Journal of Psychiatry, 196*(1), 26–30. https://doi.org/10.1192/bjp.bp.108.063347

McGinty, G., Fox, R., Ben-Ezra, M., Cloitre, M., Karatzias, T., Shevlin, M., & Hyland, P. (2021). Sex and age differences in *ICD-11* PTSD and complex PTSD: An analysis of four general population samples. *European Psychiatry, 64*(1), e66. https://doi.org/10.1192/j.eurpsy.2021.2239

Migliore, S. (1993). "Nerves": The role of metaphor in the cultural framing of experience. *Journal of Contemporary Ethnography, 22*(3), 331–360. https://doi.org/10.1177/089124193022003003

Nock, M. K., Borges, G., Bromet, E. J., Alonso, J., Angermeyer, M., Beautrais, A., Bruffaerts, R., Chiu, W. T., de Girolamo, G., Gluzman, S., de Graaf, R., Gureje, O., Haro, J. M., Huang, Y., Karam, E., Kessler, R. C., Lepine, J. P., Levinson, D., Medina-Mora, M. E., . . . Williams, D. (2008). Cross-national prevalence and risk factors for suicidal ideation, plans and attempts. *The British Journal of Psychiatry, 192*(2), 98–105. https://doi.org/10.1192/bjp.bp.107.040113

O'Connor, M., Lasgaard, M., Larsen, L., Johannsen, M., Lundorff, M., Farver-Vestergaard, I., & Boelen, P. A. (2019). Comparison of proposed diagnostic criteria for pathological grief using a sample of elderly bereaved spouses in Denmark: Perspectives on future bereavement research. *Journal of Affective Disorders, 251*, 52–59. https://doi.org/10.1016/j.jad.2019.01.056

Prigerson, H. G., Horowitz, M. J., Jacobs, S. C., Parkes, C. M., Aslan, M., Goodkin, K., Raphael, B., Marwit, S. J., Wortman, C., Neimeyer, R. A., Bonanno, G. A., Block, S. D., Kissane, D., Boelen, P., Maercker, A., Litz, B. T., Johnson, J. G., First, M. B., & Maciejewski, P. K. (2009). Prolonged grief disorder: Psychometric validation of criteria proposed for *DSM-V* and *ICD-11* [see correction at https://doi.org/10.1371/

annotation/a1d91e0d-981f-4674-926c-0fbd2463b5ea]. *PLoS Medicine, 6*(8), e1000121. https://doi.org/10.1371/journal.pmed.1000121

Prigerson, H. G., Maciejewski, P. K., Reynolds, C. F., III, Bierhals, A. J., Newsom, J. T., Fasiczka, A., Frank, E., Doman, J., & Miller, M. (1995). Inventory of Complicated Grief: A scale to measure maladaptive symptoms of loss. *Psychiatry Research, 59*(1–2), 65–79. https://doi.org/10.1016/0165-1781(95)02757-2

Reed, G. M., Mendonça Correia, J., Esparza, P., Saxena, S., & Maj, M. (2011). The WPA-WHO Global Survey of Psychiatrists' Attitudes Toward Mental Disorders Classification. *World Psychiatry, 10*(2), 118–131. https://doi.org/10.1002/j.2051-5545.2011.tb00034.x

Robles, R., Fresán, A., Evans, S. C., Medina-Mora, M. E., Lovell, A. M., Maj, M., & Reed, G. M. (2014). Problematic, absent, and stigmatizing diagnoses in current mental disorders classifications: Results from WHO-WPA and WHO-IUPsyS Global Surveys. *International Journal of Clinical and Health Psychology, 14*(3), 165–177. https://doi.org/10.1016/j.ijchp.2014.03.003

Shevlin, M., Hyland, P., Ben-Ezra, M., Karatzias, T., Cloitre, M., Vallieres, F., Bachem, R., & Maercker, A. (2020). Measuring *ICD-11* adjustment disorder: The development and initial validation of the International Adjustment Disorder Questionnaire. *Acta Psychiatrica Scandinavica, 141*(3), 265–274.

World Health Organization. (2023). *ICD-11 for mortality and morbidity statistics* (Version: 01/2023). https://icd.who.int/browse11/l-m/en#/

World Health Organization. (2024). *Clinical descriptions and diagnostic requirements for ICD-11 mental, behavioural and neurodevelopmental disorders*. https://www.who.int/publications/i/item/9789240077263

11

Dissociative Disorders

Andrew Moskowitz, Ellert Nijenhuis, Alexander Moreira-Almeida, and Roberto Lewis-Fernández

OVERARCHING LOGIC

Dissociative disorders require a truly psychologically informed approach to assessment and diagnosis. A narrow focus on presenting signs and symptoms could lead to mistaken diagnoses because some symptoms that frequently occur in dissociative disorders are also characteristic of various anxiety or fear-related disorders, depressive disorders, schizophrenia and other primary psychotic disorders, and diseases of the nervous system. Symptoms such as hearing voices or blindness, for example, may be attributed to psychosis or neurological disease if they are not recognized as part of a dissociative disorder presentation. An accurate diagnosis can only be obtained through an examination of the psychological function of the symptoms and—particularly in the case of more complex dissociative disorders such as dissociative identity disorder (DID) and partial DID—the underlying dissociative personality structure. Frequently, these symptoms represent adaptations to acute or chronic traumatizing experiences—that is, psychological attempts to protect the person from the environment.

Often, an accurate dissociative disorder diagnosis, particularly DID, may not be obtained until years after the individual's first contact with mental health services (Dell, 2009). This is partly because intensive interviews are generally required to establish a DID diagnosis, but several other factors also contribute

https://doi.org/10.1037/0000392-011
A Psychological Approach to Diagnosis: Using the ICD-11 as a Framework, G. M. Reed, P. L.-J. Ritchie, and A. Maercker (Editors)

to delays in appropriate diagnosis and treatment. These include a lack of professional awareness and knowledge of dissociative disorders (Şar & Ross, 2006), lack of training in the assessment of dissociative disorders (Dell, 2009), and even frank skepticism about their validity (Piper & Merskey, 2004). However, because dissociative disorders commonly cause considerable disability and suffering, appropriate and timely diagnosis and treatment are of crucial importance.

In the 11th revision of the *International Classification of Diseases* (*ICD-11*; World Health Organization [WHO], 2023), the grouping of dissociative disorders is placed immediately after the grouping of disorders specifically associated with stress. Dissociative disorders are usually associated with highly stressful events, but such exposure, in contrast to disorders specifically associated with stress, is not a part of their diagnostic requirements. Rather, what ties the dissociative disorders together is the phenomenon of dissociation. As conceptualized in the *Clinical Descriptions and Diagnostic Requirements for ICD-11 Mental, Behavioural and Neurodevelopmental Disorders* (*CDDR*; WHO, 2024), dissociation is an involuntary disruption or discontinuity in the normal integration of one or more of the following: identity, sensations, perceptions, affect (mood), thoughts, memories, bodily movements, or behavior. This disruption or discontinuity may be complete or partial and can vary from day to day or even from hour to hour. It is characterized as "involuntary" to exclude time-limited dissociative states that are intentionally produced, such as trance states induced as part of culturally sanctioned rituals.

A PSYCHOLOGICAL APPROACH TO DISSOCIATIVE DISORDERS

A psychological approach to dissociative disorders begins with an adequate understanding of dissociation. Dissociative disorders involve a wide range of sensory, motor, cognitive or affective symptoms; these can either involve the presence of intrusive experiences (e.g., pain without an apparent medical cause; trauma-related imagery) or the absence of normal experiences, such as memories (amnesia) or sensations (e.g., anesthesia; Nijenhuis, 2004). Many of the symptoms of dissociative disorders can occur in other *ICD-11* mental disorders or other medical conditions. For example, gaps in memory may be associated with the use of psychoactive substances, neurocognitive disorders, mood disorders, or schizophrenia and other primary psychotic disorders. However, the memory gaps in dissociative amnesia, unlike in these other disorders, generally develop after traumatizing events and can be seen as attempts at adaptation or coping. Thus, an accurate dissociative disorder diagnosis requires careful evaluation of both the relevant signs and symptoms and whether they arise from dissociated mental functions. For dissociative disorders affecting primarily a single function (memory for dissociative amnesia or specific motor or sensory functions in the case of dissociative neurological symptom disorder), the exclusion of a neurological or other medical etiology is also crucial. In addition, for the diagnosis of more complex dissociative disorders such as DID and partial DID, evidence must be gathered related to dissociative parts of the personality (also called dissociative identities or dissociative personality states) that give rise to the relevant signs and symptoms, as described later in this chapter.

GENERAL PRINCIPLES OF ASSESSING DISSOCIATIVE DISORDERS

Determining whether a symptom results from dissociative processes requires an investigation of the circumstances surrounding the onset of the symptoms, the possible meaning of the symptoms in the context of the individual's life, and evidence that such symptoms arise from nonintegrated or insufficiently integrated components of the personality. A detailed life history is essential, with particular focus on traumatizing events from childhood and adulthood, along with recent stressful events, and the full range of dissociative symptoms. Special attention should be paid to life circumstances surrounding experiences of memory gaps, depersonalization or derealization, unexplained physical complaints, and identity confusion or alteration. Reported life experiences may be stressful or traumatizing in themselves and may also be linked to earlier traumatizing experiences. Early childhood experiences of disorganized attachment (Dutra et al., 2009) or disturbing, intrusive medical experiences (Diseth, 2006) may also contribute to the etiology of dissociative disorders. With the individual's permission, interviewing knowledgeable friends or family and, if possible, previous therapists or clinicians about interpersonal conflicts, adverse and stressful events, and episodes of amnesia or apparent identity alteration can inform the diagnostic process.

There are several brief screening instruments that are freely available in multiple languages, including the Dissociative Experiences Scale (Carlson & Putnam, 1993), the Somatoform Dissociation Questionnaire–20 (Nijenhuis et al., 1996), and the Dissociative Symptoms Scale (Carlson et al., 2018). Such scales can be a valuable adjunct to careful interviewing (Müller-Pfeiffer et al., 2013) but are insufficient as a sole basis for diagnosing a dissociative disorder. Any use of measures should give careful consideration to the cultural and linguistic context of the individual patient. Measures should be culturally appropriate, administered in the preferred language of the individual to whom they are given (whether as originally developed or as a validated translation), and any standardization (e.g., *t*-scores, clinical cutoffs) should be appropriately normed for the local population. When these conditions are not met, test results must be interpreted with caution.

The Structured Clinical Interview for Dissociation Assessment in Therapy, Forensics, and Research (SCID-D; Steinberg, 2023) is designed to assess core dissociative symptoms or experiences that form the basis of dissociative disorder diagnoses in both the fifth edition of the *Diagnostic and Statistical Manual of Mental Disorders* (*DSM*) and the *ICD-11*. The SCID-D assesses for experiences of amnesia, depersonalization, derealization, identity confusion, and identity alteration, but does not address dissociative bodily symptoms. The SCID-D may be useful for differential diagnosis or as a source of information about how to ask about specific dissociative symptoms. However, it is not in the public domain, is expensive to use, and validated translations are so far available in few languages (e.g., Piedfort-Marin et al., 2022).

There are particular challenges associated with assessing for the presence of dissociative parts of the personality, the central feature of DID and partial DID.

As noted earlier, one important potential source of information is other individuals in a current or past personal or professional relationship with the individual who may be able to provide relevant evidence (e.g., striking changes in behavior, reported amnesia). Two other important sources of information come from the person themselves: (a) their report of past experiences and actions and (b) their behaviors during the actual interview(s). Familiarity with and training in the administration of a structured dissociation interview like the SCID-D can be very useful in this regard. Past experiences of losing time, finding oneself in another place without remembering how one got there, wearing clothes one doesn't remember putting on, or being with people one doesn't remember meeting all can be clues to the presence of dissociative parts of the personality.

In addition, relevant information may (but does not always) manifest during the interview through the person's speech and behavior. For example, there may be strikingly inconsistent answers (e.g., about one's childhood experiences), amnesia for questions previously asked, subtle or dramatic shifts in facial expressions and communication style, or even spontaneous identity alternations, with the newly appearing dissociative identities possibly requiring acclimatization to the interview setting and the interviewer. The person reporting hearing voices during the interview can also be an important clue, as these may represent dissociative parts that have distinct perspectives. It may be possible for the interviewer to speak with them, either directly or through the person themselves, which would provide strong evidence for the presence of dissociative parts of the personality (Moskowitz et al., 2017). However, this should not be attempted without adequate training.

DISSOCIATIVE NEUROLOGICAL SYMPTOM DISORDER

Presentations and Symptom Patterns

In the *CDDR*, dissociative neurological symptom disorder is diagnosed on the basis of involuntary disruption or discontinuity in the normal integration of motor, sensory, or cognitive functions, lasting at least several hours. The symptoms are inconsistent with a recognized disease of the nervous system or other medical condition, a neurodevelopmental or neurocognitive disorder, or another mental disorder and are not due the effects of a substance or medication. The symptoms of dissociative neurological symptom disorder manifest as either (a) intrusive sensations or movements (e.g., nonepileptic seizures or involuntary muscle movements such as chorea, myoclonus, tremor, dystonia, or dyskinesia) or (b) the loss of normal sensations or movements (e.g., blindness, anesthesia, analgesia, or motor inhibition or "freezing"). The onset of the symptoms is typically directly or symbolically linked to traumatizing or highly stressful events (Nijenhuis, 2004), and the symptoms may be viewed as expressions of insufficiently integrated emotional or other psychological difficulties. The three most prevalent types of symptoms are nonepileptic seizures, loss of consciousness, and motor symptoms. To be diagnosed, the symptoms must be severe enough to cause significant impairment in personal, family, social, educational, occupational, or other areas of functioning. Dissociative neurological symptom disorder was referred to as conversion disorder in the past, a term that has been retained in *DSM-5*, and is also sometimes referred to as functional neurological disorder. The *ICD-11* label intentionally emphasizes the underlying dissociative nature of the symptoms.

Specifiers

A range of specifiers are provided for dissociative neurological symptom disorder to describe the specific nature of the symptoms involved (e.g., visual disturbance, vertigo or dizziness, nonepileptic seizures, paresis or weakness), including an "other specified" symptoms category. In addition to the common motor and sensory disturbances such as nonepileptic seizures and inability to see, hear, or move, specific categories are provided for cognitive symptoms, such as memory or language problems.

Differential Diagnosis

The term *dissociative neurological symptom disorder* indicates the presence of symptoms that do not have a demonstrable neurological or other medical basis but rather are dissociative in nature. Symptoms of neurological origin, such as those due to temporal lobe epilepsy or a neurological sensory abnormality (e.g., blindness) must be excluded. This assessment is based on negative findings from physical exam and other relevant tests or the presence of a pattern of symptoms that is inconsistent with the recognized presentation of neurological disorders or other medical conditions. Symptoms consistent with dissociative neurological symptom disorder may also occur as part of another dissociative disorder, such as DID, and in these cases, an additional diagnosis of dissociative neurological symptom disorder should not be assigned. Other mental disorders such as hypochondriasis (health anxiety), bodily distress disorders, or factitious disorders may also be characterized by bodily symptoms that do not have a demonstrable medical basis, but in these disorders, the symptoms do not derive from dissociative processes.

Assessment

Medical evaluation is needed to rule out neurological etiologies. Establishing the dissociative nature of presenting symptoms requires detailed interviewing, which may be facilitated by instruments such as the Somatoform Dissociation Questionnaire–20 (Nijenhuis et al., 1996).

DISSOCIATIVE AMNESIA

Presentations and Symptom Patterns

In the *CDDR*, dissociative amnesia is characterized by the inability to recall important autobiographical information that is inconsistent with ordinary forgetting and is associated with significant impairment. This inability to recall—typically of groups of memories, rather than single activities, feelings, or thoughts—is assumed to be psychologically motivated as a form of protection against, or adaptation to, overwhelming cognitions and emotions deriving from personal experiences of a highly stressful or traumatic nature (Dalenberg et al., 2012). Experimental psychology research has demonstrated that traumatizing events can be associated with deficits not due to an underlying neurological disease process in both forming and accessing trauma-related memories (Staniloiu & Markowitsch, 2014). In dissociative amnesia, the difficulties involve memories of the past, related to episodic-autobiographical information (e.g., life events), not the creation of new memories. Other cognitive abilities such as intelligence and language capacities are unaffected. Implicit or general semantic memory (i.e., knowledge, information) is preserved, but procedural memory (i.e., learned actions, such as bicycle riding) is occasionally involved. Dissociative amnesia is commonly associated with difficulties in forming and sustaining satisfying interpersonal relationships and may also be associated with self-mutilation, suicide attempts, other high-risk behaviors, depression, depersonalization, and sexual problems.

Three types of dissociative amnesia have been described (Loewenstein et al., 2017). In localized amnesia, the inability to recall is circumscribed to a discrete period (e.g., 1 year of elementary school). Selective amnesia is characterized by the ability to remember some, but not all, of the events during a circumscribed period (e.g., inability to recall combat-related events but not other aspects of military deployment occurring during the same period). In generalized amnesia, individuals are unable to recall their entire life, often including their identity. This latter type is rare and most often develops after acute, traumatizing events, such as combat or rape.

The failures of recollection in dissociative amnesia are not due to the effects of a substance or medication, to a disease of the nervous system (e.g., temporal lobe epilepsy), or to head trauma. The amnesia does not occur exclusively during another dissociative disorder and cannot be better accounted for by another mental disorder (e.g., posttraumatic stress disorder [PTSD]). Many individuals with nongeneralized amnesia present for care not because of their memory loss but due to other complaints, such as physical symptoms (e.g., blindness, arm paralysis), depersonalization/derealization, or symptoms common to other disorders (e.g., depressed mood, suicidal ideation). Individuals with dissociative amnesia may be partly unaware of their memory problems, and those who are aware may minimize their importance and become uncomfortable when prompted to address them. The dissociated memories may reveal themselves in a disguised form, such as in flashbacks, nightmares, or physical symptoms.

The disorder typically has a clear-cut onset and offset, enabling the person to recognize subjective gaps in memory. Episodes typically resolve within hours to months, spontaneously or with treatment. However, the amnesia can become chronic in some circumstances, such as when there is strong motivation not to recall the memories (because of overwhelming fear of what they might contain) or when functioning is impaired and integrative capacity is severely limited (Staniloiu & Markowitsch, 2014).

Specifiers

In the *ICD-11*, a specifier of "with or without dissociative fugue" may be applied to dissociative amnesia. Dissociative fugue is defined as sudden, apparently purposeful travel away from home, work, or significant others for an extended period (days, weeks, or even months) that is accompanied by amnesia for the person's usual circumstances and even their identity that still allows them to conduct complex activities. At a later stage, the person may become aware of the amnesia or loss of identity and may develop confusion; trance-like behavior; other dissociative, mood, anxiety, or PTSD symptoms; or suicidal behavior, often accompanied by amnesia for the first stage of the fugue.

Differential Diagnosis

Dissociative amnesia must be distinguished from alternative etiologies of memory loss. These include age-associated cognitive decline, other dissociative disorders, other mental disorders (e.g., PTSD, acute and transient psychotic disorder), the direct effects of substance use, neurocognitive disorders, head trauma, and other medical conditions (e.g., a brain tumor). A general principle of the differential diagnosis of dissociative amnesia is that in patients with other physical and mental conditions, the memory loss for personal information is embedded in a broader set of cognitive, linguistic, attentional, behavioral, and memory problems (Loewenstein et al., 2017). Moreover, in nondissociative amnesia, a specific etiological factor or underlying disease process may be found (e.g., thiamine deficiency in Korsakoff syndrome). In addition, unlike in most neurocognitive disorders and substance-related memory impairments, dissociative amnesia is frequently reversible, typically through treatment.

Assessment

No single test or examination can establish whether a memory disorder has a dissociative, neurocognitive, factitious, malingered, or mixed etiology (Staniloiu & Markowitsch, 2014). Neuroimaging can help rule out disorders due to major brain injury, which is not typical of dissociative amnesia, although cases of mild traumatic brain injury have been observed. Several instruments may facilitate evaluation, including the SCID-D and the Steinberg Dissociative Amnesia Questionnaire (Şar et al., 2014; Steinberg & Schnall, 2000). It can be useful to interview family members or caretakers about recent life events, including the occurrence of stressful or traumatizing life events.

TRANCE DISORDER AND POSSESSION TRANCE DISORDER

Presentations and Symptom Patterns

Trance and possession trance disorders are characterized in the *CDDR* by a marked involuntary alteration in an individual's state of consciousness resulting in a trance state or a possession trance state (a trance state that is experienced as being controlled by another entity). These changes in consciousness occur during a single episode that lasts for at least several days or as recurrent episodes. The trance state is characterized by a narrowing of awareness of the person's surroundings or an unusually narrow and selective focus on specific environmental stimuli (e.g., an unfocused or fixed gaze, focusing only on one person or object, or unresponsiveness to pain). It is also characterized by a limited repertoire of movements, postures, and speech (Cardeña et al., 2009). Amnesia may or may not occur. In possession trance disorder, the individual's normal sense of personal identity is replaced by what is attributed to be an external "possessing" identity such as a spirit, power, deity, or other spiritual entity. Changes in consciousness and the subjective sense of being externally controlled are attributed to the possessing agent, as evidenced by phenomena such as involuntary shaking movements, talking in a different voice, or being unable to move or speak (van Duijl et al., 2013). There is typically amnesia for the episode of possession. In both trance and possession trance disorders, the observed behaviors are experienced as being beyond the individual's control.

Both possession trance disorder and trance disorder most commonly occur in the context of stressful events, or chronically stressful conditions. The personality and behaviors of the possessing entity in possession trance disorder are often consistent with local cultural patterns and beliefs. A diagnosis of trance disorder or possession trance disorder should be made only when the trance or possession trance states are unwanted, uncontrolled, and involuntary and cause significant distress or functional impairment. A diagnosis of trance disorder or possession trance disorder is not warranted when trance states occur only when falling asleep or waking up, or due to fatigue, substance use, or a disease of the nervous system.

Globally, most trance and possession trance states are experienced during collective cultural or religious practices that create little or only transient distress to the person or members of their cultural community and have no pathological sequelae and therefore should not be considered to be symptoms of a mental disorder. Some individuals (e.g., mediums), habitually enter trance or possession trance states to perform religious, spiritual, or cultural functions. Compared with individuals who enter trance or possession trance states for ritual purposes, those in whom trance is a feature of a diagnosable dissociative disorder have a higher rate of other mental disorders such as depressive disorders and disorders due to substance use, poorer social adjustment, and greater likelihood of previous exposure to trauma (Moreira-Almeida & Cardeña, 2011).

Differential Diagnosis

Although individuals with trance disorder or possession trance disorder may experience amnesia for trance or possession trance episodes, it is distinguished from dissociative amnesia in that the memory disruption involves only what happened during the period of altered states of consciousness and is accompanied by other trance or possession trance symptoms. The relationship between possession trance disorder and DID is a subject of debate. It is unclear whether possession trance disorder results from underlying dissociative states (dissociative identities), as would be the case in DID, or represents more transient and less pervasive dissociative pathology, whose expression is facilitated by cultural acceptance of the intrusion of spiritual forces into the everyday world. Longitudinal follow-up of individuals with possession trance disorder is needed to ascertain the frequency of its recurrence as a marker of pervasive dissociative vulnerability. Some individuals present with both internal and external types of identities (some alternate identities are referred to as parts of the patient's own mind and others are viewed as external possessing spirits). When this occurs, the diagnosis of DID would be more appropriate. It is worth noting that the boundary between possession trance disorder and DID is treated differently in the *ICD-11* than it is in the *DSM-5*, where possession trance experiences are treated as culturally patterned variants of DID. In *ICD-11*, possession trance disorder is a separate diagnosis, reflecting its prevalence and global distribution (Spiegel et al., 2011).

The differential diagnosis of possession trance disorder and schizophrenia or other primary psychotic disorders is crucial. While perceptual alterations, such as hearing voices, are common during episodes of possession trance, these symptoms are usually episodic, abate after the possession episodes, and appear to have a dissociative origin. Negative symptoms of schizophrenia (e.g., apathy) are uncommon in trance disorder or possession trance disorder and chronic psychotic symptoms are rare. Very transient trance or possession trance experiences (typically minutes to hours rather than several days) may occur in the context of some other mental disorders, such as an anxiety or fear-related disorders or depressive disorders. In these cases, an additional trance disorder or possession trance disorder diagnosis is not warranted.

The differentiation between nonpathological and pathological trance presents a challenge similar to other mental disorders that resemble spiritual experiences: avoiding the extremes of pathologizing normal experiences (thus causing iatrogenic harm) or considering an experience as nonpathological, which is actually better understood as a symptom of mental disorder (and thus not offering necessary treatment). Since cultural norms may mask or camouflage an actual mental disorder, cultural acceptance should not be the only criterion on which to evaluate whether a given experience is pathological. It is essential to take into consideration other criteria, such as suffering, functional impairment, lack of control over the experience, and the presence of other symptoms suggestive of a mental disorder (Moreira-Almeida & Cardeña, 2011).

Assessment

It is important to assess the family and cultural context of the trance or possession trance episodes. Key questions include the degree to which the experiences are considered odd or frightening by the person and others in their social network, to what extent the experiences are unwanted and uncontrolled, and the associated level of distress and impairment.

DISSOCIATIVE IDENTITY DISORDER

Presentations and Symptom Patterns

DID is described in the *ICD-11 CDDR* as a disruption of identity characterized by the presence of two or more distinct personality states (dissociative identities) associated with marked discontinuities in sense of self and agency. Each dissociative identity includes its own pattern of experiencing, perceiving, conceiving, and relating to the self, body, and environment; but dissociative identities may share some autobiographical memories (e.g., school events that do not evoke strong emotions) and skills (such as speaking a foreign language). At least two dissociative identities recurrently take control of the person's consciousness and functioning, including daily life functions such as parenting, work, or during specific situations perceived as threatening. These changes are accompanied by alterations in motivation, sensation, affect, perception, cognition, memory, motor control, and behavior. DID symptoms are not due to the direct effects of a substance or medication on the central nervous system, including withdrawal effects, and are not due to a disease of the nervous system or a sleep–wake disorder.

Substantial episodes of amnesia typically occur at some point in the course of the disorder. However, dissociative identities may be aware and remember the activities of other dissociative identities. Dissociative identities may also intrude on each other's thoughts, emotions, perceptions, behaviors, or bodily sensations. Beyond having different psychological characteristics, different dissociative identities appear to be associated with differential neurobiological activity (Schlumpf et al., 2014). For example, one study found that when confronted with threat cues or reminders of traumatizing events, identities focused on defending against a threat differed significantly in physiological features and brain activity from identities that normally undertake daily life activities (Reinders et al., 2016).

DID has been diagnosed more often in women than in men, with gender ratios of up to 8:1 reported (Loewenstein et al., 2017). However, it is possible that differences in help seeking or clinician bias may lead to substantial underdiagnosis of DID in men.

Differential Diagnosis

In contrast to DID, partial DID does not involve alternating dissociative identities that recurrently take executive control over consciousness and behavior. In possession trance disorder, the dissociative identities are attributed to external, usually spiritual, entities, whereas in DID they are usually interpreted as parts of the person. Individuals with PTSD and complex PTSD may experience alterations in identity and agency when reexperiencing traumatic events (e.g., flashbacks), but these alternations do not occur in other circumstances. However, DID often co-occurs with PTSD or complex PTSD, as well as with anxiety or fear-related disorders and depressive disorders.

Personality disorder is characterized by persistent disturbances in sense of identity and self-direction and often by problems with affect regulation, but it does not involve the presence of dissociative identities. While intrusion symptoms may also occur in schizophrenia or other primary psychotic disorders, individuals with DID do not exhibit formal thought disorder or negative symptoms of schizophrenia (e.g., flat affect, social withdrawal). However, some psychotic symptoms that are emphasized in the diagnosis of schizophrenia, such as auditory or verbal hallucinations and experiences of influence, passivity and control can also occur in DID as intrusive dissociative symptoms (Moskowitz & Heim, 2019). The presence of other concurrent symptoms helps to distinguish between the dissociative and psychotic disorders.

Assessment

Many individuals with DID are not correctly diagnosed for many years even when they do come into contact with mental health services. Individuals with this disorder often do not disclose their experiences out of shame, fear, or concern they will not be believed. A significant challenge to accurate assessment lies in the nature of the disorder; individuals often have apparently high-functioning parts of their personality that may be aware only of peculiar gaps in their memory or medically unexplained headaches or physical pain. A correct diagnosis may take several sessions to establish evidence for different dissociative identities (dissociative parts of the personality). Multiple sources of information, including interviews with family members and the use of diagnostic instruments, may be required. Particularly for DID and partial DID, structured diagnostic interviews such as the SCID-D can be useful.

PARTIAL DISSOCIATIVE IDENTITY DISORDER

Presentations and Symptom Patterns

Partial DID is introduced in the *ICD-11* to capture clinical presentations related to, but less complex than, those found in DID. Such presentations have long been recognized but were previously characterized as part of a residual diagnostic category (such as "other specified dissociative (conversion) disorder" in the *ICD-10* or "dissociative disorder not otherwise specified" in the *DSM*). Like DID, partial DID is characterized by two or more distinct personality states (dissociative identities), involving marked discontinuities in sense of self and agency. However, in partial DID these dissociative identities do not typically take control of the person's consciousness and functioning. Rather, the person (technically, the dominant dissociative identity) regularly experiences intrusions by other dissociative parts of the personality, in the form of voices, visions, thoughts, perceptions, movements, or emotions. These are typically aversive and are not experienced as being "owned" by the dominant dissociative identity. Episodes of amnesia are rare and usually brief.

Providing a diagnostic label for this presentation is important because it is a common form of dissociative pathology (roughly 40% of all dissociative disorders) in both inpatient and outpatient settings (Dell, 2009). The term partial DID does not imply that individuals with this condition suffer less than those with DID. Indeed, the functioning of individuals diagnosed with partial DID, whose consciousness may be intruded on frequently throughout the day and night, is typically significantly impaired.

Differential Diagnosis

The distinction between DID and partial DID, with regard to symptomatology, is largely one of degree. In contrast to DID, alternating dissociative identities are rare and transient in partial DID and are typically associated with highly stressful experiences or episodes of self-harm. Nondominant dissociative identities are also less elaborated and independent than in DID, with a more circumscribed behavioral repertoire. However, intrusions may also occur in DID, and these episodes, as in partial DID, might not be associated with amnesia. The key distinction is that episodes of executive control by alternate dissociative identities are sporadic and circumscribed in partial DID but are typically a regular and sustained occurrence in DID. Consistent with the less profound dissociation of the personality in partial DID, the severity of psychological (cognitive–emotional) and somatoform dissociative symptoms, although still high, is significantly lower than in DID (Nijenhuis, 2015).

Intrusions regularly occur in trance and possession trance disorders, but in partial DID, there is evidence of distinct personality states that are not attributed to external possessing agents. Symptoms common in psychotic disorders, such as intrusive thoughts and hearing voices, frequently occur in partial DID (Moskowitz et al., 2017) but without delusions, formal thought disorder, or the negative symptoms of schizophrenia (e.g., flat affect, social withdrawal).

Assessment

Assessment procedures for Partial DID are similar to those for DID. The use of a formal dissociative disorders interview such as the SCID-D may be required, particularly to rule out other possible diagnoses; self-report measures of dissociative symptoms can also be useful.

DEPERSONALIZATION-DEREALIZATION DISORDER

Presentations and Symptom Patterns

Depersonalization-derealization disorder is characterized by persistent or recurrent experiences of depersonalization and/or derealization. Depersonalization involves feeling that the self is strange or unreal, or one is detached from or an outside observer of one's thoughts, feelings, sensations, body, or actions. Depersonalization may take the form of emotional and/or physical numbing, a sense of watching oneself from a distance, or perceptual alterations (e.g., a distorted sense of time). Derealization is characterized by experiencing other persons, objects, or the world as strange or unreal (e.g., dreamlike, distant, foggy, lifeless, colorless, or visually distorted) or feeling detached from one's surroundings. These experiences are common during highly stressful events, typically to distance or detach oneself from overwhelming experiences, and are usually transient (Simeon, 2009). Individuals with depersonalization-derealization disorder have developed a particular pattern of emotional responses to stressful stimuli, which appears to have neurobiological correlates and manifests in hypoemotionality or numbing (Sierra & Berrios, 1998).

Depersonalization-derealization disorder symptoms may be episodic or chronic and persistent. They are experienced as distressing and typically result in significant impairment in personal, family, social, educational, occupational, or other important areas of functioning. However, the diagnosis can still be assigned when functioning is maintained through significant additional effort. For example, some individuals with depersonalization-derealization disorder may be able to avoid exhibiting or discussing their symptoms in work contexts that are highly structured or require only limited social contact.

Differential Diagnosis

Experiences of depersonalization or derealization may occur in other dissociative disorders, mood disorders, and anxiety or fear-related disorders but do not warrant a separate diagnosis unless the depersonalization or derealization symptoms become chronic after the co-occurring disorder improves. Such symptoms are also found in schizophrenia or other primary psychotic disorders but are typically associated with delusions. In depersonalization-derealization disorder, the experiences have an "as-if" quality, and the person recognizes that they are not "real" (Simeon, 2009). Limited expression of emotion (flat affect) may occur, but other symptoms of schizophrenia are absent. A diagnosis of depersonalization-derealization disorder is not warranted if the experiences are due to a substance or medication or to a medical condition.

Assessment

Depersonalization-derealization disorder commonly co-occurs with other mental disorders and may be masked by anxiety or depressive symptoms. Individuals are often reluctant to describe their apparently bizarre experiences for fear of being considered psychotic. Facial and bodily expressions of emotion may be limited as a part of the characteristic depersonalization-derealization disorder symptom of emotional numbing and can be a diagnostic clue. A dissociative disorders interview or specialized assessment tool such as the Cambridge Depersonalization Scale (Sierra & Berrios, 2000) may be useful for assessment.

DEVELOPMENTAL COURSE OF DISSOCIATIVE DISORDERS

Dissociative disorders are typically diagnosed in adulthood, but adolescent cases of DID, depersonalization-derealization disorder, or trance disorder and possession trance disorder do occur. In addition, childhood cases of DID and trance disorder and possession trance disorder have been reported.

Adverse childhood experiences, especially childhood trauma, are a major precipitant for all dissociative disorders. Although some dissociative disorders may arise in response to adult trauma, they are more typically associated with childhood physical, sexual, and emotional abuse, as well as with emotional neglect. The association between childhood trauma and dissociation is generally a dose–response relationship; the more chronic and severe the adversity, the more severe the dissociation tends to be. Exposure to multiple types of adverse events, in comparison to only one form of abuse, is associated with more severe dissociative symptoms (Nijenhuis, 2015).

DID, in particular, is strongly linked to chronic traumatizing life events, including early-onset childhood physical, sexual, and emotional abuse, along with emotional neglect and related disruptions of attachment (Dalenberg et al., 2012; Şar et al., 2017). Frequently, multiple perpetrators are involved, often including parents or other close relatives. This confronts the traumatized child with an exceptionally difficult situation: For their physical and psychological survival, they must approach and seek comfort from the very persons who harm them. Children who develop DID adjust to this situation by creating dissociative identities motivated by attachment needs and dissociative identities motivated by defensive/protective needs. Indeed, for this reason it has been argued that disorganized (fearful–avoidant) attachment, usually understood as arising from an infant coming to fear their attachment figure because of threatening behavior, contributes to the development of dissociation and is a risk factor for DID (Dutra et al., 2009; Liotti, 2004; Pasquini et al., 2002). Similar developmental factors may play a role for partial DID, but research is limited. Finally, in depersonalization-derealization disorder, reports of childhood physical or sexual abuse also occur but tend to be rated as less frequent or severe than those reported in other dissociative disorders; on the other hand, emotional abuse appears to be a common childhood precipitant of depersonalization-derealization disorder (Simeon et al., 2001).

CULTURAL CONSIDERATIONS

Clinicians are cautioned against interpreting experiences that are part of accepted cultural, religious, or spiritual practice as evidence for a dissociative disorder. Pathologizing transient dissociative experiences that are common in certain healing and religious practices around the world should be avoided. Nonetheless, specific patterns of dissociative disorder presentations may reflect local specificity. Symptoms of dissociative neurological symptom disorder, for example, may vary by region (e.g., heat and "peppery" sensations in parts of Asia and Africa). The identities and behaviors presented during the altered state in possession trance disorder vary cross-culturally, typically corresponding to the spiritual beliefs of each society.

In some contexts, individuals with trance disorder or possession trance disorder presentations may gradually learn to control and integrate these experiences through training in culturally endorsed spiritual or psychological practices. Although their initial level of distress may warrant the diagnosis, over time these experiences may become nondistressing, circumscribed to ritual settings, and even adaptive (Moreira-Almeida, & Cardeña, 2011). By contrast, intentionally induced experiences of depersonalization and derealization can be desired objectives of spiritual or meditative practices. In some societies, presentations of DID or partial DID may tend to occur after stressful precipitants (e.g., chronic parental affect dysregulation) even in the absence of known physical or sexual abuse (Şar et al., 2017). The tendency toward dissociative responses to stressors may be increased in cultures with less individualistic conceptions of the self or in circumstances of socioeconomic deprivation.

VALIDITY

The validity of some dissociative disorders, particularly those associated with amnesia and sustained personality changes (i.e., DID, partial DID, dissociative amnesia, and dissociative fugue) has been debated. Many argue that dissociative disorders are typically related to traumatizing events. However, an alternative view, often called the *sociocognitive model*, proposes that suggestive individuals are trained by therapists into believing "false memories" of abuse (about which it is claimed they previously experienced "amnesia") and coached into acting as though they experience and express multiple parts of their personality (Spanos, 1996). There is, however, strong empirical evidence arguing against the validity of the sociocognitive model. This includes evidence that (a) traumatic memories are most often recalled, after a period of years with no recollections, outside of the context of therapy; (b) such memories appear no more or less accurate than traumatic memories that have been continuously recalled; (c) persons diagnosed with DID are no more suggestible and fantasy prone than individuals with PTSD or personality disorder with borderline pattern; (d) psychological, physiological, and neurobiological functioning appears significantly different between identity states in individuals with DID but not in highly suggestible controls and actors instructed and trained to "fake" the dissociated identities of DID; and (e) the neurobiological sequelae and structural brain changes occurring after childhood abuse, and in PTSD, are broadly similar to those seen in severe dissociative disorders (Chalavi et al., 2015; Dalenberg et al., 2012; Nijenhuis, 2015; Vissia et al., 2016).

PREVALENCE

Abundant research demonstrates the global presence of dissociative disorders. General population studies show a lifetime prevalence of dissociative amnesia (primarily without fugue) of 2% to 7%, depersonalization-derealization disorder of 1% to 3%, possession trance disorder of 1% to 3.5%, DID of 1% to 1.5%, and partial DID (or *DSM-IV* dissociative disorder not otherwise specified, a previous category which overlaps with partial DID) of 2% to 8% (Loewenstein et al., 2017; Spiegel et al., 2011). Studies of patients with mental disorders show high levels of undiagnosed dissociative disorders and suggests that these patients are likely to be misdiagnosed with schizophrenia (Schäfer et al., 2019).

KEY POINTS

- Dissociative disorders are a manifestation of dissociation, the expression of nonintegrated or insufficiently integrated components of mental functioning.

- This abnormal lack of integration gives rise to six disorders: dissociative neurological symptom disorder, dissociative amnesia, trance disorder and possession trance disorder, dissociative identity disorder (DID), partial DID, and depersonalization-derealization disorder.

- Dissociative symptoms include gaps in memory, pseudo-neurological symptoms lacking a medical basis, experiences of depersonalization and derealization, and alterations of identity.

- Dissociative disorders may also include a wide range of symptoms common to other disorders, particularly anxiety or fear-related disorders, depressive disorders, and schizophrenia or other primary psychotic disorders.

- There is strong evidence that the dissociative disorders develop after adversity in a dose–response relationship; the more chronic and severe the adversity, the more complex the dissociation tends to be. Dissociation is typically, at least in part, a way to cope with or to adapt to overwhelming experiences.

- Research shows that dissociative disorders are common, that individuals with these disorders are not highly suggestible, and that instruction and motivation to simulate dissociative identities do not succeed in reproducing their phenomenological or psychobiological characteristics.

- Correct diagnosis requires establishing the dissociative nature of the presenting symptoms.

- The accurate assessment of dissociative disorders calls for a psychologically informed approach, considering the role of traumatizing and stressful experiences in symptom generation and maintenance, and may require screening instruments or dissociative disorder diagnostic interviews, along with information from family or friends.

REFERENCES

Cardeña, E., Van Duijl, M., Weiner, L. A., & Terhune, D. B. (2009). Possession/trance phenomena. In P. F. Dell & J. A. O'Neil (Eds.), *Dissociation and the dissociative disorders: DSM-V and beyond* (pp. 171–181). Routledge.

Carlson, E. B., & Putnam, F. W. (1993). An update on the Dissociative Experiences Scale. *Dissociation, 6*(1), 16–27.

Carlson, E. B., Waelde, L. C., Palmieri, P. A., Macia, K. S., Smith, S. R., & McDade-Montez, E. (2018). Development and validation of the Dissociative Symptoms Scale. *Assessment, 25*(1), 84–98. https://doi.org/10.1177/1073191116645904

Chalavi, S., Vissia, E. M., Giesen, M. E., Nijenhuis, E. R. S., Draijer, N., Cole, J. H., Dazzan, P., Pariante, C. M., Madsen, S. K., Rajagopalan, P., Thompson, P. M., Toga, A. W., Veltman, D. J., & Reinders, A. A. T. S. (2015). Abnormal hippocampal morphology in dissociative identity disorder and post-traumatic stress disorder correlates with childhood trauma and dissociative symptoms. *Human Brain Mapping, 36*(5), 1692–1704. https://doi.org/10.1002/hbm.22730

Dalenberg, C. J., Brand, B. L., Gleaves, D. H., Dorahy, M. J., Loewenstein, R. J., Cardeña, E., Frewen, P. A., Carlson, E. B., & Spiegel, D. (2012). Evaluation of the evidence for the trauma and fantasy models of dissociation. *Psychological Bulletin, 138*(3), 550–588. https://doi.org/10.1037/a0027447

Dell, P. F. (2009). The long struggle to diagnose Multiple Personality Disorder (MPD): Partial MPD. In P. F. Dell & J. A. O'Neil (Eds.), *Dissociation and the dissociative disorders: DSM-V and beyond* (pp. 403–428). Routledge.

Diseth, T. H. (2006). Dissociation following traumatic medical treatment procedures in childhood: A longitudinal follow-up. *Development and Psychopathology, 18*(1), 233–251. https://doi.org/10.1017/S0954579406060135

Dutra, L., Bureau, J. F., Holmes, B., Lyubchik, A., & Lyons-Ruth, K. (2009). Quality of early care and childhood trauma: A prospective study of developmental pathways to dissociation. *Journal of Nervous and Mental Disease, 197*(6), 383–390. https://doi.org/10.1097/NMD.0b013e3181a653b7

Liotti, G. (2004). Trauma, dissociation and disorganized attachment: Three strands of a single braid. *Psychotherapy: Theory, Research, & Practice, 41*(4), 472–486. https://doi.org/10.1037/0033-3204.41.4.472

Loewenstein, R., Frewen, P., & Lewis-Fernández, R. (2017). Dissociative disorders. In B. J. Sadock, V. A. Sadock, & R. Ruiz (Eds.), *Kaplan & Sadock's comprehensive textbook of psychiatry* (Vol. 1, pp. 1866–1952). Lippincott, Williams, & Wilkins.

Moreira-Almeida, A., & Cardeña, E. (2011). Differential diagnosis between non-pathological psychotic and spiritual experiences and mental disorders: A contribution from Latin American studies to the *ICD-11*. *The Brazilian Journal of Psychiatry, 33*(Suppl. 1), S21–S36. https://doi.org/10.1590/S1516-44462011000500004

Moskowitz, A., & Heim, G. (2019). The role of dissociation in the historical concept of schizophrenia. In A. Moskowitz, M. J. Dorahy, & I. Schäfer (Eds.), *Psychosis, trauma and dissociation: Evolving perspectives on severe psychopathology* (pp. 55–67). Wiley.

Moskowitz, A., Mosquera, D., & Longden, E. (2017). Auditory verbal hallucinations and the differential diagnosis of schizophrenia and dissociative disorders: Historical, empirical and clinical perspectives. *The European Journal of Trauma and Dissociation, 1*(1), 37–46. https://doi.org/10.1016/j.ejtd.2017.01.003

Müller-Pfeiffer, C., Rufibach, K., Wyss, D., Perron, N., Pitman, R., & Rufer, M. (2013). Screening for dissociative disorders in psychiatric out- and daycare patients. *Journal of Psychopathology and Behavioral Assessment, 35*(4), 592–602. https://doi.org/10.1007/s10862-013-9367-0

Nijenhuis, E. R. S. (2004). *Somatoform dissociation: Phenomena, measurement, and theoretical issues.* W.W. Norton & Company.

Nijenhuis, E. R. S. (2015). *The trinity of trauma: Ignorance, fragility, and control* (Vols. 1–2). Vandenhoeck & Ruprecht. https://doi.org/10.13109/9783666402470

Nijenhuis, E. R. S., Spinhoven, P., Van Dyck, R., Van der Hart, O., & Vanderlinden, J. (1996). The development and psychometric characteristics of the Somatoform Dissociation Questionnaire (SDQ-20). *Journal of Nervous and Mental Disease, 184*(11), 688–694. https://doi.org/10.1097/00005053-199611000-00006

Pasquini, P., Liotti, G., Mazzotti, E., Fassone, G., Picardi, A., & the Italian Group for the Study of Dissociation. (2002). Risk factors in the early family life of patients suffering from dissociative disorders. *Acta Psychiatrica Scandinavica, 105*(2), 110–116. https://doi.org/10.1034/j.1600-0447.2002.01062.x

Piedfort-Marin, O., Tarquinio, C., Steinberg, M., Azarmsa, S., Cuttelod, T., Piot, M.-E., Wisler, D., Zimmermann, E., & Nater, J. (2022). Reliability and validity study of the French-language version of the SCID-D semi-structured clinical interview for diagnosing *DSM-5* and *ICD-11* dissociative disorders. *Annales Médico-Psychologiques, Revue Psychiatrique, 180*(6S), S1–S9. https://doi.org/10.1016/j.amp.2020.12.012

Piper, A., & Merskey, H. (2004). The persistence of folly: A critical examination of dissociative identity disorder: Part 1. The excesses of an improbable concept. *Canadian Journal of Psychiatry, 49*(9), 592–600. https://doi.org/10.1177/070674370404900904

Reinders, A. A. T. S., Willemsen, A. T. M., Vissia, E. M., Vos, H. P. J., den Boer, J. A., & Nijenhuis, E. R. S. (2016). The psychobiology of authentic and simulated dissociative personality states: The full Monty. *Journal of Nervous and Mental Disease, 204*(6), 445–457. https://doi.org/10.1097/NMD.0000000000000522

Şar, V., Alioğlu, F., Akyuz, G., & Karabulut, S. (2014). Dissociative amnesia in dissociative disorders and borderline personality disorder: Self-rating assessment in a college population. *Journal of Trauma & Dissociation, 15*(4), 477–493. https://doi.org/10.1080/15299732.2014.902415

Şar, V., Dorahy, M. J., & Krüger, C. (2017). Revisiting the etiological aspects of dissociative identity disorder: A biopsychosocial perspective. *Psychology Research and Behavior Management, 10,* 137–146. https://doi.org/10.2147/PRBM.S113743

Şar, V., & Ross, C. (2006). Dissociative disorders as a confounding factor in psychiatric research. *The Psychiatric Clinics of North America, 29*(1), 129–144. https://doi.org/10.1016/j.psc.2005.10.008

Schäfer, I., Aderhold, V., Freyberger, H. J., Spitzer, C., & Schroeder, K. (2019). Dissociative symptoms in schizophrenia-spectrum disorders. In A. Moskowitz, M. J. Dorahy, & I. Schäfer (Eds.), *Psychosis, trauma and dissociation: Evolving perspectives on severe psychopathology* (pp. 179–194). Wiley.

Schlumpf, Y. R., Reinders, A. A. T. S., Nijenhuis, E. R. S., Luechinger, R., van Osch, M. J. P., & Jäncke, L. (2014). Dissociative part-dependent resting-state activity in dissociative identity disorder: A controlled fMRI perfusion study. *PLoS One, 9*(6), e98795. https://doi.org/10.1371/journal.pone.0098795

Sierra, M., & Berrios, G. E. (1998). Depersonalization: Neurobiological perspectives. *Biological Psychiatry, 44*(9), 898–908. https://doi.org/10.1016/S0006-3223(98)00015-8

Sierra, M., & Berrios, G. E. (2000). The Cambridge Depersonalization Scale: A new instrument for the measurement of depersonalization. *Psychiatry Research, 93*(2), 153–164. https://doi.org/10.1016/S0165-1781(00)00100-1

Simeon, D. (2009). Depersonalization disorder. In P. F. Dell & J. A. O'Neil (Eds.), *Dissociation and the dissociative disorders:* DSM-V *and beyond* (pp. 435–444). Routledge.

Simeon, D., Guralnik, O., Schmeidler, J., Sirof, B., & Knutelska, M. (2001). The role of childhood interpersonal trauma in depersonalization disorder. *The American Journal of Psychiatry, 158*(7), 1027–1033. https://doi.org/10.1176/appi.ajp.158.7.1027

Spanos, N. P. (1996). *Multiple identities and false memories: A sociocognitive perspective.* American Psychological Association. https://doi.org/10.1037/10216-000

Spiegel, D., Loewenstein, R. J., Lewis-Fernández, R., Şar, V., Simeon, D., Vermetten, E., Cardeña, E., & Dell, P. F. (2011). Dissociative disorders in *DSM-5. Depression and Anxiety, 28*(9), 824–852. https://doi.org/10.1002/da.20874

Staniloiu, A., & Markowitsch, H. J. (2014). Dissociative amnesia. *The Lancet Psychiatry, 1*(3), 226–241. https://doi.org/10.1016/S2215-0366(14)70279-2

Steinberg, M. (2023). *The SCID-D Interview: Dissociation assessment in therapy, forensics, and research.* American Psychiatric Association.

Steinberg, M., & Schnall, M. (2000). *The stranger in the mirror.* Cliff Street Books.

van Duijl, M., Kleijn, W., & de Jong, J. (2013). Are symptoms of spirit possessed patients covered by the *DSM-IV* or *DSM-5* criteria for possession trance disorder? A mixed-method explorative study in Uganda. *Social Psychiatry and Psychiatric Epidemiology, 48*(9), 1417–1430. https://doi.org/10.1007/s00127-012-0635-1

Vissia, E. M., Giesen, M. E., Chalavi, S., Nijenhuis, E. R. S., Draijer, N., Brand, B. L., & Reinders, A. A. T. S. (2016). Is it trauma- or fantasy-based? Comparing dissociative identity disorder, post-traumatic stress disorder, simulators, and controls. *Acta Psychiatrica Scandinavica, 134*(2), 111–128. https://doi.org/10.1111/acps.12590

World Health Organization. (2023). *ICD-11 for mortality and morbidity statistics* (Version: 01/2023). https://icd.who.int/browse11/l-m/en#/

World Health Organization. (2024). *Clinical descriptions and diagnostic requirements for ICD-11 mental, behavioural and neurodevelopmental disorders.* https://www.who.int/publications/i/item/9789240077263

12

Feeding and Eating Disorders

Kathleen M. Pike, Robyn Sysko, and Rachel Bryant-Waugh

OVERARCHING LOGIC

The grouping of feeding and eating disorders in the 11th revision of the *International Classification of Diseases* (*ICD-11*; World Health Organization [WHO], 2023) brings together disturbances in patterns of behavior related to feeding and eating that were variously categorized in the *ICD-10* as feeding disorders, other emotional and behavioral disorders with onset usually occurring in childhood and adolescence, and eating disorders. The feeding disorders included in the new *ICD-11* grouping are pica, rumination-regurgitation disorder, and avoidant-restrictive food intake disorder. The eating disorders included in this grouping are anorexia nervosa, bulimia nervosa, and binge eating disorder. This grouping also includes the residual category "other specified feeding or eating disorder," a diagnosis for patterns of abnormal feeding and eating behaviors that are not fully consistent with the clinical descriptions of the specified feeding and eating disorders in the grouping. Three of the disorders in this grouping—binge eating disorder, avoidant-restrictive food intake disorder, and rumination-regurgitation disorder—are new categories in the *ICD-11*, although they have been recognized in clinical practice for a long time.

Feeding and eating disorders were merged into a single grouping in *ICD-11* because these disorders have in common essential behavioral disturbances in food intake and eating behavior. Moreover, the *ICD-11* takes a lifespan approach to diagnosis; grouping feeding and eating disorders together better

https://doi.org/10.1037/0000392-012
A Psychological Approach to Diagnosis: Using the ICD-11 as a Framework, G. M. Reed, P. L.-J. Ritchie, and A. Maercker (Editors)

captures the related nature of these disorders across the developmental trajectory. All the disorders in this grouping can emerge and occur across childhood, adolescence, or adulthood. Diagnostic requirements in this grouping have been updated to reflect the current research and clinical evidence base (Al-Adawi et al., 2013; Claudino et al., 2019), particularly for anorexia nervosa and bulimia nervosa. The additions and refinements in the *ICD-11* were designed to improve clinical utility and global relevance by providing greater clarity regarding disturbances in feeding and eating disorders, enhancing representation of cultural variations in the *Clinical Descriptions and Diagnostic Requirements for ICD-11 Mental, Behavioural and Neurodevelopmental Disorders* (*CDDR*; WHO, 2024), and reflecting greater appreciation for a lifespan approach to understanding these disorders (Al Adawi et al., 2013). These changes were tested in a global field study (Claudino et al., 2019). Ultimately, the changes in the classification of feeding and eating disorders should aid in public health estimates of prevalence and incidence, early identification of clinical cases, and development of tailored clinical interventions to improve therapeutic care and outcomes for individuals with feeding and eating disorders.

A PSYCHOLOGICAL APPROACH TO FEEDING AND EATING DISORDERS

Feeding and eating disorders are multidetermined disturbances that involve dysregulation in eating behaviors and nutritional intake. They are not due to another medical condition and the behaviors are considered inappropriate for the individual's age, culture, and developmental history. Although feeding and eating disorders share this common behavioral phenomenology, they differ fundamentally in terms of the factors that drive the behavioral disturbances. Feeding disorders are characterized by behavioral disturbances in food intake that are not related to concerns about body shape and weight. In contrast, preoccupation with food and distress associated with body shape and weight play a central role in eating disorders, particularly anorexia nervosa and bulimia nervosa. Marked distress about the pattern of eating or significant impairment in functioning is also an essential feature aspect of binge eating disorder.

The psychological model of eating disorders incorporates cognitive, emotional, and environmental factors that increase risk. Cognitive disturbances involving overconcern for eating, shape, and weight and behavioral disturbances that affect eating and weight control behavior interact in ways that both increase risk for the development of an eating disorder and the maintenance of the symptoms of the disorder over time. Cultural factors are also significant in setting the stage for risk. To varying degrees across anorexia nervosa, bulimia nervosa, and binge eating disorder, low self-esteem, anxiety, and mood disturbances can predispose individuals to be especially vulnerable to internalizing sociocultural ideals about appearance and the importance of thinness. Adopting these sociocultural ideals and developing an internal mindset or schema that attaches primary value to shape, weight, and control over eating increases the risk for these disturbances and serves to perpetuate these eating disturbances when they occur.

PRESENTATIONS, SYMPTOM PATTERNS, AND SPECIFIERS

Anorexia Nervosa

Anorexia nervosa is diagnosed when an individual has a significantly low body weight for height, age, and developmental stage, which is not due to unavailability of food and is not better accounted for by another medical condition (e.g., rapid weight loss due to chemotherapy for cancer). *ICD-11* provides guidance on the threshold for low weight status, but clinical judgment should also be exercised in considering weight status in relation to cultural context and stage of development. The *ICD-11* indicates that a commonly used threshold for low body weight is a body mass index (BMI, calculated as kilograms per square meter, or kg/m^2) of less than 18.5 in adults or one that falls below the fifth percentile by gender and age (BMI-for-age) in children and adolescents. Low weight status may be the result of weight loss or a failure to gain weight as expected based on the individual's developmental trajectory. The inclusion of enhanced guidance in *ICD-11* regarding what is intended by "significantly low body weight" reflects an appreciation for the diversity of developmental experiences and cultural contexts. In Japan, for example, normative body mass index is significantly lower than in the United States such that low body mass for anorexia nervosa is often lower in Japan compared with the United States (Pike & Dunne, 2015). Two specifiers for anorexia nervosa describe the severity of underweight status: *significantly low body weight* and *dangerously low body weight* (< 14.0 kg/m^2). Severely low BMI is associated with more health complications, greater need for clinical services (such as hospitalization), and substantially increased mortality risk (Sullivan, 1995).

Two circumstances are recognized in which individuals would still be diagnosed with anorexia nervosa despite not having low body mass. The first occurs in the context of rapid weight loss (e.g., more than 20% of total body weight within 6 months), as long as all other diagnostic features are present. In the second case, the *ICD-11* recommends the retention of the diagnosis of anorexia nervosa until a full and lasting recovery—not just weight restoration—has been achieved (e.g., for at least 1 year after intensive treatment is withdrawn). In this circumstance, a specifier for "in recovery with normal body weight" may be applied to the diagnosis of anorexia nervosa. This guidance facilitates appropriate continuity of clinical care in the recovery of anorexia nervosa, which is critical to relapse prevention and long-term recovery (Pike et al., 2003).

Another core feature exhibited by individuals with anorexia nervosa is a pattern of food restriction and other behaviors such as fasting, spitting out food, purging, medication misuse, and exercise that lead to, or maintain, abnormally low body weight. Two specifiers with implications for treatment planning may be applied to describe these patterns: "restricting pattern" and "binge-purge pattern." These behaviors are predominantly motivated by an overvaluation of low body weight and extreme fear of weight gain. In most cases, individuals with anorexia nervosa will explicitly describe their fears associated with weight gain and intense concerns about body weight and shape. However, even if it is not explicitly reported, preoccupation with weight and shape can also be inferred from behaviors such as repeatedly checking body weight or shape using scales, tape measures, or mirrors; constantly monitoring caloric intake; or extreme avoidant behaviors, such as refusal to have mirrors at home or refusal to know one's weight. Individuals with anorexia nervosa often fail to recognize that they are underweight and may dismiss objective evidence regarding their actual weight or shape or the seriousness of their condition.

The *ICD-11* diagnostic requirements for anorexia nervosa are likely to result in a larger proportion of individuals receiving this diagnosis, including individuals who in *ICD-10* were diagnosed with atypical anorexia nervosa, which has been eliminated in *ICD-11*, and "other eating disorder." These include individuals who have gained weight but who are still in early stages of treatment recovery and individuals whose weight and shape concerns are not explicitly reported but can be inferred from their behavior. All these changes facilitate identification of behavior patterns that underlie anorexia nervosa and the rapid implementation of evidence-informed treatment strategies.

Bulimia Nervosa

Bulimia nervosa is characterized by the hallmark features of recurrent episodes of binge eating coupled with engaging in inappropriate compensatory behaviors such as vomiting, laxative misuse or excessive exercise to prevent weight gain. The *ICD-11 CDDR* for the diagnosis of bulimia nervosa specify frequent, recurrent episodes of binge eating and provide guidance that this would typically be a minimum threshold of binge eating an average of once per week over the course of a minimum duration of 1 month. This relatively low threshold of binge frequency is based on clinical and empirical data indicating that individuals who binge eat at an average frequency of once a week are comparable to those who do so more frequently (Wilson & Sysko, 2009) and is also intended to enable early implementation of treatment.

The construct of binge eating has historically depended on two dimensions: eating an objectively large quantity of food and experiencing concomitant loss of control over the type or amount of food eaten. Whereas eating an objectively large amount of food is typical for most individuals with bulimia nervosa, clinical observation and empirical data indicate that individuals who describe binge eating on lesser quantities of food report impairment and distress comparable to those who engage in objective binge eating (Palavras et al., 2013; Thompson et al., 2022; Watson et al., 2013). For many individuals, violating one's rules about type of food (e.g., a typical binge food vs. diet food) or eating plans (e.g., was not planning to eat lunch because of an anticipated big dinner, but then eats an afternoon snack) can lead to significant experience of loss of control over their own eating behavior, which is highly salient for many individuals (Wolfe et al., 2009). Subjective binge eating occurs when an individual experiences a loss of control over eating but consumes an amount of food that is objectively within normal limits (e.g., a bowl of ice cream). Individuals who report subjective binge episodes have similar levels of psychopathology, comorbidity, and clinical service utilization as those who report objective binge eating episodes (Fitzsimmons-Craft et al., 2014; Mond et al., 2010). Thus, according to *ICD-11 CDDR*, it is not necessary to consume an objectively large amount of food during a binge eating episode; a subjective amount of food in the context of loss of control is sufficient to satisfy this requirement. This innovation in *ICD-11* is likely to reduce the number of individuals classified with an "other eating disorder" diagnosis compared with *ICD-10*, while preserving similarities in presentation and treatment response among diagnosed individuals (Walsh & Sysko, 2009).

In addition to binge eating, individuals with bulimia nervosa engage in diverse, recurrent, inappropriate compensatory behaviors to prevent weight gain. The most typical compensatory behavior is vomiting immediately following binge eating. Other compensatory behaviors include diuretic or laxative misuse, fasting, and excessive exercise. Clinical judgment is necessary to evaluate the intensity and duration of exercise that might constitute inappropriate compensatory behavior. In many cases, individuals with bulimia nervosa engage in both purging and non-purging behaviors. Similar to the *ICD-11* guidance for the binge eating frequency threshold, repeated, inappropriate compensatory behaviors are described as typically occurring at a minimum of once per week over the course of a minimum duration of 1 month.

Preoccupation with body weight and shape that excessively influences self-evaluation is an essential feature of bulimia nervosa. As with anorexia nervosa, this can be self-reported or inferred from behaviors (e.g., repeatedly checking body weight on a scale, checking mirrors, refusal to know one's weight). Preoccupation with weight and shape is associated with negative self-esteem and overall self-assessment. The cycle of engaging in binge eating followed by inappropriate compensatory behaviors is associated with marked distress or significant impairment in other areas of one's life such as personal, family, social, educational, and occupational areas of functioning.

Although individuals with both anorexia nervosa and bulimia nervosa can report binge eating and/or purging behaviors, a diagnosis of anorexia nervosa should be assigned when the patient is significantly underweight. When binge eating occurs in the absence of compensatory behaviors, the appropriate diagnosis is binge eating disorder.

Binge Eating Disorder

Individuals with binge eating disorder report recurrent episodes of binge eating (e.g., once a week or more over a period of 3 months). As with bulimia nervosa, binge eating episodes in binge eating disorder include both objectively and subjectively large amounts of food accompanied by loss of control. The *ICD-11* includes subjective binge episodes in the diagnosis of binge eating disorder because individuals who have all the other symptoms of binge eating disorder, but report only subjective binge episodes, describe similar levels of impairment, distress, and psychopathology as those whose binges are described as objectively large (Wolfe et al., 2009). As with bulimia nervosa, loss of control during binge eating episodes is a highly salient clinical dimension for individuals with binge eating disorder.

The distinction between bulimia nervosa and binge eating disorder is that individuals with binge eating disorder do not report regular compensatory behaviors to prevent weight gain following binge eating episodes. Overvaluation of body shape and weight may be endorsed by individuals with binge eating disorder, but this symptom is not required for a diagnosis. Some studies suggest that individuals exhibiting overvaluation of shape or weight may have a more severe form of binge eating disorder; however, requiring it for a diagnosis would exclude a meaningful proportion of individuals with clinically significant pathology. Individuals with binge eating disorder describe marked distress about their pattern of binge eating or significant impairment in other areas of life such as personal, family, social, educational, and occupational areas of functioning.

Binge eating disorder is a newly introduced category in *ICD-11* that describes a syndrome previously included in a heterogeneous, residual category of "other eating disorders." The inclusion of binge eating disorder should reduce the number of individuals who receive a residual diagnosis and thereby improve capacity to deliver tailored prevention and treatment efforts for the disorder. Binge eating disorder is often associated with weight gain and obesity. However, individuals with binge eating disorder may also be of normal or low weight; the diagnosis of binge eating disorder is not dependent on any particular weight status. Because obesity is a common presenting complaint among individuals seeking treatment for binge eating disorder, it is important to distinguish between a pattern of dysregulated eating characterized by binge eating as already described and one characterized by other forms of overeating that involve consuming an excess of calories over the course of the day. In making this distinction, assessing the following additional clinical features that commonly occur in binge eating disorder can be useful: eating much more rapidly than normal; eating until feeling uncomfortably full; eating large amounts of food when not feeling physically hungry; eating alone due to feeling embarrassed of how much one is eating; or feeling disgusted with oneself, depressed, or very guilty after overeating. Finally, infrequent or occasional overeating, even of large amounts of food, or culturally sanctioned feasting (e.g., during specific holidays or celebrations) would not be consistent with assigning a diagnosis of binge eating disorder.

Avoidant-Restrictive Food Intake Disorder

The inclusion of the new diagnosis of avoidant-restrictive food intake disorder in *ICD-11* reflects a growing body of clinical evidence and aims to improve clinical recognition of this behavioral disturbance across the developmental continuum. Individuals with avoidant-restrictive food intake disorder engage in avoidant or restrictive food intake in terms of quantity and/or variety of foods, which results in a failure to meet adequate energy or nutritional requirements and is associated with significant impairment in important areas of functioning. Commonly observed types of food restriction include erratic eating with long periods between food consumption; general absence of eating avidity (enthusiasm); food avoidance based on the sensory features of food (e.g., texture, smell, appearance); and fear-based avoidance, often associated with a previous adverse experience (e.g., exclusive consumption of liquids due to a fear of choking).

In individuals with avoidant-restrictive food intake disorder, limited food intake is not due to preoccupation with body shape or weight or significant body dissatisfaction, lack of food availability, another mental disorder or medical condition (e.g., schizophrenia or another primary psychotic disorder, a gastrointestinal disorder), or the effects of a medication or substance. Avoidant-restrictive food intake disorder often co-occurs with other conditions (e.g., autism spectrum disorder, anxiety and fear-related disorders, food allergies); where this is the case, the eating disturbance exceeds that explained by the co-occurring condition or has negatively affected the physical health of the individual or is associated with levels of distress and impairment that require clinical intervention specifically focused on the eating behaviors. Avoidant eating or feeding behaviors often begin during childhood but can occur throughout the life span. For most individuals, there is no specific precipitating event, and eating difficulties are long-standing. In what appears to be a minority of cases, the onset of food avoidance may follow a traumatic incident such as witnessing someone choking or an individual choking themselves.

The restriction of food intake in avoidant-restrictive food intake disorder contributes to several possible, sometimes co-occurring, outcomes. These include (a) significant weight loss, (b) a failure to gain weight as expected in childhood or pregnancy, (c) clinically significant deficiencies of specific nutrients, (d) other impacts on the physical health of the individual (e.g., reliance on enteral feeding), or (e) impairments in psychosocial functioning (e.g., avoidance of social experiences involving eating). Individuals with unusual patterns of eating or who are picky eaters should not be diagnosed with avoidant-restrictive food intake disorders in the absence of significant impact on weight (weight loss) or negative health (e.g., anemia) or psychosocial consequences (e.g., impaired friendships due to avoidance or distress related to participating in social experiences that involve eating).

Pica

The diagnosis of pica requires the regular consumption of nonnutritive substances (e.g., clay, soil, chalk, plaster, plastic, metal, paper) at a level that is persistent or severe enough to require clinical attention. That is, the eating behavior causes damage or significant risk to health or impairment in functioning due to the frequency, amount, or type of substances ingested. Pica can occur throughout the life span. Because it is normative for infants and very young children to place nonfood objects in their mouths for sensory exploration, it is recommended that pica should only be diagnosed after 2 years of age (or equivalent level of intellectual development), after which children are typically able to distinguish between edible and nonedible substances. During pregnancy, women may desire and consume nonnutritive substances such as chalk or ice, but this does not typically warrant a diagnosis unless the eating behavior is extreme and has the potential to cause harm. A diagnosis of pica is not appropriate when eating nonnutritive substances is a culturally sanctioned behavior (e.g., eating of soil or clay in parts of Africa), the result of a medically explained nutritional deficiency, or explained by another mental disorder (e.g., autism spectrum disorder, schizophrenia, trichotillomania), unless clinical intervention is required due to the nature or quantity of the substances ingested.

Rumination-Regurgitation Disorder

Individuals with rumination-regurgitation disorder repeatedly bring up previously swallowed food into the mouth (i.e., regurgitation), which may be rechewed and reswallowed (i.e., rumination) or may be deliberately spat out (in contrast to vomiting). The regurgitation of food is frequent (at least several times per week) over a period of at least several weeks, is volitional, and occurs with relative ease. The recurrent regurgitation may be maintained by a reduction of anxiety, feeling of pleasure, or self-soothing derived from the behavior and is not better explained by a medical condition (e.g., esophageal blockages or gastrointestinal thickening). A diagnosis of rumination-regurgitation disorder may not be given to individuals with a developmental age of less than 2 years. The regurgitation in rumination-regurgitation disorder must be volitional and intentional and can occur in response to high levels of anxiety or emotional distress. Rumination-regurgitation disorder should be differentiated from vomiting as part of a culturally sanctioned practice (e.g., yogic practitioners, vomiting without an organic pathology, or vomiting as a somatic expression of distress as noted in South Asia; Pike et al., 2013). As the disorder progresses, regurgitation may become more automatic and more difficult to distinguish from vomiting. In addition, rumination-regurgitation disorder may either be episodic, with more frequent symptoms accompanying greater anxiety, or continuous. The symptoms are typically accompanied by feelings of shame and embarrassment, attempts to keep the behavior secret because it is known to be socially unacceptable, and a reluctance to seek treatment. It is also associated with significant physical health impact—most notably, tooth decay, esophageal damage, and significant weight loss because people avoid eating rather than ruminating in public.

BOUNDARY WITH NORMALITY AND DIFFERENTIAL DIAGNOSIS

Most of the cardinal features of feeding and eating disorders are extreme versions of behaviors that are commonplace in the general population. Avoiding certain foods, dieting, eating large amounts of food at one time, body dissatisfaction, limited interest in food, and compensating for overconsumption, for example, are widespread. Most people have some foods they dislike and avoid eating. Certain situations and emotional experiences can affect most people's eating to some extent. Some people are "picky eaters," "comfort eaters," or "big eaters." To meet the threshold for a clinical diagnosis of a feeding or eating disorder, symptoms must be sufficiently problematic that they are associated with significant distress and impairment. Impairment may occur in a range of domains, such as personal, family, social, educational, occupational, and other areas of health.

Because the disorders in this grouping have multiple features in common, differentiating among them can sometimes be difficult. Individuals with anorexia nervosa are distinguished from those with bulimia nervosa based on their very low body weight, even if they binge and purge. If someone with anorexia nervosa is in recovery and has gained weight, they should still retain the diagnosis of anorexia nervosa until a full and lasting recovery is achieved rather than switching to bulimia nervosa or other specified feeding eating disorders. Anorexia nervosa and avoidant-restrictive food intake disorder can sometimes be difficult to distinguish because individuals with anorexia nervosa do not always verbalize concerns about weight or fears of gaining weight. If body shape and weight concerns can be inferred based on the individual's behavior, even if not explicitly reported by the patient, the diagnosis of anorexia nervosa is warranted. If no evidence exists that the individual is concerned about weight or afraid of gaining weight, avoidant-restrictive food intake disorder is the appropriate diagnosis.

There are also important differential diagnoses with disorders outside the grouping. In the case of pica, individuals who have specific nutritional deficiencies associated with the ingestion of related nonnutritive substances may cease their abnormal eating behaviors if the primary nutritional deficiency is successfully treated. It is not uncommon for individuals with disorders of intellectual development to consume nonnutritive substances; the diagnosis of pica is appropriate only if the individual is able to distinguish between nutritive foods and nonnutritive substances.

It is common for individuals with feeding and eating disorders to have anxiety and mood symptoms that are intimately and integrally tied to their feeding or eating disorder. Co-occurring mood disorders and anxiety and fear-related disorders are also common. Differential diagnosis in these cases can be complicated. If the anxiety or mood-related symptoms only exist as part of the feeding and eating disorder syndrome (e.g., beliefs of low self-worth related to body weight or shape, worry about binge eating), it is not appropriate to assign an additional diagnosis. For example, changes in appetite or weight can be a feature of major depressive disorder, however, in most cases of feeding and eating disorders, these symptoms are better explained by the feeding or eating disorder and should not be considered a feature of a distinct mood disorder. If the mood or anxiety symptoms also relate to other domains or are independent of episodes of eating disturbance, a separate diagnosis should be assigned if other diagnostic requirements are met. The key determination in the differential diagnosis is whether the symptom extends beyond and exists independent of the eating disorder.

Moreover, individuals with feeding and eating disorders may hold beliefs that are demonstrably untrue or not shared by others (e.g., an individual with anorexia nervosa claiming to be overweight at a BMI of 14 kg/m^2 or an individual with avoidant-restrictive food intake disorder fearing that a food causes extreme illness). At the extreme, they may appear to be delusional about their weight, shape, or eating behavior. When these fixed ideas are limited to symptoms related to the presenting eating disturbances, an additional diagnosis of delusional disorder or another primary psychotic disorder is not warranted. Individuals with feeding and eating disorders often report obsessive and perseverative thinking about weight and shape, may experience such thoughts as intrusive, and may also engage in compulsive behaviors such as vomiting or excessive exercise. If these thoughts and behaviors are limited to the core features of the feeding or eating disorder, an additional diagnosis of obsessive-compulsive disorder is not warranted. Body dysmorphic disorder is characterized by persistent preoccupation with one or more perceived defects or flaws in appearance that are either unnoticeable or only slightly noticeable to others. It is distinguished from the eating disorders in that no disturbance in eating is present and these concerns are focused on features other than overall weight, shape, and body size.

CO-OCCURRING DISORDERS

Feeding disorders are common among individuals with disorders of intellectual development and autism spectrum disorder. Current evidence suggests that the most common co-occurring disorders for avoidant-restrictive food intake disorder are autism spectrum disorder and attention deficit hyperactivity disorder. Anxiety and fear-related disorders and mood disorders are common among individuals across all feeding and eating disorders. The majority of individuals who present for mental health treatment have co-occurring conditions associated with the distress and impairment that brought them to care. In all cases, the central question is whether the symptom patterns are sufficiently distinct and independent to warrant two diagnoses (WHO, 2024).

DEVELOPMENTAL COURSE

Feeding and eating disorders occur across the life span, with feeding disorders most commonly emerging in childhood and eating disorders in later childhood and adolescence. The vast majority of cases of eating disorders emerge before 25 years (Ward et al., 2019). The extent to which early feeding disorders increase risk for subsequent eating disorders is unknown. Prognosis for individuals with feeding and eating disorders varies across diagnostic categories, with anorexia nervosa associated with the highest mortality rate of all mental disorders (Zipfel et al., 2015). However, individuals with anorexia nervosa who are younger or receive treatment after a short duration of symptoms appear to have better treatment outcomes compared with adults and those with a longer course of the disorder (Forsberg & Lock, 2015). As with most health conditions, prognosis is better the sooner individuals secure appropriate treatment.

ASSESSMENT

Accurate diagnosis enhances the likelihood that individuals will be referred to appropriate and evidence-informed care because much of our knowledge base about clinical care is built on results from studies evaluating treatments for individuals based on their clinical diagnosis. Given the multidetermined risk across all the feeding and eating disorders and the potential consequences for health and even mortality, a comprehensive multicomponent—and ideally multidisciplinary—assessment is vital.

The four dimensions of eating behavior, compensatory behavior, associated cognitions, and body weight are essential to inform the diagnosis of eating and feeding disorders. Because these dimensions are differentially relevant across disorders, because there is some continuity of symptom patterns across disorders, and because many individuals with eating disorders do not fit the well-defined syndromes of anorexia nervosa, bulimia nervosa, or binge eating disorder, Walsh and Sysko (2009) have argued that a broad dimensional approach to the diagnosis (and therefore assessment) of feeding and eating disorders is useful. The proposed broad categories for diagnosis of eating disorders consists of three broad categories, in a hierarchical relationship, anorexia nervosa and behaviorally similar disorders, bulimia nervosa and behaviorally similar disorders, binge eating disorder and behaviorally similar disorders, and a residual category of "eating disorder not otherwise specified." Although this approach to diagnosis has not been officially adopted by the *ICD-11*, the conceptual underpinnings informed its development, and the focus on these dimensions is useful in the assessment process as described here.

Body weight is most crucial for deciding between diagnoses like anorexia nervosa with a binge-purge pattern versus bulimia nervosa, as similar behavioral symptoms are present in both disorders. Obtaining the patient's weight and calculating BMI (weight in kg/height in m²) or BMI percentile in the case of younger patients ensures an accurate diagnosis. Calculators for assessing BMI and BMI-for-age are available online.

Before initiating treatment, a complete health assessment should be conducted for individuals who present with possible feeding and eating disorders. Many other health conditions can lead to symptoms that might appear to be part of a feeding or eating disorder. Ongoing assessment of medical complications that may emerge during the course of treatment is also good practice. This is especially true for individuals who are at very low weight and for individuals with binge eating and purging behaviors who are at risk for electrolyte disturbances. Individuals who seek treatment who are overweight (BMI > 25 kg/m²) or obese (BMI > 30 kg/m²), which includes the majority of individuals presenting with binge eating disorder, should be assessed for important medical sequelae such as type 2 diabetes, sleep apnea, and hypertension.

Assessing eating behaviors, preoccupation with food, and related weight and shape concerns are essential to developing an accurate diagnosis. First, it is essential to assess the specific disturbances in eating behavior in terms of the eating behavior and the associated experience of loss of control. Assessing the eating behavior will provide clarity in terms of the ways in which the eating behavior is problematic. The typical patterns of disturbance are eating too little food, eating only a few kinds of foods, eating excessively slowly, binge eating, chewing, spitting, and eating nonnutritive substances. Individuals with eating disorders do not typically consume nonnutritive substances, which is the defining feature of pica. The extent to which individuals describe loss of control over eating and distress related to their eating behavior is central to the assessment of binge eating. In addition to assessing disturbances in food intake, ascertaining whether and which compensatory behaviors are present is essential. Compensatory behaviors to explore include purging and non-purging behaviors. Typical purging behaviors are self-induced vomiting and the misuse of laxatives, diuretics, and enemas. Typical nonpurging compensatory behavior are excessive exercise and excessive physical activity throughout the day in the form of fidgeting and hyperactivity. Assessing the frequency of these behaviors will inform diagnosis and help frame treatment priorities.

One of the distinguishing features between feeding and eating disorders is that individuals with eating disorders describe obsessions and compulsions about food, eating, shape, and weight, whereas these disturbances are typically absent for individuals suffering from feeding disorders. Preoccupation with eating and body shape and weight concerns are commonly linked to larger issues of perfectionism, body dissatisfaction, impulse dysregulation, and internalized ideals of thinness—factors that are generally understood to be relevant in both the development and maintenance of eating disorder syndromes. Thus, distinguishing anorexia nervosa from avoidant-restrictive food intake disorder requires careful assessment of motivation and thoughtful probing to identify the intent behind the altered feeding or eating behavior. Because feeding and eating disorders can develop in early childhood and adolescence, some individuals have limited insight into their behavior. In these cases, it can be helpful to gather information from a reliable and trusted informant, typically a parent or caregiver, to assist in the differential diagnosis.

CULTURAL AND CONTEXTUAL CONSIDERATIONS

Cultural preoccupation with body shape and weight, and population increases in overweight and obesity globally, set a cultural stage that contributes significantly to risk for eating disorders. Anorexia nervosa tends to be more prevalent in high-income communities, with comparable rates across many Western and non-Western high-income countries. Bulimia nervosa and binge eating disorder have also been described globally; however, prevalence varies more widely than for anorexia nervosa, suggesting that sociocultural factors may play an even greater role in terms of risk for these disorders than anorexia nervosa. Rapid and significant trends in industrialization and globalization that contribute to changing gender roles, employment norms, food supply, and lifestyle appear to be the most salient sociocultural risk factors for eating disorders.

Despite the significant disability associated with feeding and eating disorders and their global prevalence, a substantial proportion of these disorders go undetected or untreated, even in high-resource countries and health systems. Many general health providers have limited knowledge, do not assess for feeding and eating disorders, or assume these disturbances are rare conditions that afflict only a narrow segment of the population (Hudson et al., 2007). The *ICD-11* provides clinical descriptions of a wider range of expression of eating disorders across cultures with the aim of increasing recognition and diagnosis of these disorders globally.

Differences exist in the prevalence of feeding and eating disorders, detection in clinical settings, and expression across cultures. When assessing eating disturbances, familiarity with cultural norms and practices will ensure that culturally sanctioned practices are not misunderstood or misconstrued as disorders. Certain cultures are vegetarian, some avoid pork and shellfish, some have holidays in which fasting plays a role in the religious practice, some eat soil or other nonfoods. Of course, when such practices are culturally sanctioned by an individual's family or community group (e.g., fasting during Ramadan or following the laws of kashruth), a diagnosis of a feeding or eating disorder is inappropriate unless the diagnostic threshold is met—that is, the disturbance is over and above what would be considered normative under the circumstances in that individual's cultural group. In practice, if clinicians are not familiar with an individual's cultural or religious practices, it can be helpful to obtain information from other family members to assess normative and disordered eating behaviors accurately.

GENDER-RELATED CONSIDERATIONS

Feeding disorders appear to occur at approximately equal rates across gender. When avoidant-restrictive food intake disorder co-occurs with autism spectrum disorder, there is a higher prevalence among males. This largely reflects the fact that males are more likely to receive a diagnosis of autism spectrum disorder. In the case of anorexia nervosa and bulimia nervosa, in most countries, women are at elevated risk compared with men, but the data are limited by the fact that most estimates of prevalence have been conducted in Western Europe and North America. Data based on previous diagnostic requirements provide lifetime estimates for anorexia nervosa, bulimia nervosa, and binge eating disorder of .9%, 1.5%, and 3.5% among women, and .3% .5%, and 2.0% among men (Hudson et al., 2007).

Although anorexia nervosa is more prevalent among females, it appears to be increasing among men globally, with some data suggesting that weight concerns and eating disturbances are more prevalent among men in some Asian and Eastern Mediterranean societies than in the Americas (Pike et al., 2013). In addition to the differential risk for developing an eating disorder for women versus men, some clinical differences exist by gender as well. The existing clinical conceptualization for eating disorders, particularly anorexia nervosa and bulimia nervosa, centers on the role of drive for thinness, and when men and boys preoccupied with achieving thinness with limited muscularity present for treatment, they are more readily recognized as having an eating disorder. For those males who have significant body image disturbance that is centered on an extreme desire for muscularity and low body fat, the differential diagnosis between anorexia nervosa and body dysmorphic disorder can be challenging in clinical practice (Hildebrandt et al., 2006).

PREVALENCE

The Global Burden of Disease Study (https://www.healthdata.org/gbd) has dramatically enhanced our understanding of the worldwide distribution and burden of anorexia nervosa and bulimia nervosa. It provides an estimate of burden of a given health condition based on an algorithm that incorporates years lived with the disorder, years of life lost due to the disorder, and associated degree of impairment. Within high-income countries, anorexia nervosa and bulimia nervosa combined have been ranked consistently as the 12th leading cause of disability adjusted life years (DALYs) for females aged 15 to 19. Within low- and middle-income countries, DALYs associated with anorexia nervosa and bulimia nervosa increased from a ranking of 58th to 46th place between 1990 to 2013 (Erskine et al., 2016). Despite lower prevalence rates, given the large population of India and China, along with the United States, these countries have the highest contributions of total DALYs caused by anorexia nervosa and bulimia nervosa among women aged 15 to 49 (Thomas et al., 2016).

Epidemiologic estimates are largely derived from studies in Western Europe and North America. Epidemiological data from Asia and Pacific Island countries remain scarce; the same holds true for Latin America and even more so for Africa. The rate of anorexia nervosa appears to be relatively stable in high-income countries, with the exception of a notable increase among females aged 15 to 19 (Smink et al., 2013). The most recent studies in Europe show that anorexia nervosa affects 1% to 4% of women in Europe; in the United States, the prevalence rate is approximately 0.8% in adults and 0.3% in adolescents (Swanson et al., 2011; Udo & Grilo, 2018). Rates of anorexia nervosa remain low in Africa (van Hoeken et al., 2016). The aggregated prevalence rate of bulimia nervosa is approximately 1% (range: 0.0–4.5%;

Hoek & van Hoeken, 2003). Men make up a slightly higher percentage of individuals with bulimia nervosa (Swanson et al., 2011; Udo & Grilo, 2018). Bulimia nervosa has been described in a variety of non-Western cultures (Nobakht & Dezhkam, 2000; Pike & Mizushima, 2005). Binge eating disorder is estimated to affect 1.6% of adolescents and between 0.8% and 2.8% of adults (Swanson et al., 2011; Udo & Grilo, 2018) and is more common among males than either anorexia nervosa or bulimia nervosa. Relative to other eating disorders, binge eating disorder is more prevalent across a variety of racial and ethnic groups (Wonderlich et al., 2009). Epidemiological research on avoidant-restrictive food intake disorder is scarce, and the data that exist report widely diverse estimates of prevalence. Even less is known about the prevalence of avoidant-restrictive food intake disorder across different racial and ethnic groups. Reliable prevalence estimates of pica and rumination-regurgitation disorder do not exist.

Given the prevalence of eating disorders and the diversity of individuals who experience these disturbances, it is good clinical practice to include a few questions regarding eating and weight concerns in primary care and when conducting all initial psychological assessments. Because many individuals feel embarrassed or ashamed about their eating or weight concerns, they may not initially volunteer this important clinical information. Early and routine assessment of these possible issues will help identify individuals for whom eating and weight concerns are a source of significant distress and impairment, which will be useful in developing a formulation and treatment plan.

KEY POINTS

- The *ICD-11* feeding and eating disorders grouping brings together disorders that share a common phenomenological foundation of disturbances in eating behaviors that are distinguished from each other by diverse patterns related to preoccupation with food, elevated body weight and shape concerns, eating, and compensatory behaviors.

- The inclusion of binge eating disorder, avoidant-restrictive food intake disorder, and rumination-regurgitation disorder in the *ICD-11* feeding and eating disorders grouping permits the identification of three specific syndromes not previously systematically described.

- The *ICD-11* explicitly relaxes requirements related to weight for anorexia nervosa and binge eating for bulimia nervosa and binge eating disorder. These changes are likely to result in more individuals being diagnosed with these disorders who experience substantial distress and dysfunction and could benefit from treatment.

- The lifespan approach to diagnosis of feeding and eating disorders captures the related and developmental nature of these disorders, with avoidant-restrictive food intake disorder and pica being more likely to develop in childhood and anorexia nervosa, bulimia nervosa, and binge eating disorder more commonly emerging in adolescence and early adulthood. The vast majority of individuals who develop a feeding or eating disorder in their lifetime will have done so by the age of 25.

- Global data suggest that feeding and eating disorders exist around the world. Population-based estimates are limited, but the extant data suggest that gender and cultural issues contribute substantially to eating disorders. Women from high-income countries continue to be at greatest risk, but rates appear to be increasing in non-Western and middle-income countries and among men.

REFERENCES

Al-Adawi, S., Baks, B., Bryant-Waugh, R., Claudino, A. M., Hay, P., Monteleone, P., Norring, C., Pike, K. M., Pilon, D. J., Herscovici, C. R., Reed, G. M., Rydelius, P.-A., Sharan, P., Thiels, C., Treasure, J., & Uher, R. (2013). Revision of *ICD*: Status update on feeding and eating disorders. *Advances in Eating Disorders: Theory, Research and Practice, 1*(1), 10–20. https://doi.org/10.1080/21662630.2013.742971

Claudino, A. M., Pike, K. M., Hay, P., Keeley, J. W., Evans, S. C., Rebello, T. J., Bryant-Waugh, R., Dai, Y., Zhao, M., Matsumoto, C., Herscovici, C. R., Mellor-Marsá, B., Stona, A. C., Kogan, C. S., Andrews, H. F., Monteleone, P., Pilon, D. J., Thiels, C., Sharan, P., . . . Reed, G. M. (2019). The classification of feeding and eating disorders in the *ICD-11*: Results of a field study comparing proposed *ICD-11* guidelines with existing *ICD-10* guidelines. *BMC Medicine, 17*(1), 93. https://doi.org/10.1186/s12916-019-1327-4

Erskine, H. E., Whiteford, H. A., & Pike, K. M. (2016). The global burden of eating disorders. *Current Opinion in Psychiatry, 29*(6), 346–353. https://doi.org/10.1097/YCO.0000000000000276

Fitzsimmons-Craft, E. E., Ciao, A. C., Accurso, E. C., Pisetsky, E. M., Peterson, C. B., Byrne, C. E., & Le Grange, D. (2014). Subjective and objective binge eating in relation to eating disorder symptomatology, depressive symptoms, and self-esteem among treatment-seeking adolescents with bulimia nervosa. *European Eating Disorders Review, 22*(4), 230–236. https://doi.org/10.1002/erv.2297

Forsberg, S., & Lock, J. (2015). Family-based treatment of child and adolescent eating disorders. *Child and Adolescent Psychiatric Clinics of North America, 24*(3), 617–629. https://doi.org/10.1016/j.chc.2015.02.012

Hildebrandt, T., Schlundt, D., Langenbucher, J., & Chung, T. (2006). Presence of muscle dysmorphia symptomology among male weightlifters. *Comprehensive Psychiatry, 47*(2), 127–135. https://doi.org/10.1016/j.comppsych.2005.06.001

Hoek, H. W., & van Hoeken, D. (2003). Review of the prevalence and incidence of eating disorders. *International Journal of Eating Disorders, 34*(4), 383–396. https://doi.org/10.1002/eat.10222

Hudson, J. I., Hiripi, E., Pope, H. G., Jr., & Kessler, R. C. (2007). The prevalence and correlates of eating disorders in the National Comorbidity Survey Replication. *Biological Psychiatry, 61*(3), 348–358. https://doi.org/10.1016/j.biopsych.2006.03.040

Mond, J. M., Latner, J. D., Hay, P. H., Owen, C., & Rodgers, B. (2010). Objective and subjective bulimic episodes in the classification of bulimic-type eating disorders: Another nail in the coffin of a problematic distinction. *Behaviour Research and Therapy, 48*(7), 661–669. https://doi.org/10.1016/j.brat.2010.03.020

Nobakht, M., & Dezhkam, M. (2000). An epidemiological study of eating disorders in Iran. *International Journal of Eating Disorders, 28*(3), 265–271. https://doi.org/10.1002/1098-108X(200011)28:3<265::AID-EAT3>3.0.CO;2-L

Palavras, M. A., Morgan, C. M., Borges, F. M., Claudino, A. M., & Hay, P. J. (2013). An investigation of objective and subjective types of binge eating episodes in a clinical sample of people with co-morbid obesity. *Journal of Eating Disorders, 1,* 26. https://doi.org/10.1186/2050-2974-1-26

Pike, K. M., & Dunne, P. E. (2015). The rise of eating disorders in Asia: A review. *Journal of Eating Disorders, 3,* 33. https://doi.org/10.1186/s40337-015-0070-2

Pike, K. M., Dunne, P. E., & Addai, E. (2013). Expanding the boundaries: Reconfiguring the demographics of the "typical" eating disordered patient. *Current Psychiatry Reports, 15*(11), 411. https://doi.org/10.1007/s11920-013-0411-2

Pike, K. M., & Mizushima, H. (2005). The clinical presentation of Japanese women with anorexia nervosa and bulimia nervosa: A study of the Eating Disorders Inventory-2. *International Journal of Eating Disorders, 37*(1), 26–31. https://doi.org/10.1002/eat.20065

Pike, K. M., Walsh, B. T., Vitousek, K., Wilson, G. T., & Bauer, J. (2003). Cognitive behavior therapy in the posthospitalization treatment of anorexia nervosa. *American Journal of Psychiatry, 160*(11), 2046–2049. https://doi.org/10.1176/appi.ajp.160.11.2046

Smink, F. R., van Hoeken, D., & Hoek, H. W. (2013). Epidemiology, course, and outcome of eating disorders. *Current Opinion in Psychiatry, 26*(6), 543–548. https://doi.org/10.1097/YCO.0b013e328365a24f

Sullivan, P. F. (1995). Mortality in anorexia nervosa. *The American Journal of Psychiatry, 152*(7), 1073–1074. https://doi.org/10.1176/ajp.152.7.1073

Swanson, S. A., Crow, S. J., Le Grange, D., Swendsen, J., & Merikangas, K. R. (2011). Prevalence and correlates of eating disorders in adolescents: Results from the national comorbidity survey replication adolescent supplement. *Archives of General Psychiatry, 68*(7), 714–723. https://doi.org/10.1001/archgenpsychiatry.2011.22

Thomas, J. J., Lee, S., & Becker, A. E. (2016). Updates in the epidemiology of eating disorders in Asia and the Pacific. *Current Opinion in Psychiatry, 29*(6), 354–362. https://doi.org/10.1097/YCO.0000000000000288

Thompson, K. A., DeVinney, A. A., Goy, C. N., Kuang, J., & Bardone-Cone, A. M. (2022). Subjective and objective binge episodes in relation to eating disorder and depressive symptoms among middle-aged women. *Eating and Weight Disorders, 27,* 1687–1694. https://doi.org/10.1007/s40519-021-01305-2

Udo, T., & Grilo, C. M. (2018). Prevalence and correlates of *DSM-5*–defined eating disorders in a nationally representative sample of U.S. adults. *Biological Psychiatry, 84*(5), 345–354. https://doi.org/10.1016/j.biopsych.2018.03.014

van Hoeken, D., Burns, J. K., & Hoek, H. W. (2016). Epidemiology of eating disorders in Africa. *Current Opinion in Psychiatry, 29*(6), 372–377. https://doi.org/10.1097/YCO.0000000000000274

Walsh, B. T., & Sysko, R. (2009). Broad categories for the diagnosis of eating disorders (BCD-ED): An alternative system for classification. *International Journal of Eating Disorders, 42*(8), 754–764. https://doi.org/10.1002/eat.20722

Ward, Z. J., Rodriguez, P., Wright, D. R., Austin, S. B., & Long, M. W. (2019). Estimation of eating disorders prevalence by age and associations with mortality in a simulated nationally representative U.S. cohort. *JAMA Network Open, 2*(10), e1912925–e1912925. https://doi.org/10.1001/jamanetworkopen.2019.12925

Watson, H. J., Fursland, A., Bulik, C. M., & Nathan, P. (2013). Subjective binge eating with compensatory behaviors: A variant presentation of bulimia nervosa. *International Journal of Eating Disorders, 46*(2), 119–126. https://doi.org/10.1002/eat.22052

Wilson, G. T., & Sysko, R. (2009). Frequency of binge eating episodes in bulimia nervosa and binge eating disorder: Diagnostic considerations. *International Journal of Eating Disorders, 42*(7), 603–610. https://doi.org/10.1002/eat.20726

Wolfe, B. E., Baker, C. W., Smith, A. T., & Kelly-Weeder, S. (2009). Validity and utility of the current definition of binge eating. *International Journal of Eating Disorders, 42*(8), 674–686. https://doi.org/10.1002/eat.20728

Wonderlich, S. A., Gordon, K. H., Mitchell, J. E., Crosby, R. D., & Engel, S. G. (2009). The validity and clinical utility of binge eating disorder. *International Journal of Eating Disorders, 42*(8), 687–705. https://doi.org/10.1002/eat.20719

World Health Organization. (2023). *ICD-11 for mortality and morbidity statistics* (Version: 01/2023). https://icd.who.int/browse11/l-m/en#/

World Health Organization. (2024). *Clinical descriptions and diagnostic requirements for ICD-11 mental, behavioural and neurodevelopmental disorders.* https://www.who.int/publications/i/item/9789240077263

Zipfel, S., Giel, K. E., Bulik, C. M., Hay, P., & Schmidt, U. (2015). Anorexia nervosa: Aetiology, assessment, and treatment. *The Lancet Psychiatry, 2*(12), 1099–1111. https://doi.org/10.1016/S2215-0366(15)00356-9

13

Bodily Distress Disorder

Oye Gureje and Akin Ojagbemi

OVERARCHING LOGIC

We are all aware at times of bodily or somatic sensations or symptoms, including bodily discomfort or mildly painful sensations. Unless these are associated
with an ongoing physical illness, these sensations are typically transient and
fairly easily ignored or forgotten. When such bodily concerns become a source
of persistent worry or bother (in excess of what can be attributed to a medical
condition that may be causing or contributing to the symptoms), they can
become a source of suffering and disability. The diagnosis of bodily distress
disorder in the 11th revision of the *International Classification of Diseases* (*ICD-11*;
World Health Organization [WHO], 2023) is intended to differentiate between
persons with distressing bodily symptoms to which excessive attention is
directed and who may benefit from mental health treatment from those with
somatic experiences that are less disabling and of less personal significance
(Gureje & Reed, 2016). In bodily distress disorder, somatic symptoms are
thought to represent an expression of emotional and cognitive disturbances,
for which a range of therapeutic responses may be indicated.

The immediate precursors of bodily distress disorder are several diagnostic
categories in the *ICD-10* grouping of somatoform disorders. In fact, bodily
distress disorder replaces nearly the entire *ICD-10* grouping of somatoform
disorders (except for hypochondriacal disorder, which has been moved to
the *ICD-11* grouping of obsessive-compulsive and related disorders). The main

https://doi.org/10.1037/0000392-013
A Psychological Approach to Diagnosis: Using the ICD-11 as a Framework, G. M. Reed,
P. L.-J. Ritchie, and A. Maercker (Editors)

common features of somatoform disorders in *ICD-10* were repeated presentation of physical symptoms, together with persistent requests for medical investigations despite repeated negative findings and reassurances by doctors that the symptoms have no physical basis. The nature and extent of the symptoms or the distress and the preoccupation of the patient were not explained by any medical condition that might be present. To a large extent, *ICD-11* bodily distress disorder also replaces neurasthenia, which was a specific category in *ICD-10*. The central feature of neurasthenia was a distressing feeling of persistent exhaustion commonly accompanied by a range of other symptoms, such as muscular pain, headache, sleep problems, and irritability. The concept of neurasthenia also had significant overlap with depressive disorders.

Many of the different categories included under the *ICD-10* grouping of somatoform disorders (i.e., somatization disorder, undifferentiated somatoform disorder, somatoform autonomic dysfunction, persistent somatoform pain disorder) were difficult to distinguish from one another due to their imprecise boundaries. The overlapping features of these disorders meant that even though different labels were given to them, clinicians did not distinguish among them in terms of management. Moreover, disorders of somatic distress most commonly present in general health care settings where providers who are not mental health specialists had difficulty making what may amount to subtle, or even trivial, distinctions among them. This appears to have been partly responsible for finding that the utility of the *ICD-10* somatoform disorder categories was generally poor (Dimsdale et al., 2011). In developing the *ICD-11*, bringing these categories together under a single diagnostic rubric in a way that emphasizes the behaviors involved and their functional consequences was a logical way of responding to a real need for improved clinical utility.

Previously, diagnosis of somatoform disorders was largely premised on the notion that the somatic symptoms could not be ascribed to the presence of a physical or medical disorder. Thus being "medically unexplained" was the defining feature of the disorders, and especially of the prototypical condition of the grouping: somatization disorder. One problem with this premise is the separation it suggests between mental and physical conditions as distinct and non-overlapping states of ill health. However, the reality is that medical conditions and mental disorders, including mental disorders with somatic expressions, do co-occur, and making the diagnosis of one does not exclude the need to consider the other. Indeed, this dichotomy was frequently communicated to patients, and the implied doubt that their illness was "real" often led patients with somatoform disorders to resent the diagnosis, undermining their trust in the health care professionals who made it. A related problem with basing somatoform disorder diagnoses on the "medically unexplained" nature of the symptoms is that it is not always possible to exclude, reliably and definitively, the possibility that a comorbid or undetected medical condition is causing the symptoms. In fact, evidence suggests that whether bothersome somatic symptoms are medically explained or unexplained is unrelated to either subsequent health care utilization or to health status at 6-month follow-up (Creed, 2011b).

A major focus of *ICD-11* has therefore been to define and classify bodily distress disorder based on the presence of specific psychological and behavioral features rather than the absence of a medical explanation for the individual's experience. This also allows the threshold for the condition to be set in a way that encompasses persons with distressing but mild symptoms and associated functional impairment while avoiding the medicalization of commonly occurring but relatively nontroubling somatic concerns (Creed & Gureje, 2012). It also avoids the rather simplistic approach of labeling somatic symptoms as either specifically associated with a physical illness or the result of a psychological condition or state (Sharpe & Carson, 2001). The *Clinical Descriptions and Diagnostic Requirements for ICD-11 Mental, Behavioural and Neurodevelopmental Disorders* (*CDDR*; WHO, 2024) acknowledge that bodily or somatic symptoms may be common manifestations of some other mental disorders, especially mood disorders and anxiety and fear-related disorders, and that these other mental disorders may co-occur with disorders of bodily or somatic symptoms. Bodily distress disorder in the *ICD-11* is thus a distinct clinical entity that may co-occur with either other mental disorders or with other medical conditions. This conceptualization avoids unhelpful mind–body dualism and therefore provides a more constructive basis for collaboration between the health care provider and the patient. The new *ICD-11* category of bodily distress disorder appears to have good predictive validity, outperforming the diagnosis of somatic symptom disorder in the fifth edition of the *Diagnostic and Statistical Manual of Mental Disorders* in being able to differentiate disordered from nondisordered persons (Schumacher et al., 2017). An *ICD-11* field study also indicated that mental health professionals were able to use the *ICD-11* category of bodily distress disorder more accurately and rated it as having greater clinical utility than *ICD-10* somatoform disorders (Keeley et al., 2023).

A PSYCHOLOGICAL APPROACH TO BODILY DISTRESS DISORDER

The presence of bothersome somatic symptoms is an essential feature of bodily distress disorder. Moreover, as a mental disorder, there are also important psychological features that must be present for a diagnosis to be made (Rief & Isaac, 2007). The key psychological features of bodily distress disorder are distress and excessive attention to bodily sensations and worry and fear about the import of the somatic sensation or that any physical activity may damage the body. Distress is a state of emotional pain and anxiety that, in the context of a somatic symptom, is associated with fear of what the symptom may indicate or what it forebodes. There is excessive worry or fear that the symptoms may become more troubling and may result in greater negative impact on the persons' life. There may be catastrophic interpretations or attributions, with the affected persons ascribing many difficulties to the symptoms and expressing fears that those difficulties are going to get worse if there is no relief from the symptoms. Indeed, the tendency to make such catastrophic interpretations of somatic sensations is a risk factor for developing diagnosable disorders of somatic preoccupation (Woud et al., 2016).

Persons with bodily distress disorder may entertain the fear that an underlying disease, even a serious one, may be producing the symptoms, but they are not fixated on that fear and can generally be reassured that no serious disease is present. What is more persistent in bodily distress disorder is the fear that the symptoms will continue or perhaps get worse. In seeking medical attention or help, the person with the disorder is looking for specific treatment of the symptoms and may or may not be reassured in the short term that their fear that the symptoms may persist or get worse is misplaced and not supported by clinical examination or investigations and that no specific medical treatment is indicated. If they are reassured, however, this is generally temporary as the symptoms tend to persist or recur.

In persons with bodily distress disorder, a consequence of the preoccupation with the symptoms, the unreasonable fear attached to them, and the related worry about the course of the symptoms is a disturbance in carrying out usual activities (Gureje et al., 1997)—that is, there are limitations in functioning. Typically, the degree of functional impairment is disproportional to what would be expected based on the somatic symptoms alone but rather reflect the psychological attributes of the disorder. This catastrophic or exaggerated reaction to the reported symptoms is often an important observation that may help in the decision of whether to make a diagnosis of bodily distress disorder even when a medical condition that may have similar somatic manifestations is known to be present. The presence of the psychological features of the disorder and their association with functional limitations are the characteristics that make bodily distress disorder a mental disorder (Rief & Isaac, 2007). Bodily distress disorder, defined using the presence of cognitive, affective, and behavioral symptoms, along with the bothersome somatic symptoms, provides a more reliable basis for the assessment of patients with physical complaints and therefore increases the likelihood that those who experience it will receive appropriate treatment (Rief et al., 2010).

A diagnosis of bodily distress disorder requires the presence of one or more distressing bodily symptoms. Although it is common to find that individuals affected by burdensome somatic problems may have multiple symptoms that vary over time, some may have only one nagging symptom, usually pain or fatigue (Fröhlich et al., 2006). The affected person is preoccupied with the symptoms, with their attention constantly or intermittently directed at the distraction or limitations imposed by the symptoms. The experience tends to last for at least several months, during which the person may seek help repeatedly from health care providers whose reassurance tends to provide, at best, only temporary relief to the patient. The bodily symptoms and related distress and preoccupation result in significant impairment in personal, family, social, educational, occupational, or other important areas of functioning (Gureje et al., 1997). A comorbid medical condition that potentially explains or contributes to the bodily symptoms may or may not be present. In the presence of such a medical condition, for bodily distress disorder to be diagnosed, the individual must exhibit greater distress, preoccupation with symptoms, and functional impairment than would be expected for individuals with a medical condition that is similar in nature and severity.

Bodily distress disorder encompasses a range of severity, emphasizing its underlying dimensional nature (Creed, 2011a). A determination of whether the appropriate diagnosis is mild, moderate, or severe bodily distress disorder is based on an evaluation of the severity of the specific problems presented. Severity is assessed along the embedded dimensional features of the disorder. These include the degree of associated distress or preoccupation with the bodily symptoms, the amount of time and energy the individual devotes to focusing on the symptoms and their consequences, and the extent of functional limitation that can be ascribed to the disorder. By assessing these features and forming an overall impression of their intensity, the clinician is able to place the affected individual along the severity continuum both at the point of initial diagnosis as well as during the course of the disorder when a determination of the degree of improvement or lack thereof is desired (Creed, 2011a).

The provision of categories corresponding to different levels of severity for bodily distress disorder in the *ICD-11* is intended partly to enhance clinical utility in diverse health care settings. In general health care settings, patients with bothersome somatic concerns are more likely to present when their condition is at an early stage of development and therefore more likely to be of mild to moderate severity. Almost 50% of persons with burdensome somatic symptoms presenting in general health care settings will continue to be troubled by the condition over a 12-month period (Gureje & Simon, 1999; Rief et al., 2010). By the time these individuals are referred to a mental health professional, there has often been a series of unproductive interactions with the health care system that have been frustrating for both the patient and the health professionals involved. The psychological and behavioral features of the disorder are often well entrenched by that time, and the condition is more likely to be severe, with a narrowing of interests such that the bodily symptoms and their consequences may have become the nearly exclusive focus of the individual's life, with pervasive and severe functional consequences.

PRESENTATION AND SYMPTOM PATTERNS

The most common somatic symptoms associated with bodily distress disorder include pain (e.g., musculoskeletal pain, backache, headaches), fatigue, gastrointestinal symptoms, and respiratory symptoms, although patients may be preoccupied with any other bodily symptoms. For example, symptoms related to sexual organs, such as loss of semen and vaginal discharge, have been described in some cultural groups (Patel et al., 2008). The individual may provide a rather vague description of the symptoms or may be able to describe the symptoms quite specifically, even though it may be difficult for the clinician to account for the symptoms in precise anatomical or physiological terms.

Once the presence of burdensome somatic symptoms is established, it is essential to elicit the associated psychological features, such as worry, unreasonable fear, anxiety, preoccupation, and catastrophic interpretation, as well as the extent to which the problems being experienced interfere with the performance of usual activities. Preoccupation with the symptoms is indicated by the amount of attention the individual gives to them both in terms of cognitive ruminations and behaviors or in terms of efforts to find solutions to the problems, most frequently by seeking repeated clinical examinations and investigations so intervention can be provided that would get rid of the symptoms. The repeated help-seeking often results in more clinical assessments than are warranted, and whatever treatment is given fails to provide sufficient or permanent relief to the individual. The search for a solution or an alleviation of the symptom is typical of persons with bodily distress disorder in contrast to hypochondriasis, where affected persons make repeated clinical contacts to disconfirm their fears that the symptoms they experience may be indicative of a serious, progressive, or life-threatening disease.

The level of severity should be established based on the degree of distress or preoccupation with bodily symptoms, the amount of time and energy the individual devotes to focusing on the symptoms and their consequences, and the degree of functional impairment (WHO, 2024). These dimensions tend to run in parallel: As one becomes more severe, the others tend to become more severe as well, however, this is not always the case. For example, even though the presence of multiple symptoms is likely to be associated with a higher level of distress than a single somatic symptom, in some instances a single symptom may be associated with extreme distress and considerable limitations in functioning.

Therefore, it is important for clinicians, in making a judgment about severity, to consider the total clinical picture and make a global rating. This rating will be informed by the prominence of any of the main clinical features of bodily distress disorder, such as symptom intensity, distress, fear, and limitation in functioning. History of health care seeking related the presenting somatic symptoms and other somatic symptoms should be assessed carefully (Tomenson et al., 2012), as well as the individual's reaction to the responses received from health care professionals, which they often experience as highly negative and blaming.

Persons with **mild bodily distress disorder** pose the greatest challenge in differentiating their symptoms from somatic experiences and concerns that are within the rage of normal functioning (WHO, 2024). Individuals with a mild form of bodily distress disorder will meet the diagnostic requirements for the disorder and have bodily symptoms that have been present for most days during a period of at least 3 months. They may have single or multiple symptoms, the location or nature of which may have changed during the period. What marks the disorder as mild is that, even though the symptoms are distressing, the individual spends only a limited amount of time focusing on them (e.g., no more than 1 or 2 hours per day) and is able to focus on other unrelated topics. Associated functional impairment is also mild (e.g., strain in relationships, less effective academic or occupational functioning, abandonment of specific leisure activities). The affected person may be reassured by the explanation provided by a health care provider that the symptoms are not indicative of an undetected serious illness. Sometimes, the affected person may themselves be able to attribute the experience of the symptoms to stressful life events or circumstances.

Unlike mild bodily distress disorder, **moderate bodily distress disorder** is clearly outside the range of normal somatic experience. Affected persons tend to have a greater fear and anxiety about the impact the untreated symptoms may have on their lives and greater efforts are therefore required by the health care provider to reassure them. The individual's preoccupation with the distressing symptoms and their consequences (e.g., limitations in activities) consumes a substantial amount of time and energy (e.g., several hours per day) and is typically associated with frequent medical visits to seek a solution. There is sufficient functional impairment to have a marked effect on the individual's life (e.g., relationship conflict, performance problems at work, abandonment of a range of social and leisure activities; WHO, 2024).

In **severe bodily distress disorder**, there is pervasive and persistent preoccupation with the distressing symptoms and their consequences such that the individual's interests may have narrowed to the extent that the bodily symptoms and their consequences become the nearly exclusive focus of the individual's life (WHO, 2024). Worry about the impact of the symptoms is typically obvious. The individual often describes their symptoms in great detail, with attempts to justify their catastrophic reactions to them. The affected person is clearly suffering and is more likely to seek care from multiple health providers, finding the reassurance provided by one unsatisfactory and so seeking for more investigations and the "correct" diagnosis from another. Multiple areas of functioning are severely impaired (e.g., the individual is unable to work, has alienated all or nearly all friends and family, and has abandoned nearly all social and leisure activities).

CLINICAL CASES

The following three example clinical cases are intended to illustrate typical presenting features of bodily distress disorder at different levels of severity. These case examples are based on the authors' real experiences, but they are composites that do not represent specific individuals. The identities of any individual patients involved in these examples have been properly disguised to protect their confidentiality.

Case Example: Mild Bodily Distress Disorder

Ms. Clement, a 40-year-old married female, was referred by her general practitioner for psychological assessment. She explains that she has had pain on the soles of her feet for about 6 months. She remembers that the pain started when she first visited a fertility clinic with her husband. Ms. Clement and her husband have been married for 4 years and want to start a family, but she has not become pregnant despite all their efforts. She describes the pain as limited to the soles of her feet and as a dull pain that sometimes also feels like pins and needles. The pain gets worse when she has to walk a distance of more than 100 meters or has to stand for more than about 15 minutes. She takes four 200-mg tablets of ibuprofen when she needs to take a much longer walk and reports that she gets temporary relief from the pain. She is reassured that her pain is likely not due to anything serious, although she has been somewhat distressed that the tests her doctor has conducted have not been able to identify its cause. She notes that her pain does not really interfere with her work as she is still able to continue with her usual activities except those that involve walking long distances or standing for long periods. Ms. Clement and her husband agree that the stress associated with trying to become pregnant and being unsuccessful might be contributing to her pain.

Case Example: Moderate Bodily Distress Disorder

Mr. Lewis is a 41-year-old unmarried man who works as an office clerk. He was referred for evaluation by a gastroenterologist from whom he sought care because of abdominal discomfort and changes in bowel habits. He described a persistent feeling of bloating and the need to visit the toilet frequently without passing much stool. He reports that his symptoms started just over 3 years ago. He is distressed by the symptoms, especially because his frequent visits to the toilet sometimes affects his ability to carry out his work as an office clerk, and his supervisor has complained about his spending so much time away from his desk. His symptoms have gotten worse during the past 2 months, and he has called in sick twice to have time to empty his bowels properly. He takes multiple doses of an over-the-counter laxative on his days off. He has consulted three physicians and has undergone several investigations. He had felt reassured that nothing showed up in the abdominal scans and stool tests, but his relief did not last long. He has recently taken interest in watching medical documentaries, which led him to inquire about exploratory laparotomy surgery, which he hopes might lead to proper identification of the cause of the problem, enabling effective treatment. Apart from his preoccupation and worries about his symptoms, Mr. Lewis complains that he feels fatigued easily and has sometimes been uninterested in going out or seeing friends. Mr. Lewis explains that his hesitancy to participate in social events is related to his need to have access to a toilet. He does not report other symptoms of depression. He says that he is happy with his life, and everything would be fine if he could just resolve his bowel problems.

Case Example: Severe Bodily Distress Disorder

Ms. Johnson is a 34-year-old unmarried woman who works as a cashier at a nearby supermarket. She was referred by her primary care physician because of persistent pain and discomfort during the past 5 years. Looking very worried, she explains that she feels a dull pain that radiates from both of her upper limbs to her chest and then to her lower limbs. She also complains of a sensation of crawling just under her scalp. She experiences episodes of dizziness at work, which often necessitate frequent breaks. She has missed work due to these symptoms several times during the past few weeks and is now concerned that she might lose her job. She is preoccupied by her symptoms and distressed by the effects they are having on her ability to carry out her daily activities. She has visited more than 10 doctors during the past 5 years, including an expert in Chinese medicine, to try to find out what is causing her symptoms and to get some relief. During this time, she has had numerous investigations that failed to detect any disease that could explain her symptoms. She has so far not been reassured by the visits to the doctors and the negative findings of the investigations and says she is sure they are missing something that could be treated and provide relief from her pain. Ms. Johnson has no previous history of mental health consultation, and apart from the episodes of dizziness, she had no other symptoms suggestive of anxiety and depression. Ms. Johnson says she has so far had very difficult relationships with men, which she blames on her undiagnosed medical problems. She is not currently in a relationship. She says she would definitely be unable to handle a relationship with a man when she is constantly having to cope with her pain and discomfort. She used to be part of a group of close friends who went out together on a regular basis, but she does not have time to see them anymore because she has to focus on finding out what is wrong with her; she therefore feels like they no longer have much in common. She has stopped exercising, which she used to do an almost daily basis, because she is afraid that this will make her symptoms worse.

ASSESSMENT

For individuals presenting with bothersome and distressing bodily symptoms, a detailed assessment by interview is required. In general, assessment should include a history of the symptoms, their number, their duration, and any associated pain or discomfort. The assessment should determine whether the symptoms are examples of commonly occurring somatic concerns that are often transient and do not generally lead to clinical encounters or, if they do, rarely to repeated encounters. It is important to note what factors may have been noticed by the individual that aggravate or relieve the symptoms. Individuals with bodily distress disorder may be able to indicate whether their symptoms occur in relation to any type of activity, stressor, or recent life event. The interpretation the individual gives to the symptoms should be obtained, as well as whether previous medical help has been sought and investigations conducted.

It is important to establish a therapeutic alliance with these patients, and clinicians must frame interview questions in a nonstigmatizing and non-embarrassing way to increase patient comfort and enhance their engagement in the diagnostic process. In being referred to a psychologist or other mental health professional by a general practitioner or other medical professional, the idea that these patients' symptoms are not real or are "all in their head" will often have been communicated, even if unintentionally. Therefore, these individuals may approach the encounter with a mental health professional in a negative and defensive way, which must be overcome. The clinician should communicate that they take the symptoms seriously and are not doubting the patient's experience. It is important to use familiar language, avoiding as much as possible the use of technical terminology. For example, it would be more understandable to the average person to say "physical symptoms" rather than "somatic symptoms" or to say "your thoughts about these symptoms" rather than "negative cognitions." The clinician should allow the patient to provide details about all symptoms they may have. A family member or significant other may also be available to provide information that helps to understand the extent to which the symptoms have been a source of concern, distress, or worry as well as the pathway of help seeking. The clinician should pay attention to verbal and nonverbal behaviors that may provide indications of the patient's level of distress, preoccupation, and fears. Particular attention should be paid to requests for investigations by the patient because they may indicate beliefs about possible causation.

Other than establishing the presence of somatic symptoms, making a diagnosis of bodily distress disorder also requires the elicitation of associated distress, worry, or preoccupation. Thus, the patient should be asked how much worry or distress is associated with each of the symptoms, using their own assessment of whether the worry or distress has been mild, moderate, or severe. A detailed description is required about the level and length of psychological distress and how much attention the symptoms have elicited. It is sometimes possible to get a sense of the patient's level of worry or fear about the symptoms and what they may indicate through facial expression, general comportment, and tone of voice. Preoccupation is indicated by attention being frequently or constantly directed toward the symptoms. The individual may find it difficult to switch their attention away from the symptoms, irrespective of the activity at hand.

Fear and preoccupation may be related to the manner in which the symptoms are being interpreted. Rather than seeing a particular pain or other bodily sensation as merely troubling, the patient may fear that it is going to get much worse or that it is indicative of cancer. Even if examinations and investigations conducted by the clinician and other health professionals convince the patient that the attribution of the pain to possible cancer is incorrect, the patient may nevertheless continue to fear that the symptom will get worse and may therefore seek more investigations or treatment from another clinician. The extent to which the patient continues to be troubled by the symptoms or to harbor the fear that they may get worse will determine how often or how many times the patient seeks further investigations or the help of other clinicians.

Patients should be interviewed to get a full picture of the ways in which the symptoms and associated psychological factors have led to any decline in the performance of roles or functions. The severity of symptoms, the intensity of the worry or fear and preoccupation, and the extent to which time and resources are devoted to seeking investigations into the cause of the symptoms all influence the extent to which other activities are given up and the level of functional impairment that accompanies the bodily symptoms. The consequence may vary from mild impairment to relatively severe disability, especially among patients with numerous somatic symptoms. As the case of Ms. Clement shows, mild impairment is often limited to failing to perform an expected social role because the mind is distracted by a preoccupation with the bodily symptoms. On the other hand, and as exemplified in the case of Mr. Lewis, moderate impairment may be indicated by several days of calling off sick as a result of the symptoms and abandonment of significant social and leisure activities. Persons with severe impairment may, like Mr. Johnson, give up their work as a result of the symptoms or have experienced great difficulties in performing usual activities across several domains. There is some evidence for a dose–response relationship between number of symptoms and extent of disability (Harris et al., 2009). In assessing severity, it is important for the clinician to make use of all information available from the clinical assessment to make a global rating of severity. This will include a consideration of symptom intensity, distress, fear, and limitation in functioning.

The adoption of a dimensional approach to conceptualizing bodily distress disorder, encompassing the number of somatic concerns as well as behavioral and cognitive features, helps to avoid medicalization of innocuous and relatively nontroubling somatic symptoms, which are common. This dimensional approach encompasses the broad spectrum of burdensome somatic concerns, from mild to very severe, without the need to create discrete categories based on the specific symptomatic presentation, as in the *ICD-10*. Although these dimensions tend to run in parallel—as one becomes more severe, so do the others—this is not always the case. For example, although severe bodily distress disorder tends to be associated with numerous distressing bodily symptoms, some individuals experience extreme distress about a single somatic symptom.

Detailed history is required about the occurrence of any other mental health condition, especially mood disorders and anxiety and fear-related disorders. If any other conditions are present, it is important to establish their temporal relationship to the burdensome somatic concerns and whether the two conditions only occur together or have occurred at different times as well. If mood and anxiety symptoms are present, the clinician needs to determine whether they meet the diagnostic requirements for a mood disorder or an anxiety and fear-related disorder. Establishing the temporal relationship of the occurrence of mood or anxiety symptoms and of burdensome somatic concerns is important in determining whether the diagnosis of a mood disorder or an anxiety or fear-related disorder is sufficient to account for the patient's problems or whether a co-occurring diagnosis of bodily distress disorder is also appropriate. When another mental health condition is present concurrently with bodily distress disorder, it may be difficult to determine which of them accounts for functional impairment that may be noted. It is likely that one condition makes the impact of the other worse. However, some understanding of the impact of one or the other may be possible if a clear temporal relationship can be established.

In view of the importance of excluding any possible physical health causation of the symptoms, assessment by a physician is generally important. The result of any investigations conducted as part of such assessment may be available in the patient's medical records or may be obtained from the physician. Clear information should be provided to the patient about why these assessments and investigations are being conducted. However, it is also important not to request that investigations that have already been properly conducted be repeated or to order fresh ones that are not relevant or essential just because the patient demands them. Unnecessary investigations sometimes only serve to reinforce the patient's belief that there is indeed an underlying physical health condition yet to be detected. When the results of investigations are negative, they should be presented and explained to the patient in a way to provide relief and not as an indication of failure of the tests. The presence of a comorbid medical condition, even one with similar symptoms with those of the presenting somatic concerns, does not exclude the possibility of a diagnosis of bodily distress disorder. For example, a patient may have a pain condition for which there is some radiological evidence of underlying pathology. However, the diagnosis of bodily distress disorder may be justified if the clinician determines that the psychological symptoms of distress, worry, fear, and preoccupation shown by the patient are in excess of what would be expected as a result of the pain that may be solely due to the pathology shown on the radiological evidence.

COMMON CO-OCCURRING DISORDERS AND DIFFERENTIAL DIAGNOSIS

Persons with mood disorders or those with anxiety and fear-related disorders often have multiple somatic complaints as manifestations of their condition. Such persons may be preoccupied with the somatic symptoms, and, especially in primary care settings (Goldberg et al., 2017), the symptoms may be their main presenting complaints. On the other hand, patients with bodily distress disorder will commonly be afraid, have worry and preoccupation, and may also have depressed mood as a result of their burdensome somatic concerns. For these reasons, it is important to conduct a full assessment to decide whether somatic symptoms occur exclusively in the context of the mood or anxiety symptoms or at other times as well. If the former is the case, and sufficient symptoms are present to establish the diagnosis of a mood disorder or an anxiety or fear-related disorder, then a diagnosis of bodily distress disorder is generally not justified. If burdensome somatic concerns occur when mood and anxiety symptoms are absent or insufficient to make a diagnosis and seem to be a part of the psychological manifestations of the somatic concerns, then a diagnosis of bodily distress disorder is typically appropriate.

There is evidence that a dose–response relationship exists between number of somatic symptoms and prevalence of mood disorders or anxiety and fear-related disorders. However, several lines of evidence support the distinction between bodily distress disorder and both mood disorders and anxiety and fear-related disorders. Only 50% to 60% of patients with somatoform disorders have co-occurring mood disorders or anxiety and fear-related disorders (Kato et al., 2010), and there is evidence that when patients with somatoform disorders benefit from either psychological or antidepressant treatment, the benefit is not mediated through a reduction of depressive or anxiety symptoms (Escobar et al., 2010; Kato et al., 2010; Kroenke, 2007; Kroenke & Swindle, 2000). When both sets of symptoms are present in a patient, it is important to establish whether, on the basis of temporally distinct onset of each disorder, a co-occurring diagnosis of the appropriate mood or anxiety or fear-related disorder and bodily distress disorder is indicated. When somatic symptoms are a part of a mood or anxiety disorder, the treatment of the latter should result in a relief from the former. On the other hand, when bodily distress disorder is clearly present, even in the context of a mood or anxiety disorder, it is important to develop a treatment plan that addresses both conditions. This is because, as earlier indicated, the effective treatment of one does not always translate to a relief from the other (Escobar et al., 2010; Kato et al., 2010; Kroenke, 2007; Kroenke & Swindle, 2000).

During panic attacks, patients may experience a range of anxiety and somatic symptoms. The temporal clustering of the symptoms and their rapid onset should make it possible to differentiate those episodes from bodily distress disorder, where the somatic symptoms will generally have occurred over a much longer period. The symptom pattern may also help the clinician to differentiate the conditions because panic attacks are typically characterized by somatic symptoms related to autonomic arousal.

Hypochondriasis, which in *ICD-10* was classified as a somatoform disorder, is classified in *ICD-11* in the grouping of obsessive-compulsive and related disorders. In addition to frequent co-occurrence (Fink et al., 2004), hypochondriasis shares several features with bodily distress disorder. These include similar cognitive perceptual styles and several risk factors (Noyes et al., 2006; Rief et al., 1998). Nevertheless, hypochondriasis, also referred to as health anxiety disorder, is differentiated from bodily distress disorder by a greater focus of affected persons on the possibility of having one or more serious, progressive, or life-threatening illnesses rather than on specific symptoms and their impact. Whereas patients with bodily distress disorder are preoccupied with their symptoms and seek medical attention to remove the symptoms, those with hypochondriasis have persistent fear about the presence of an underlying disease and therefore seek medical investigations to disconfirm its presence. Patients with bodily distress disorder are eager for a solution that will result in the alleviation of the symptoms; in contrast, those with hypochondriasis may paradoxically be so fearful of the import of their symptoms and what may be found through clinical examination that they avoid medical appointments. Making the distinction is important because there is some indication that hypochondriasis may be more likely than bodily distress disorder to respond to certain classes of antidepressants (Stein et al., 2016; van den Heuvel et al., 2014).

Persons with body dysmorphic disorder are concerned about defects in some part of their bodies rather than fear of having a disease, as may be indicated by somatic symptoms. When individuals with body dysmorphic disorder seek medical attention, it is typically a surgical intervention or other treatment to alter the defect and not because of concern about specific symptoms or for the possible detection and treatment of an underlying disease.

Complaints about somatic symptoms are central to conditions such as irritable bowel syndrome and fibromyalgia. However, persons with these conditions may not display a high level of preoccupation and unreasonable fear regarding the symptoms they experience and can thus be distinguished from persons with bodily distress disorder. There are also specific symptom patterns that are more characteristic of these conditions. For example, in addition to abdominal pains, patients with irritable bowel syndrome will commonly have constipation or diarrhea as the focus of their concerns. In fibromyalgia, even though other symptoms such as fatigue and mood disturbance may be present, the focus is most commonly on multiple musculoskeletal pains. For both conditions, symptom-based treatments are often helpful. As indicated earlier, if medical conditions with somatic manifestations are nevertheless accompanied by disproportionate fear and preoccupations, an additional diagnosis of bodily distress disorder may be appropriate.

DEVELOPMENTAL COURSE

Bothersome somatic symptoms may occur in children (Garralda, 2011). These are most commonly gastrointestinal symptoms, such as abdominal pain, nausea, or vomiting. Children are more likely to have recurrent single rather than persistent multiple symptoms. The clinician should assess any associated emotional difficulties carefully and also consider whether these behaviors are being reinforced by parental responses, including excessive worry, overprotectiveness, and overinvolvement.

Somatic complaints are common among older adults. The clinical challenge is to be able to distinguish somatic concerns that indicate bodily distress disorder from those that could be manifestations of a medical condition and also not to dismiss such concerns based on the idea that aches and pains are simply part of the aging process. Pain conditions or multiple complaints across several body parts are the most common presentations of bodily distress disorder in older adults. When multiple pains are in fact related to problems associated with age, most older adults can be helped to find coping strategies rather than the pains becoming a focus of persistent concerns and worry. Elderly patients with multiple burdensome somatic symptoms more suggestive of bodily distress disorder are likely to seek more frequent primary care consultation, have poorer health status, more likely to be hospitalized, and have an increased mortality rate (Hausteiner-Wiehle et al., 2011). Although persistence of burdensome somatic symptoms among individuals presenting in general health care settings is common (approximately 50% over 1 year), it is more common among older persons (Gureje & Simon, 1999; Rief et al., 2010).

CULTURAL CONSIDERATIONS

It is important to consider culture in the assessment and treatment of bodily distress disorder (Gureje et al., 2019). Distressing or concerning somatic symptoms that are strongly related to emotional problems have been found to be present in every culture in which they have been studied. Differences in the prevalence of these experiences have been commonly reported, but there is no clear evidence that some cultures are more at risk than others. The specific somatic symptoms commonly presented to the clinician differ from one culture to another, probably reflecting the cultural views and understandings attached to the working or functioning of different parts of the body. Thus, while abdominal symptoms (such as feeling bloated) may be common in one culture, symptoms relating to the functioning of the sexual organs may be more likely in another. Culture may also influence the meaning or attribution attached to the symptoms, including interpretations along traditional, religious, spiritual, and personal lines, and this may influence both the extent of the distress experienced and help-seeking behaviors. It is important that clinicians attending to persons with somatic concerns have an understanding of these cultural influences to arrive at an accurate diagnosis and a way of framing the clinical problem and treatment options so that they are most likely to be acceptable to the patient.

GENDER-RELATED FEATURES

Bothersome and distressing somatic concerns are more commonly reported by females (Gureje & Simon, 1999; Schäfer et al., 2010), and it is therefore likely that bodily distress disorder has a higher prevalence among females than males, although epidemiological studies based on the *ICD-11* diagnosis of bodily distress disorder have not yet been done. Specific patterns of symptoms or complaints may be related to gender—for example, specific cultural presentations believed to be due to loss of semen in males and symptoms related to the menstrual cycle reported by females.

PREVALENCE

Somatic concerns that are associated with distress are common and constitute a high burden among patients consulting primary care (Fink et al., 2007; Goldberg et al., 2017). There are few population-based studies of the prevalence of burdensome somatic symptoms. Findings from such studies indicate that the median prevalence of *ICD-10* somatization disorder, which requires many symptoms from diverse areas of the body and is closer to severe bodily distress disorder in the *ICD-11*, is approximately 0.4% (range: 0.03%–0.84%). In contrast to these low figures, the reported rates for the *ICD-10* undifferentiated somatoform disorder are much higher, ranging between 9.1% to 19.7% (Creed & Gureje, 2012). Like bodily distress disorder, the diagnosis of undifferentiated somatoform disorder does not require the presence of multiple somatic symptoms, but the accompanying psychological symptoms are less well articulated than they are for bodily distress disorder in the *ICD-11*. The prevalence of *ICD-10* somatization disorder is still very low in primary care settings, whereas the prevalence of less restrictively defined forms of somatic concerns is much higher (Gureje et al., 1997). The inference to be drawn from these epidemiological studies is that the threshold for defining somatization disorder was too high, and that for the undifferentiated forms *ICD-10* somatoform disorders was too low. In the context of the revised definition of bodily distress disorder, especially with greater emphasis on the presence of core psychological symptoms, it is likely that the prevalence of bodily distress disorder in general health care settings will be approximately 4% to 6%— much higher than was commonly reported for somatization disorder with its multisymptom requirement but lower than that of undifferentiated somatoform disorder in which psychological features may be less pronounced. As shown in cross-country studies of somatoform disorders, it is likely that the prevalence rate of bodily distress disorder will vary across settings.

KEY POINTS

- Somatic concerns that are associated with distress are common and constitute a high burden among patients consulting primary care. Bodily distress disorder in the *ICD-11* is a new category that has been specifically conceptualized to enhance its clinical utility and support the delivery of appropriate care to affected persons, especially in general health care settings where the condition most commonly presents.

- The single diagnosis of bodily distress disorder replaces all the previous grouping of somatoform disorders in *ICD-10*, with the exception of hypochondriasis. Detailed consideration has been given to the many problems in the ways that disorders of burdensome somatic concerns had previously been defined. Bodily distress disorder represents a major reformulation of the way in which these disorders should be assessed and diagnosed in clinical settings and studied in research settings that is more in line with current evidence and clinical practice.

- Bodily distress disorder is defined in a way that gives prominence to the psychological features that make it a mental disorder and avoids the simplistic mind–body dichotomy implied by the notion of "unexplained medical symptoms." Thus, for the diagnosis to be assigned, along with bothersome somatic symptoms, the presence of core psychological symptoms such as distress, preoccupation, worry, and fear is required, as is evidence of functional impairment.

- Bodily distress disorder is a distinct mental disorder even though it has overlapping features and often co-occurs with other mental disorders, particularly mood disorders and anxiety and fear-related disorders. For a diagnosis of bodily distress disorder to be made, the somatic symptoms should not occur exclusively during and be entirely explainable by episodes of a mood disorder or an anxiety or fear-related disorder.

- The presence of a potentially explanatory or contributory medical conditions does not exclude a diagnosis of bodily distress disorder. In this context, the clinician should establish that the psychological features (e.g., preoccupation, worry, fear) and functional impairment associated with the somatic symptoms are substantially in excess of what would be expected based on the medical condition alone.

- Culture may affect the specific symptoms of bodily distress disorder as well as how those symptoms are experienced, interpreted, and responded to. For this reason, it is important that clinicians take cultural views into consideration in the assessment and treatment planning of bodily distress disorder.

REFERENCES

Creed, F. (2011a). Psychosocial factors as predictors of outcome in the medically ill. *Journal of Psychosomatic Research, 70*(5), 392–394. https://doi.org/10.1016/j.jpsychores.2011.02.010

Creed, F. (2011b). The relationship between somatic symptoms, health anxiety, and outcome in medical out-patients. *Psychiatric Clinics of North America, 34*(3), 545–564. https://doi.org/10.1016/j.psc.2011.05.001

Creed, F., & Gureje, O. (2012). Emerging themes in the revision of the classification of somatoform disorders. *International Review of Psychiatry, 24*(6), 556–567. https://doi.org/10.3109/09540261.2012.741063

Dimsdale, J., Sharma, N., & Sharpe, M. (2011). What do physicians think of somatoform disorders? *Psychosomatics, 52*(2), 154–159. https://doi.org/10.1016/j.psym.2010.12.011

Escobar, J. I., Cook, B., Chen, C.-N., Gara, M. A., Alegría, M., Interian, A., & Diaz, E. (2010). Whether medically unexplained or not, three or more concurrent somatic symptoms predict psychopathology and service use in community populations. *Journal of Psychosomatic Research, 69*(1), 1–8. https://doi.org/10.1016/j.jpsychores.2010.01.001

Fink, P., Ørnbøl, E., Toft, T., Sparle, K. C., Frostholm, L., & Olesen, F. (2004). A new, empirically established hypochondriasis diagnosis. *The American Journal of Psychiatry, 161*(9), 1680–1691. https://doi.org/10.1176/appi.ajp.161.9.1680

Fink, P., Toft, T., Hansen, M. S., Ørnbøl, E., & Olesen, F. (2007). Symptoms and syndromes of bodily distress: An exploratory study of 978 internal medical, neurological, and primary care patients. *Psychosomatic Medicine, 69*(1), 30–39. https://doi.org/10.1097/PSY.0b013e31802e46eb

Fröhlich, C., Jacobi, F., & Wittchen, H. U. (2006). *DSM-IV* pain disorder in the general population. An exploration of the structure and threshold of medically unexplained pain symptoms. *European Archives of Psychiatry and Clinical Neuroscience, 256*(3), 187–196. https://doi.org/10.1007/s00406-005-0625-3

Garralda, M. E. (2011). Unexplained physical complaints. *Child and Adolescent Pediatric Clinics of North America, 58*(4), 803–813, ix. https://doi.org/10.1016/j.chc.2010.01.002

Goldberg, D. P., Reed, G. M., Robles, R., Minhas, F., Razzaque, B., Fortes, S., Mari, J. J., Lam, T. P., Garcia, J. Á., Gask, L., Dowell, A. C., Rosendal, M., Mbatia, J. K., & Saxena, S. (2017). Screening for anxiety, depression, and anxious depression in primary care: A field study for *ICD-11* PHC. *Journal of Affective Disorders, 213*, 199–206. https://doi.org/10.1016/j.jad.2017.02.025

Gureje, O., Lewis-Fernandez, R., Hall, B. J., & Reed, G. M. (2019). Systematic inclusion of culture-related information in *ICD-11. World Psychiatry, 18*(3), 357–358. https://doi.org/10.1002/wps.20676

Gureje, O., & Reed, G. M. (2016). Bodily distress disorder in *ICD-11*: Problems and prospects. *World Psychiatry, 15*(3), 291–292. https://doi.org/10.1002/wps.20353

Gureje, O., & Simon, G. E. (1999). The natural history of somatization in primary care. *Psychological Medicine, 29*(3), 669–676. https://doi.org/10.1017/S0033291799008417

Gureje, O., Simon, G. E., Ustun, T. B., & Goldberg, D. P. (1997). Somatization in cross-cultural perspective: A World Health Organization study in primary care. *The American Journal of Psychiatry, 154*(7), 989–995. https://doi.org/10.1176/ajp.154.7.989

Harris, A. M., Orav, E. J., Bates, D. W., & Barsky, A. J. (2009). Somatization increases disability independent of comorbidity. *Journal of General Internal Medicine, 24*(2), 155–161. https://doi.org/10.1007/s11606-008-0845-0

Hausteiner-Wiehle, C., Grosber, M., Bubel, E., Groben, S., Bornschein, S., Lahmann, C., Eyer, F., Eberlein, B., Behrendt, H., Löwe, B., Henningsen, P., Huber, D., Ring, J., & Darsow, U. (2011). Patient–doctor interaction, psychobehavioural characteristics and mental disorders in patients with suspected allergies: Do they predict "medically unexplained symptoms"? *Acta Dermato-Venereologica, 91*(6), 666–673. https://doi.org/10.2340/00015555-1147

Kato, K., Sullivan, P. F., & Pedersen, N. L. (2010). Latent class analysis of functional somatic symptoms in a population-based sample of twins. *Journal of Psychosomatic Research, 68*(5), 447–453. https://doi.org/10.1016/j.jpsychores.2010.01.010

Keeley, J., Reed, G. M., Rebello, T., Brechbiel, J., Garcia-Pacheco, J. A., Adebayo, K., Esan, O., Majekodunmi, O., Ojagbemi, A., Onofa, L., Robles, R., Matsumoto, C., Medina-Mora, M. E., Kogan, C. S., Kulygina, M., Gaebel, W., Zhao, M., Roberts, M. C., Sharan, P., . . . Gureje, O. (2023). Case-controlled field study of the *ICD-11* clinical descriptions and diagnostic requirements for bodily distress disorders. *Journal of Affective Disorders, 333*, 271–277. https://doi.org/10.1016/j.jad.2023.04.086

Kroenke, K. (2007). Efficacy of treatment for somatoform disorders: A review of randomized controlled trials. *Psychosomatic Medicine, 69*(9), 881–888. https://doi.org/10.1097/PSY.0b013e31815b00c4

Kroenke, K., & Swindle, R. (2000). Cognitive-behavioral therapy for somatization and symptom syndromes: A critical review of controlled clinical trials. *Psychotherapy and Psychosomatics, 69*(4), 205–215. https://doi.org/10.1159/000012395

Noyes, R., Stuart, S., Watson, D. B., & Langbehn, D. R. (2006). Distinguishing between hypochondriasis and somatization disorder: A review of the existing literature. *Psychotherapy and Psychosomatics, 75*(5), 270–281. https://doi.org/10.1159/000093948

Patel, V., Andrew, G., & Pelto, P. J. (2008). The psychological and social contexts of complaints of abnormal vaginal discharge: A study of illness narratives in India. *Journal of Psychosomatic Research, 64*(3), 255–262. https://doi.org/10.1016/j.jpsychores.2007.10.015

Rief, W., Hiller, W., & Margraf, J. (1998). Cognitive aspects of hypochondriasis and the somatization syndrome. *Journal of Abnormal Psychology, 107*(4), 587–595. https://doi.org/10.1037/0021-843X.107.4.587

Rief, W., & Isaac, M. (2007). Are somatoform disorders "mental disorders"? A contribution to the current debate. *Current Opinion in Psychiatry, 20*(2), 143–146. https://doi.org/10.1097/YCO.0b013e3280346999

Rief, W., Mewes, R., Martin, A., Glaesmer, H., & Braehler, E. (2010). Are psychological features useful in classifying patients with somatic symptoms? *Psychosomatic Medicine, 72*(7), 648–655. https://doi.org/10.1097/PSY.0b013e3181d73fce

Schäfer, I., von Leitner, E. C., Schön, G., Koller, D., Hansen, H., Kolonko, T., Kaduszkiewicz, H., Wegscheider, K., Glaeske, G., & van den Bussche, H. (2010). Multimorbidity patterns in the elderly: A new approach of disease clustering identifies complex interrelations between chronic conditions. *PLoS One, 5*(12), e15941. https://doi.org/10.1371/journal.pone.0015941

Schumacher, S., Rief, W., Klaus, K., Brähler, E., & Mewes, R. (2017). Medium- and long-term prognostic validity of competing classification proposals for the former somatoform disorders. *Psychological Medicine, 47*(10), 1719–1732. https://doi.org/10.1017/S0033291717000149

Sharpe, M., & Carson, A. (2001). "Unexplained" somatic symptoms, functional syndromes, and somatization: Do we need a paradigm shift? *Annals of Internal Medicine, 134*(9 Pt. 2), 926–930. https://doi.org/10.7326/0003-4819-134-9_Part_2-200105011-00018

Stein, D. J., Kogan, C. S., Atmaca, M., Fineberg, N. A., Fontenelle, L. F., Grant, J. E., Matsunaga, H., Reddy, Y. C. J., Simpson, H. B., Thomsen, P. H., van den Heuvel, O. A., Veale, D., Woods, D. W., & Reed, G. M. (2016). The classification of obsessive-compulsive and related disorders in the *ICD-11*. *Journal of Affective Disorders, 190*, 663–674. https://doi.org/10.1016/j.jad.2015.10.061

Tomenson, B., McBeth, J., Chew-Graham, C. A., MacFarlane, G., Davies, I., Jackson, J., Littlewood, A., & Creed, F. H. (2012). Somatization and health anxiety as predictors of health care use. *Psychosomatic Medicine, 74*(6), 656–664. https://doi.org/10.1097/PSY.0b013e31825cb140

van den Heuvel, O. A., Veale, D., & Stein, D. J. (2014). Hypochondriasis: Considerations for *ICD-11*. *Brazilian Journal of Psychiatry, 36*(Suppl. 1), 21–27. https://doi.org/10.1590/1516-4446-2013-1218

World Health Organization. (2023). *ICD-11 for mortality and morbidity statistics* (Version: 01/2023). https://icd.who.int/browse11/l-m/en#/

World Health Organization. (2024). *Clinical descriptions and diagnostic requirements for ICD-11 mental, behavioural and neurodevelopmental disorders*. https://www.who.int/publications/i/item/9789240077263

Woud, M. L., Zhang, X. C., Becker, E. S., Zlomuzica, A., & Margraf, J. (2016). Catastrophizing misinterpretations predict somatoform-related symptoms and new onsets of somatoform disorders. *Journal of Psychosomatic Research, 81*, 31–37. https://doi.org/10.1016/j.jpsychores.2015.12.005

14

Disruptive Behavior and Dissocial Disorders and Attention Deficit Hyperactivity Disorder

Spencer C. Evans, Francisco R. de la Peña, Walter Matthys, and John E. Lochman

OVERARCHING LOGIC

Disruptive behavior and dissocial disorders, along with attention deficit hyperactivity disorder (ADHD), are among the most common and impairing psychological conditions in children and adolescents. Clinicians and researchers increasingly recognize these conditions as relevant across the life span, with great heterogeneity in presentation, variation across settings and informant perspectives, and links to other important clinical and functional concerns. For these reasons, effective psychological assessment in this area is both a key skill set for clinicians to possess and a challenging one to implement in practice.

Taxonomically, oppositional defiant disorder and conduct-dissocial disorder comprise the two major disorder categories in the disruptive behavior and dissocial disorders grouping of 11th revision of the *International Classification of Diseases (ICD-11*; World Health Organization [WHO], 2023), whereas ADHD is an important category in the neurodevelopmental disorders grouping. Clinically, oppositional defiant disorder and conduct-dissocial disorder include different clusters of problematic oppositional or antisocial behaviors that differ in type, severity, and frequency, whereas ADHD is characterized by persistent symptoms of inattention and/or hyperactivity-impulsivity that have a direct negative impact on academic, occupational, or social functioning.

https://doi.org/10.1037/0000392-014
A Psychological Approach to Diagnosis: Using the ICD-11 as a Framework, G. M. Reed, P. L.-J. Ritchie, and A. Maercker (Editors)

Despite being classified in different sections of the *ICD-11*, disruptive behavior or dissocial disorders and ADHD are addressed together in this volume for several reasons. First, oppositional defiant disorder, conduct-dissocial disorder, and ADHD all typically have their first onset in childhood or adolescence. Second, these symptoms and diagnoses commonly co-occur, either simultaneously or over the course of development. Third, clinical assessment of any of these problems should entail a differential diagnosis of the others. Finally, even when different diagnoses are applied (e.g., oppositional defiant disorder vs. ADHD), the focus and methods of treatment are often quite similar (e.g., behavioral parent training, cognitive behavior therapy). In light of this overlap, we adopt a comprehensive approach to the psychological assessment of disruptive behavior and dissocial disorders and ADHD in youth. In doing so, we emphasize principles and practices common to all three disorders whenever possible, while also offering guidance on the individual disorders.

A PSYCHOLOGICAL APPROACH TO DISRUPTIVE BEHAVIOR AND DISSOCIAL DISORDERS AND ADHD

Attention to social and developmental context is of utmost importance for the understanding, assessment, and treatment of oppositional defiant disorder, conduct-dissocial disorder, and ADHD. These disorders are somewhat unique in that they are defined less by the experience of distress and more by whether one's behavior aligns with the norms and expectations of the social environment and sociocultural context. A young child exhibiting hyperactive, impulsive, and strong-willed behaviors might be considered unremarkable in a family care setting during early childhood, but these same behaviors could cause considerable impairment, disruption, and learning challenges upon entering primary school. Similarly, it is important for clinicians to have some appreciation of both typical and atypical development because differentiating the two is central to diagnosis. Disruptive features (e.g., temper outbursts, arguing, high-energy behaviors) are somewhat normative in young children but can warrant clinical attention if they are especially severe, persistent, or impairing relative to same-age peers.

For these reasons, the focus of assessment should include the child's social environment in all its forms (e.g., family, peers, school, community) in addition to individual factors in the identified patient. Correspondingly, the methods of assessment should not rely solely on any one person or tool. What is needed is a developmentally informed, hypothesis-driven, comprehensive approach that considers multiple informants across settings (Matthys & Powell, 2018; McMahon & Frick, 2005; Pelham et al., 2005; Rohde et al., 2020). Put differently, assessment requires a psychological conceptualization, seeking to answer a few key questions: What is the nature of the concern? How did it come about? What factors are maintaining the problem? How might these be modified through treatment? Although etiology is beyond the scope of this chapter, these disorders are influenced by genetic and environmental factors (and interactions thereof). In sum, the assessment process is very much just that: a process. It involves developing and testing hypotheses using multiple types and sources of data to shed light on competing explanations.

PRESENTATIONS AND SYMPTOM PATTERNS

Oppositional defiant disorder, conduct-dissocial disorder, and ADHD share common characteristics, including a persistent pattern of symptoms that is inconsistent with developmental level and sociocultural expectations and is associated with functional impairment (WHO, 2024). For example, youths who often argue, defy instructions, and become angry (features of oppositional defiant disorder) are prone to experience impairment in their functioning with parents and teachers. Those who skip school, start fights, and shoplift (as in conduct-dissocial disorder) will likely face significant difficulties in their environment. And a child who has a hard time paying attention and waiting their turn (features of ADHD) will likely experience behavioral, academic, and social problems at school. Thus, all three disorders are necessarily linked to functional impairment, although there is substantial variability among individuals with the same diagnosis (Frick & Nigg, 2012; Lochman & Matthys, 2018; Loeber et al., 2000).

Oppositional Defiant Disorder

In oppositional defiant disorder, the pattern is predominantly disruptive in character, including markedly noncompliant, defiant, and disobedient behavior. This description characterizes the individual's behavior through its impact on the environment, and different types of behaviors can fit this description. As described in the *Clinical Descriptions and Diagnostic Requirements for ICD-11 Mental, Behavioural and Neurodevelopmental Disorders* (*CDDR*; WHO, 2024), these behaviors include (a) difficulty getting along with others, especially authority figures and peers; (b) antagonistic or spiteful/vindictive behavior; or (c) emotional dysregulation including severe irritability and anger. The developmental and relational context is critical. It should be established that the presenting concerns do not arise from a relationship with a single authority figure (e.g., just one parent or teacher) or from an unreasonable set of demands being placed on the child (relative to their age and ability). These situations are not sufficient for diagnosis; instead, they might argue for a clinical focus on the social environment, such as consulting with a teacher or caregiver.

Conduct-Dissocial Disorder

Conduct-dissocial disorder is defined by a pattern of problematic behaviors resulting in violating the basic rights of others or significant violations of age-appropriate social or cultural norms, rules, or laws. The four major domains include (a) aggression toward people or animals, such as bullying or sexual assault; (b) destruction of property, such as setting fires or breaking other children's toys; (c) deceitfulness or theft, such as persistent lying or shoplifting; and

(d) serious violations of rules, such as repeatedly running away from home or skipping school or work. Typically, multiple such behaviors must occur over a relatively long period of time. Depending on their severity, however, a large constellation of many problems may not be required for clinical diagnosis and care. For example, fewer instances of cruelty toward animals or deliberate fire setting would be needed for the diagnosis, whereas behaviors such as lying may require greater evidence of their severity and atypicality (e.g., a recurrent pattern of lying to mislead and cheat others). Note that these behaviors often require other forms of intervention outside the mental health domain. For example, fighting, truancy, and theft may necessitate attention from educational or legal authorities before a persistent pattern could be documented for diagnosis. Conversely, a pattern of lying and cheating others could justify a conduct-dissocial disorder diagnosis without constituting any particular crime or rule violation.

Attention Deficit Hyperactivity Disorder

ADHD is characterized by a persistent pattern of inattention and/or hyperactivity-impulsivity that is outside the limits of normal variation expected for age and level of intellectual development. Symptoms must be severe enough to have a negative effect on functioning in multiple settings (e.g., home, academic, social, occupational). There are three ADHD presentations (inattentive, hyperactive-impulsive, and combined) based on the two symptom clusters (inattention, hyperactivity-impulsivity). Inattention includes difficulty sustaining attention to tasks that do not provide a high level of stimulation or reward or require sustained mental effort; being easily distracted by extraneous stimuli or thoughts not related to the task at hand; and difficulty with planning, managing, and organizing schoolwork, tasks, and other activities. Hyperactivity-impulsivity includes excessive motor activity (e.g., a child leaving their seat or running about when expected to sit still); difficulty waiting one's turn or interrupting or intruding on others in conversation, games, or activities; and a tendency to act in response to immediate stimuli without consideration of the risks and consequences. Knowledge of typical development is key to identifying what is atypical at what ages. Consider the meaning of "difficulty sitting still" in a 4-year-old versus a 10-year-old or "makes impulsive decisions" in a 15-year-old versus a 30-year-old.

SPECIFIERS

Oppositional Defiant Disorder and Conduct-Dissocial Disorder

If the essential features in the *CDDR* for oppositional defiant disorder are met, the clinician specifies whether the presentation is (a) "without chronic irritability-anger," a common, predominantly oppositional-defiant pattern, not accompanied by severe emotion dysregulation; or (b) "with chronic irritability-anger," characterized by a prevailing, persistently angry/irritable mood, which can include feeling angry or resentful, being touchy or easily annoyed, and often losing one's temper. On the basis of substantial research on the irritability dimension of oppositional defiant disorder and on syndromes of severe/disruptive mood dysregulation, the *ICD-11* designated chronic irritability-anger as a subtype of oppositional defiant disorder rather than as a new standalone diagnosis (Evans et al., 2017; Lochman et al., 2015). The presence of chronic irritability-anger is linked to risk for depressive disorders, anxiety and fear-related disorders, suicidality, and school, relational, and occupational challenges.

If the *CDDR* essential features for conduct-dissocial disorder are met, the clinician indicates whether it is (a) "childhood onset" or (b) "adolescent onset." This distinction—based on whether any features were clearly present and persistent before the beginning of adolescence (or about 10 years of age)—is clinically and developmentally meaningful. Early-onset conduct-dissocial disorder tends to predict greater severity and persistence of antisocial behavior over time, whereas onset in adolescence can often be a function of deviant peer affiliation and is more likely to remit as youths enter young adulthood. However, these specifiers should not be interpreted to mean that either presentation is less clinically important or less amenable to change than the other.

If conduct-dissocial disorder and/or oppositional defiant disorder is present, the clinician should indicate whether the condition occurs (a) "with typical prosocial emotions" or (b) "with limited prosocial emotions." This specifier derives from research on callous-unemotional traits, primarily in the context of conduct-dissocial disorder (Frick et al., 2014). Limited prosocial emotions are defined by limited or absent empathy or sensitivity; limited remorse, guilt, or shame; limited concern over one's own poor/problematic performance; and limited or shallow expression of emotions or positive/loving feelings toward others. These features typically emerge before adolescence and predict a trajectory of more severe antisocial behavior. Research has supported the validity of callous-unemotional traits among younger children with and without oppositional defiant disorder (e.g., Ezpeleta et al., 2015). Such findings suggest that detecting limited prosocial emotions within oppositional defiant disorder could help facilitate early identification and treatment of children at greatest risk for a severe antisocial trajectory. Still, diagnostic decisions should be guided by evidence that only a small minority of youth with either disorder would be expected to have limited prosocial emotions (Frick & Nigg, 2012).

Attention Deficit Hyperactivity Disorder

If the requirements for ADHD are met, the clinician has already ascertained that there is an impairing pattern of inattention and/or hyperactivity-impulsivity; the purpose of the specifiers is to designate the nature of that pattern from among three options: (a) predominantly inattentive presentation, (b) predominantly hyperactive-impulsive presentation, or (c) combined presentation. The ADHD symptom dimensions are well established (Willcutt et al., 2012) and could have important clinical implications. For example, youth with hyperactive-impulsive symptoms may require attention for aggressive, inappro-priate, and disruptive behavior. Those with severe inattention may be less disruptive and therefore less likely to be identified but are at greater risk for aca-demic difficulties and depressive disorders (Meinzer et al., 2014).

ASSESSMENT

Clinical assessment can be considered a hypothesis-generating and hypothesis-testing decision-making process in which the clinician assesses for the presence (or absence) of one or more disorders, considers the underlying etiology, and plans treatment. In addition to producing an *ICD-11* diagnosis, assessment should produce a case formulation that includes risk and protective factors that play a role in the development of the disorder. This decision process can be described in eight steps (Matthys & Lochman, 2017; Matthys & Powell, 2018).

First, during an initial screening phase before the first interview, it may be appropriate to provide comprehensive standardized rating scales to be com-pleted by the parents and the youth's teacher or, in the case of young children, their daycare provider. Examples of widely used, well-validated, comprehensive rating scales available in several languages include the Achenbach System of Empirically Based Assessment (Achenbach & Rescorla, 2001) and the Strengths and Difficulties Questionnaire (SDQ; Goodman & Scott, 1999). Both instrument suites are copyrighted and can be administered in electronic or other formats at some cost (although the SDQ permits paper administration at no cost). Numerous free youth mental health scales are available, especially for paper administration (for reviews of measures that are freely available, often in multiple languages, see Becker-Haimes et al., 2020, and Wikiversity, 2020). Ideally, at least one gen-eral measure could be administered to adults with different perspectives on the child, to obtain a quick view on whether the youth functions within the clinical or normal range of various domains according to their parent(s) and teacher(s). Of course, a diagnosis cannot be made based on any single test result. Moreover, any use of measures should take careful account of cultural and linguistic con-text. Measures should be culturally appropriate, administered in the preferred language of the individual(s) to whom they are given (whether as originally developed or as a validated translation), and any standardization (e.g., *t*-scores, clinical cutoffs) should be appropriately normed for the local population. When these conditions are not met, test results must be interpreted with caution.

Second, in the initial interview with the youth and caregiver, information is obtained on the onset and development of the problems and their progression over time. The clinician asks at what age the various symptoms first occurred, in which settings, and with whom (parents, other adults, teachers, siblings, peers). The developmental course of each symptom is discussed in terms of frequency, interactions with particular individuals, and consequences on overall func-tioning (e.g., peer relations, academic achievement). Also, potential risk and protective factors are explored. Risk factors may include prenatal/perinatal birth complications, child temperament, co-occurring disorders, low parental moni-toring and harsh parenting, affiliation with delinquent peers, and low engage-ment with school and community. Protective factors could include the presence of supportive adults, resources for care, extracurricular activities, and child social skills, friendships, problem-solving, intelligence, and academic achievement.

Third, based on the information gathered, the clinician generates a differen-tial diagnosis while considering boundaries with other possible diagnoses with similar symptoms as well as co-occurring conditions. The differential diagnosis is considered as a clinical hypothesis to be tested during the next steps of the assessment. Fourth, this hypothesis helps the clinician decide what issues they need to look for or focus on in the clinical interview with the youth. Clinicians should generally not expect to observe directly all the problems reported by parents or all the essential features of any particular diagnosis, but they may want to observe the core disruptive behaviors at least to some degree. Although there may be a presumption of the presence of a disorder based on information from parents and teachers, the clinical interview may be used to support or refute this diagnostic presumption. Fifth, an evaluation is made of whether additional assessments are needed such as standardized assessment of intellec-tual ability or neuropsychological testing.

Sixth, the clinician carefully checks each symptom separately with the parents, asking for specific examples of behaviors and probing for the frequency, duration, severity, context (settings in which symptoms occur), and conse-quences. Additional information is gathered in view of hypotheses about the questions noted previously (What is the problem? How did it come about? etc.). These hypotheses can incorporate what is known about risk and protective fac-tors and targets for intervention. For example, if the clinician's view is that indi-vidual and transactional characteristics of parent and child have evolved into a cycle of coercion, then behavioral parent training might be indicated. Seventh, the clinician integrates the information from different sources (e.g., parents, teachers, interview, observation) at the level of each symptom or group of symp-toms and decides whether the essential features are present. Through this pro-cess, the clinician obtains a final categorical *ICD-11* diagnosis, plus a working case formulation and treatment recommendations. In generating a treatment plan, priority should be given to factors that seem to play a role in maintaining the disorder(s), perhaps above those that may have played an initiating role, because the former will help guide intervention. Eighth, the clinician discusses the diagnosis and treatment plan with the parents and the child or adolescent.

DIFFERENTIAL DIAGNOSIS

Oppositional defiant disorder, conduct-dissocial disorder, and ADHD must first be distinguished from behaviors that are within the typical range considering the individual's age, gender, and sociocultural context. If the behavior problems are transient or do not result in significant impairment, they are viewed as normative difficulties. If the behavior problems emerged shortly after a significant stressor, the differential diagnosis should include adjustment disorder and possibly other disorders specifically associated with stress.

Oppositional defiant disorder and conduct-dissocial disorder are both related to and distinct from each other (Lahey & Waldman, 2012). Both are characterized by symptoms that disrupt interactions and relations with others but reflect a continuum of severity. For example, arguing, annoying others, and losing temper are less maladaptive than initiating physical fights, destroying property, and stealing. Elementary school children with oppositional defiant disorder are at elevated risk for developing conduct-dissocial disorder, but most do not. Symptoms of ADHD may also disrupt interactions and relations with others. Hyperactive-impulsive behaviors (e.g., blurting out, difficulty waiting turn, interrupting) are often very disruptive and require differentiation from oppositionality. Inattention can also be interpreted as noncompliance; children who have difficulty attending to rules and instructions are less likely to follow them. However, many ADHD symptoms are unique to ADHD, such as being easily distracted and difficulty remaining still. Importantly, ADHD and oppositional defiant disorder or conduct-dissocial disorder often co-occur. When these disorders are present together, ADHD is likely to have come first. Compared with either diagnosis alone, co-occurrence of ADHD with oppositional defiant disorder or conduct-dissocial disorder is associated with greater impairment, therefore requiring a more comprehensive treatment plan.

Severe temper outbursts that may occur in oppositional defiant disorder with chronic irritability-anger can be similar to symptoms of intermittent explosive disorder (see impulse control disorders). However, the explosive episodes in intermittent explosive disorder involve verbal or physical aggression and may result in significant damage to property or physical injury to others. Individuals with oppositional defiant disorder, on the other hand, less often exhibit physical aggression, although verbal and reactive aggression is common. Likewise, although both ADHD and intermittent explosive disorder are characterized by impulsive behavior that may be aggressive, aggression is not a core feature of ADHD.

Noncompliance is common in youth psychopathology and can be seen in the context of both depression (e.g., due to diminished interest and pleasure) and anxiety disorders (e.g., if functioning to help avoid an anxiety-provoking stimulus). Similarly, irritability occurs in more than a dozen mental disorders affecting youth (Evans et al., 2017), notably including depressive, bipolar, anxiety, and stress-related disorders, as well as oppositional defiant disorder. Generally, youth with disruptive behavior or dissocial disorders are at risk for depression and anxiety. For these reasons, mood and anxiety disorders should generally be considered for differential diagnosis when oppositionality or irritability is prominent, with careful attention given to whether these features are more episodic (characteristic of mood disorders) or chronic in nature (characteristic of oppositional defiant disorder and non-mood disorders).

Similarly, youth with ADHD, particularly the inattentive presentation, are at risk for depressive disorders, which may be increased by negative experiences with parents, teachers, and peers (Meinzer et al., 2014). Problems with attention in ADHD can also resemble depressed/withdrawn behavior. ADHD and depressive disorders can be distinguished insofar as ADHD inattention persists over time and is not episodically tied to depressive disorders. Fidgeting, restlessness, and difficulties maintaining concentration characteristic of ADHD may also occur in the context of anxiety and fear-related disorders, which can co-occur with ADHD.

Noncompliance, irritability-anger, and aggression are common among children and adolescents with autism spectrum disorder. However, in individuals with autism spectrum disorder, these behaviors are typically associated with a trigger, such as a sudden change in routine or aversive sensory stimulation, or with social communication deficits in interactions with peers. Likewise, attention problems such as being overly focused, hyperactive, and impulsive may occur in individuals with autism spectrum disorder. However, individuals with oppositional defiant disorder, conduct-dissocial disorder, or ADHD do not have the social communication deficits and restricted, repetitive, and inflexible patterns of behavior, interests, or activities that are the core features of autism spectrum disorder.

CO-OCCURRING DISORDERS

Among individuals with any mental disorder, roughly half will at some point meet the diagnostic requirements for a second disorder; of these, about half will meet the diagnostic requirements for a third disorder (Caspi & Moffitt, 2018). Thus, it is critical to consider the possibility of co-occurring disorders when assessing for ADHD, oppositional defiant disorder, or conduct-dissocial disorder. The most common co-occurrence patterns involve pairs of these three disorders co-occurring with one another. The *ICD-11* addresses this by allowing any combination of these diagnoses to be applied simultaneously when all diagnostic requirements for each are met. Traditionally, co-occurrence within disruptive behavior and dissocial disorders has been viewed hierarchically and developmentally, with oppositional defiant disorder seen as a precursor to conduct-dissocial disorder (Burke et al., 2002). However, it is important to note that a large percentage of youths with oppositional defiant disorder never develop conduct-dissocial disorder. In addition, ADHD commonly co-occurs with, and is a risk factor for, oppositional defiant disorder and conduct-dissocial disorder (Frick & Nigg, 2012). Individuals with developmental learning disorder or with disorders of intellectual development often have attention problems and may also warrant an ADHD diagnosis if all requirements are met.

Some useful data on co-occurrence come from Costello et al. (2003), who collected 3-month prevalence estimates of emotional and behavioral disorders in a representative population of 1,420 youths ages 9 to 13. Similar patterns of co-occurrence emerged for oppositional defiant disorder, conduct-dissocial disorder, and ADHD. The presence of any one of these disorders was linked to substantially increased risk for any other of these disorders, especially among boys. Generally, oppositional defiant disorder, conduct-dissocial disorder, and ADHD also carried increased risk for depressive disorders, anxiety and fear-related disorders, and disorders due to substance use. Rates of co-occurrence tended to follow the developmental and gender trends of the associated disorders. For example, among individuals with a disruptive behavior or dissocial disorder or ADHD diagnosis, risk for co-occurring depressive disorders or disorders due to substance use increases during adolescence and young adulthood. As for gender, girls with oppositional defiant disorder, conduct-dissocial disorder, and/or ADHD showed higher co-occurrence with anxiety and fear-related disorders and depressive disorders and lower co-occurrence with externalizing disorders compared to boys (Costello et al., 2003).

Oppositional defiant disorder, conduct-dissocial disorder, and ADHD have also been linked to other health concerns. Sleep disturbance is common in disruptive behavior and dissocial disorders and in ADHD. There is a link between ADHD and epilepsy that warrants attention both for their elevated co-occurrence and for differential diagnosis given the possibility of absence (petit mal) seizures— brief "staring-spell" seizures lasting a few seconds—that can masquerade as inattention in settings such as classrooms. ADHD is associated with obesity and overweight status, which may not be clinically significant until adolescence or adulthood (Nigg et al., 2016). Similarly, unintentional injuries (e.g., burns, poisoning, fractures, head injuries) are associated with mental disorders generally and uniquely linked to ADHD, oppositional defiant disorder, and conduct-dissocial disorder (Rowe et al., 2004). It is not difficult to imagine how these disorders' features (e.g., sensation-seeking, impulsivity, hyperactivity, risk-taking, lowered sensitivity to punishment, aggression, delinquent peer affiliation, rule violations) could place youths at risk for various adverse health outcomes. Clinicians should consider safety and physical health implications as part of a biopsychosocial conceptualization of disruptive behavior and dissocial disorders and ADHD. Finally, given documented associations of externalizing behavior with various forms of life adversity (Frick & Nigg, 2012), it is important to assess for a history of, and risk for, various forms of maltreatment and trauma.

DEVELOPMENTAL COURSE

Developmentally, oppositional defiant disorder is thought to emerge most often within the family environment. As children develop and peers play an increasingly influential role, youths may transition from argumentative, defiant, and oppositional behavior at home to exhibiting similarly difficult behaviors in the peer and school context. Problems with emotion regulation and social-cognitive processes are often present. Youth with oppositional defiant disorder and conduct-dissocial disorder tend to be rejected by their peers and form affiliations with more delinquent peers. They may victimize, be victimized, or both (bully-victims). In school, youth with these conditions often encounter academic challenges and may be at greater risk for dropping out. Some of this may be due to co-occurring ADHD, which is more specifically linked to academic problems. The stability of oppositional defiant disorder and conduct-dissocial disorder is relatively low, meaning that youth who meet requirements for the diagnosis at one point may experience a decline of symptoms and return to a typical trajectory. However, the emergence of both oppositional defiant disorder and conduct-dissocial disorder earlier in childhood (rather than later in adolescence) is a robust predictor of mental health and functional problems into adulthood, and those who also show limited prosocial emotions tend to have most severe and persistent patterns (Frick et al., 2014). Finally, although oppositional defiant disorder and conduct-dissocial disorder have been considered disorders of childhood and adolescence, they remain relevant, common, and clinically important in adulthood. Thus, the *ICD-11* allows both diagnoses to be given to adults when applicable. Adults who would have received a diagnosis of dissocial personality disorder in the *ICD-10* or antisocial personality disorder according to the fifth edition of the *Diagnostic and Statistical Manual of Mental Disorders* (*DSM-5*) may best be diagnosed with conduct-dissocial disorder in the *ICD-11*, as this represents essentially the same pattern from a lifespan perspective.

Regarding ADHD, inattention and hyperactivity-impulsivity are present in many typically developing individuals during early to middle childhood. What indicates ADHD is the greater severity, persistence, and pervasiveness of these symptoms and the degree of associated impairment. In young children, the combined presentation is most common. With increasing age, hyperactivity-impulsivity tends to decrease, and inattentive presentations become more common. This may reflect a true developmental pattern or a difficulty in measurement across the life span. The *ICD-11* has taken steps to address the latter issue by incorporating specific additional behaviors as symptoms (e.g., reckless driving). Most preschool cases of ADHD persist into childhood and adolescence, with the combined subtype showing the strongest stability; however, it is common for an individual's symptom presentation subtype to shift over time. For an ADHD diagnosis to be made in adolescents and adults, there must be evidence of significant inattention and/or hyperactivity-impulsivity in childhood (e.g., before age 12). For example, this evidence could be obtained by interviewing a family member or reviewing school records. In the absence of such evidence, an ADHD diagnosis in adults should be made with caution.

Early childhood ADHD symptoms and executive function are significant predictors of ADHD persistence and impairment, whereas inadequate parenting practices predict problems in emotional and behavioral adjustment and co-occurring oppositional defiant disorder. Parent and child behaviors are bidirectionally related, with parenting practices influencing child behavior and vice versa. In school-age children, ADHD symptom severity and related impairment, cognitive functioning, and family factors continue to be important predictors of ADHD persistence and functional outcomes later in life. Co-occurrence with oppositional defiant disorder and conduct-dissocial disorder emerges as an additional important predictor of both ADHD persistence and impaired functioning in adolescence and adulthood. Adults with any of these conditions may show impairments in the educational, occupational, relational, family, and community domains. At any developmental stage, effective intervention can be an important factor in determining the course and outcome of these conditions.

PREVALENCE

The best evidence concerning the prevalence of oppositional defiant disorder, conduct-dissocial disorder, and ADHD comes from large epidemiological surveys and meta-analyses. The National Comorbidity Survey Replication–Adolescent Supplement (Merikangas et al., 2010) collected a representative sample of 10,123 of adolescents in the United States. Results showed that 12.6% of youth had a lifetime history of oppositional defiant disorder (13.9% in males, 11.3% in females), and 6.8% had conduct-dissocial disorder (7.9% in males, 5.8% in females). For ADHD, lifetime prevalence was 8.7% (13.1% of males, 4.2% of females). Overall, approximately one in five youths (19.6%; 23.5% in males, 15.5% in females) had any history of the three disorders. By synthesizing results from many similar studies, a more robust and internationally representative picture begins to emerge. The most comprehensive global meta-analysis of ADHD prevalence used data from 175 studies and estimated that 7.2% (95% confidence interval: [6.7%, 7.8%]) of youth in the population had ADHD at any given time (Thomas et al., 2015). To our knowledge, similar data are not available for oppositional defiant disorder and conduct-dissocial disorder, but epidemiological research has generally suggested that rates of ADHD, oppositional defiant disorder, and conduct-dissocial disorder do not vary substantially over time or across global regions—that is, these are not "American disorders" nor are they rapidly increasing in prevalence (Canino et al., 2010; Thomas et al., 2015; Willcutt, 2012).

However, prevalence estimates do not speak to the cross-cultural variations in clinical practices and social perceptions of diagnosing and treating ADHD, oppositional defiant disorder, and conduct-dissocial disorder. There is evidence in the United States, for example, that rates of ADHD diagnoses have increased since the 1990s, with regional variations in diagnosis and medication prescription (Centers for Disease Control and Prevention, 2020). Such developments for ADHD—and perhaps also for oppositional defiant disorder and conduct-dissocial disorder—have not been without controversy and do not seem to be unfolding in the same manner across countries. These observations are somewhat anecdotal, underscoring the need for more research. In particular, research is needed in low- and middle-income countries.

Prevalence estimates hold useful clinical implications. For example, these data suggest that within a classroom of 20 to 30 students, there are probably three to six students—more often boys—who at some point will be affected by ADHD and/or disruptive behavior or dissocial disorders. At any given time, approximately one to three of these students might show all the essential features for one or more of these disorders. This knowledge provides a frame of reference for clinicians attempting to draw accurate diagnostic formulations about a referred youth's reported difficulties. However, epidemiological estimates only go so far. They do not describe disorder prevalence the settings where clinical care is provided, such as the local clinic or hospital. Thus, we encourage clinicians to investigate the "local base rates" periodically for these diagnoses in their settings because this provides an actuarial baseline to guide evidence-based assessment (Youngstrom et al., 2017).

VALIDITY AND OTHER KEY SCIENTIFIC ISSUES

Substantial evidence supports the validity of oppositional defiant disorder, conduct-dissocial disorder, and ADHD in children and adolescents (Frick & Nigg, 2012). As one indicator of this validity, oppositional defiant disorder and conduct-dissocial disorder in childhood predict many common forms of psychopathology later in adolescence and adulthood. Differential outcomes have been found for ADHD, oppositional defiant disorder (more predictive of anxiety and depression), and conduct-dissocial disorder (more predictive of delinquency and antisocial outcomes) in early adulthood. These diagnoses may also be validly made in earlier developmental periods. In preschool, oppositional defiant disorder and conduct-dissocial disorder show good evidence of validity, including relations to teacher-rated impairment and stability over time into the early school years.

Recent changes in the *ICD-11* are expected to enhance the validity and clinical utility of these diagnoses, permitting more finely tuned treatment planning. One key classification decision has been to include a subtype of chronic irritability-anger within oppositional defiant disorder in the *ICD-11* rather than as a standalone disorder (Evans et al., 2017; Lochman et al., 2015). In global field trials, this formulation led to greater accuracy in diagnosing youth irritability and oppositionality, compared with the *DSM-5* and *ICD-10* (Evans et al., 2021). Another decision involved adding a specifier of "limited prosocial emotions" to conduct-dissocial disorder and oppositional defiant disorder diagnoses, largely based on research on callous-unemotional traits in youth. Callous-unemotional traits have been found to predict criminal and antisocial behavior outcomes in adults, even after controlling for oppositional defiant disorder and conduct-dissocial disorder symptoms. However, callous-unemotional traits show only moderate stability during childhood and are affected by family and peer interactions (Frick et al., 2014).

MAJOR DIFFERENCES WITH *DSM-5*

Research has indicated that children with severe anger and irritability are at considerable risk for particular negative outcomes, including depressive disorders and anxiety and fear-related disorders. Consequently, concern arose that irritability had not been adequately classified in prior diagnostic systems, and changes were made to address this concern in both the *DSM-5* and the *ICD-11*. The *DSM-5* added a new childhood depressive disorder diagnosis, disruptive mood dysregulation disorder. This decision was met with several concerns, however, including that it was based on only limited research and that the new syndrome was not clearly distinct from existing disorders (especially oppositional defiant disorder). Based on recommendations from a working group and a comprehensive literature review (Evans et al., 2017), the *ICD-11* did not include disruptive mood dysregulation disorder but instead added a specifier for oppositional defiant disorder with "chronic irritability-anger." This seems to be the most parsimonious, scientifically supported option for better identifying and treating children with this maladaptive form of emotional dysregulation (Evans et al., 2021; Lochman et al. 2015).

A second distinction between the *ICD-11* and *DSM-5* involves the decision to use the specifier limited prosocial emotions for both oppositional defiant disorder and conduct-dissocial disorder. It was concluded that there were insufficient data to justify restricting the limited prosocial emotions specifier to conduct-dissocial disorder alone. Indeed, much of the research on the predictive effects of callous-unemotional traits has emerged from samples of youth with and without externalizing problems, broadly defined (e.g., Ezpeleta et al., 2015).

CULTURAL AND CONTEXTUAL CONSIDERATIONS

Oppositional defiant disorder, conduct-dissocial disorder, and ADHD are mental health diagnoses with evidence for validity and applicability at a global level (Bauermeister et al., 2010; Evans et al., 2021). Youth mental health symptom dimensions share structural similarities across countries—for example, with specific internalizing problems (e.g., worries, sad) being more strongly correlated with one another than with specific externalizing problems (e.g., argues, gets angry; Lahey & Waldman, 2012; Rescorla et al., 2012). Culture and context affect the presentation, perception, and implications of mental health symptoms, however. Societies have varying thresholds for separating normative from clinical behaviors (Rescorla et al., 2012), with important implications for clinicians. When evaluating youths from cultural backgrounds in which average problem scores are lower than those of their current community, common assessment practices (e.g., one-size-fits-all cutoff scores) could cause oppositional defiant disorder, conduct-dissocial disorder, or ADHD to go undetected. Conversely, youths from racial/ethnic minority groups are sometimes disproportionately identified for behavior problems; they might be inappropriately referred for treatment when a disorder is not present or receive discipline rather than care when a disorder is present. Thus, clinicians should consider individual, family, and community cultural factors to promote appropriate and effective care.

GENDER-RELATED CONSIDERATIONS

In the *ICD-11*, the requirements for oppositional defiant disorder, conduct-dissocial disorder, and ADHD are the same irrespective of gender, but gender is a key consideration for assessment and conceptualization. All three conditions show a male preponderance, and this can help calibrate clinicians' expected base rates to guide evidence-based assessment. However, the extent to which gender imbalances reflect true sex-differences or gender bias in diagnostic instruments and practices is unclear. When gender-based expectancies are held by parents, teachers, and professionals, boys could be overidentified and girls underidentified.

Generally, boys and girls with disruptive behavior or dissocial disorders or ADHD exhibit similar symptoms, impairment, and developmental trajectories. However, there are some gender-related patterns clinicians should know. The associations of oppositional defiant disorder, conduct-dissocial disorder, and ADHD with depressive disorders and anxiety and fear-related disorders are especially pronounced in females. The symptoms of disruptive behavior or dissocial disorders and ADHD can be less overt in females, such as lower levels of externalizing problems across these disorders and greater symptoms of inattention and lower hyperactivity-impulsivity in ADHD. Among youths with externalizing behaviors, boys with disruptive behavior or dissocial disorders are more likely than girls to show aggressive and destructive behavior and severe rule violations. Girls seem to exhibit more nonviolent and covert aggression. As a result, antisocial behaviors among girls are more likely to go undetected longer and be diagnosed at a later age. Risk for sexual abuse and early pregnancy warrants special attention. Finally, it is important for clinicians to monitor "subclinical" or "borderline" cases, which might be especially common in girls, because this can lead to clinically significant long-term outcomes. The flexibility of the *ICD-11 Clinical Descriptions and Diagnostic Requirements* allows clinicians to exercise professional judgment in identifying such individuals.

KEY POINTS

- In the *ICD-11*, oppositional defiant disorder and conduct-dissocial disorder are classified in the grouping of disruptive behavior and dissocial disorders, and ADHD is classified as a neurodevelopmental disorder.

- These conditions are common, typically emerge in childhood and adolescence, and often co-occur with one another and with other conditions.

- Clinical assessment in this area is a multistep hypothesis-testing process involving data from multiple informants and methods to develop a formulation and plan.

- Comprehensive evaluation for any one concern should assess for all three as well as other disorders and normality, considering environment, development, gender, and culture.

- There is meaningful symptom heterogeneity within and across conditions and over development, with subtypes and specifiers communicating this information clinically.

- This chapter and the *ICD-11* can help guide effective diagnostic assessment and case formulation for disruptive behavior and dissocial disorders and ADHD.

REFERENCES

Achenbach, T. M., & Rescorla, L. A. (2001). *Manual for the ASEBA school age forms and profiles*. University of Vermont. https://store.aseba.org/MANUAL-FOR-THE-ASEBA-SCHOOL-AGE-FORMS-PROFILES/productinfo/505/

Bauermeister, J. J., Canino, G., Polanczyk, G., & Rohde, L. A. (2010). ADHD across cultures: Is there evidence for a bidimensional organization of symptoms? *Journal of Clinical Child and Adolescent Psychology, 39*(3), 362–372. https://doi.org/10.1080/15374411003691743

Becker-Haimes, E. M., Tabachnick, A. R., Last, B. S., Stewart, R. E., Hasan-Granier, A., & Beidas, R. S. (2020). Evidence base update for brief, free, and accessible youth mental health measures. *Journal of Clinical Child and Adolescent Psychology, 49*(1), 1–17. https://doi.org/10.1080/15374416.2019.1689824

Burke, J. D., Loeber, R., & Birmaher, B. (2002). Oppositional defiant disorder and conduct disorder: A review of the past 10 years, part II. *Journal of the American Academy of Child & Adolescent Psychiatry, 41*(11), 1275–1293. https://doi.org/10.1097/00004583-200211000-00009

Canino, G., Polanczyk, G., Bauermeister, J. J., Rohde, L. A., & Frick, P. J. (2010). Does the prevalence of CD and ODD vary across cultures? *Social Psychiatry and Psychiatric Epidemiology, 45*(7), 695–704. https://doi.org/10.1007/s00127-010-0242-y

Caspi, A., & Moffitt, T. E. (2018). All for one and one for all: Mental disorders in one dimension. *The American Journal of Psychiatry, 175*(9), 831–844. https://doi.org/10.1176/appi.ajp.2018.17121383

Centers for Disease Control and Prevention. (2020, September). *Attention-deficit hyperactivity disorder (ADHD): Data and statistics*. U.S. Department of Health and Human Services. https://www.cdc.gov/ncbddd/adhd/data.html

Costello, E. J., Mustillo, S., Erkanli, A., Keeler, G., & Angold, A. (2003). Prevalence and development of psychiatric disorders in childhood and adolescence. *Archives of General Psychiatry, 60*(8), 837–844. https://doi.org/10.1001/archpsyc.60.8.837

Evans, S. C., Burke, J. D., Roberts, M. C., Fite, P. J., Lochman, J. E., de la Peña, F. R., & Reed, G. M. (2017). Irritability in child and adolescent psychopathology: An integrative review for *ICD-11*. *Clinical Psychology Review, 53*, 29–45. https://doi.org/10.1016/j.cpr.2017.01.004

Evans, S. C., Roberts, M. C., Keeley, J. W., Rebello, T. J., de la Peña, F., Lochman, J. E., Burke, J. D., Fite, P. J., Ezpeleta, L., Matthys, W., Youngstrom, E. A., Matsumoto, C., Andrews, H. F., Medina-Mora, M.-E., Ayuso-Mateos, J. L., Khoury, B., Kulygina, M., Robles, R., Shartan, P., . . . Reed, G. M. (2021). Diagnostic classification of irritability and oppositionality in youth: A global field study comparing *ICD-11* with *ICD-10* and *DSM-5*. *Journal of Child Psychology and Psychiatry, and Allied Disciplines, 62*(3), 303–312.

Ezpeleta, L., Granero, R., de la Osa, N., & Domènech, J. M. (2015). Clinical characteristics of preschool children with oppositional defiant disorder and callous-unemotional traits. *PLoS One, 10*(9), e0139346. https://doi.org/10.1371/journal.pone.0139346

Frick, P. J., & Nigg, J. T. (2012). Current issues in the diagnosis of attention deficit hyperactivity disorder, oppositional defiant disorder, and conduct disorder. *Annual Review of*

Clinical Psychology, 8(1), 77–107. https://doi.org/10.1146/annurev-clinpsy-032511-143150

Frick, P. J., Ray, J. V., Thornton, L. C., & Kahn, R. E. (2014). Annual research review: A developmental psychopathology approach to understanding callous-unemotional traits in children and adolescents with serious conduct problems. *Journal of Child Psychology and Psychiatry, and Allied Disciplines, 55*(6), 532–548. https://doi.org/10.1111/jcpp.12152

Goodman, R., & Scott, S. (1999). Comparing the Strengths and Difficulties Questionnaire and the Child Behavior Checklist: Is small beautiful? *Journal of Abnormal Child Psychology, 27*(1), 17–24. https://doi.org/10.1023/A:1022658222914

Lahey, B. B., & Waldman, I. D. (2012). Annual research review: Phenotypic and causal structure of conduct disorder in the broader context of prevalent forms of psychopathology. *Journal of Child Psychology and Psychiatry, and Allied Disciplines, 53*(5), 536–557. https://doi.org/10.1111/j.1469-7610.2011.02509.x

Lochman, J. E., Evans, S. C., Burke, J. D., Roberts, M. C., Fite, P. J., Reed, G. M., de la Peña, F. R., Matthys, W., Ezpeleta, L., Siddiqui, S., & Garralda, M. E. (2015). An empirically based alternative to *DSM-5*'s disruptive mood dysregulation disorder for *ICD-11. World Psychiatry, 14*(1), 30–33. https://doi.org/10.1002/wps.20176

Lochman, J. E., & Matthys, W. (Eds.). (2018). *The Wiley handbook of disruptive and impulse-control disorders.* Wiley Blackwell.

Loeber, R., Burke, J. D., Lahey, B. B., Winters, A., & Zera, M. (2000). Oppositional defiant and conduct disorder: A review of the past 10 years, part I. *Journal of the American Academy of Child & Adolescent Psychiatry, 39*(12), 1468–1484. https://doi.org/10.1097/00004583-200012000-00007

Matthys, W., & Lochman, J. E. (2017). *Oppositional defiant disorder and conduct disorder in childhood* (2nd ed.). John Wiley & Sons.

Matthys, W., & Powell, N. P. (2018). Problem-solving structure of assessment. In J. E. Lochman & W. Matthys (Eds.), *The Wiley handbook of disruptive and impulsive-control disorders* (pp. 373–389). John Wiley & Sons.

McMahon, R. J., & Frick, P. J. (2005). Evidence-based assessment of conduct problems in children and adolescents. *Journal of Clinical Child and Adolescent Psychology, 34*(3), 477–505. https://doi.org/10.1207/s15374424jccp3403_6

Meinzer, M. C., Pettit, J. W., & Viswesvaran, C. (2014). The co-occurrence of attention-deficit/hyperactivity disorder and unipolar depression in children and adolescents: A meta-analytic review. *Clinical Psychology Review, 34*(8), 595–607. https://doi.org/10.1016/j.cpr.2014.10.002

Merikangas, K. R., He, J. P., Burstein, M., Swanson, S. A., Avenevoli, S., Cui, L., Benjet, C., Georgiades, K., & Swendsen, J. (2010). Lifetime prevalence of mental disorders in U.S. adolescents: Results from the National Comorbidity Survey Replication–Adolescent Supplement (NCS-A). *Journal of the American Academy of Child & Adolescent Psychiatry, 49*(10), 980–989. https://doi.org/10.1016/j.jaac.2010.05.017

Nigg, J. T., Johnstone, J. M., Musser, E. D., Long, H. G., Willoughby, M. T., & Shannon, J. (2016). Attention-deficit/hyperactivity disorder (ADHD) and being overweight/obesity: New data and meta-analysis. *Clinical Psychology Review, 43*, 67–79. https://doi.org/10.1016/j.cpr.2015.11.005

Pelham, W. E., Jr., Fabiano, G. A., & Massetti, G. M. (2005). Evidence-based assessment of attention deficit hyperactivity disorder in children and adolescents. *Journal of Clinical Child and Adolescent Psychology, 34*(3), 449–476. https://doi.org/10.1207/s15374424jccp3403_5

Rescorla, L., Ivanova, M. Y., Achenbach, T. M., Begovac, I., Chahed, M., Drugli, M. B., Emerich, D. R., Fung, D. S., Haider, M., Hansson, K., Hewitt, N., Jaimes, S., Larsson, B., Maggiolini, A., Marković, J., Mitrović, D., Moreira, P., Oliveira, J. T., Olsson, M., . . . Zhang, E. Y. (2012). International epidemiology of child and adolescent psychopathology ii: Integration and applications of dimensional findings from 44 societies.

Journal of the American Academy of Child & Adolescent Psychiatry, 51(12), 1273–1283.e8. https://doi.org/10.1016/j.jaac.2012.09.012

Rohde, L., Coghgil, D., Asherson, P., & Banaschewski, T. (2020). ADHD assessment across the life span. In L. A. Rohde, J. K. Buitelaar, M. Gerlach, & S. V. Faraone (Eds.), *The World Federation of ADHD guide* (pp. 42–62). World Federation of ADHD/ARTMED EDITORA.

Rowe, R., Maughan, B., & Goodman, R. (2004). Childhood psychiatric disorder and unintentional injury: Findings from a national cohort study. *Journal of Pediatric Psychology, 29*(2), 119–130. https://doi.org/10.1093/jpepsy/jsh015

Thomas, R., Sanders, S., Doust, J., Beller, E., & Glasziou, P. (2015). Prevalence of attention-deficit/hyperactivity disorder: A systematic review and meta-analysis. *Pediatrics, 135*(4), e994–e1001. https://doi.org/10.1542/peds.2014-3482

Wikiversity. (2020, June 25). *Evidence-based assessment/assessment center/clinician resources.* https://en.wikiversity.org/wiki/Evidence-based_assessment/Assessment_Center/Clinician_resources

Willcutt, E. G. (2012). The prevalence of *DSM-IV* attention-deficit/hyperactivity disorder: A meta-analytic review. *Neurotherapeutics, 9*(3), 490–499. https://doi.org/10.1007/s13311-012-0135-8

Willcutt, E. G., Nigg, J. T., Pennington, B. F., Solanto, M. V., Rohde, L. A., Tannock, R., Loo, S. K., Carlson, C. L., McBurnett, K., & Lahey, B. B. (2012). Validity of *DSM-IV* attention deficit/hyperactivity disorder symptom dimensions and subtypes. *Journal of Abnormal Psychology, 121*(4), 991–1010. https://doi.org/10.1037/a0027347

World Health Organization. (2023). *ICD-11 for mortality and morbidity statistics* (Version: 01/2023). https://icd.who.int/browse11/l-m/en#/

World Health Organization. (2024). *Clinical descriptions and diagnostic requirements for ICD-11 mental, behavioural and neurodevelopmental disorders.* https://www.who.int/publications/i/item/9789240077263

Youngstrom, E. A., Van Meter, A., Frazier, T. W., Hunsley, J., Prinstein, M. J., Ong, M. L., & Youngstrom, J. K. (2017). Evidence-based assessment as an integrative model for applying psychological science to guide the voyage of treatment. *Clinical Psychology: Science and Practice, 24*(4), 331–363. https://doi.org/10.1111/cpsp.12207

15

Disorders Due to Substance Use

Jason P. Connor and John B. Saunders

OVERARCHING LOGIC

Disorders due to substance use rank among the leading causes of death and disability worldwide (Rehm & Shield, 2019). At the same time, psychoactive substances have been used by human societies throughout history. Laws and social norms have developed in different societies to distinguish between appropriate use and substance misuse in an attempt to minimize harmful consequences to the individual, the family, the community, and society as a whole. These laws and norms attempt to counteract the appealing nature and marketability of psychoactive substances. Because they typically increase pleasure temporarily, there are individual and commercial incentives for their use, even in unhealthy amounts (Saunders, 2016).

Health professionals have several important roles related to psychoactive substance use. These include (a) ensuring that health considerations related to psychoactive substance use are understood and approaches are applied to minimize harm; (b) ensuring that persons who are using psychoactive substances in a hazardous way have effective information to help them avoid harmful consequences of that use; and (c) ensuring that individuals who have diagnosable disorders related to their substance use have access to appropriate, evidence-based treatments and are supported in recovering from their disorders and/or minimizing the substance-related harm. To minimize risk to the individual substance user and to other affected persons, assessment

https://doi.org/10.1037/0000392-015
A Psychological Approach to Diagnosis: Using the ICD-11 as a Framework, G. M. Reed,
P. L.-J. Ritchie, and A. Maercker (Editors)

of substance use—including its pattern, problematic features, and severity—should be included within routine history taking in health care settings.

The classification of disorders due to substance use in the 11th revision of the *International Classification of Diseases* (*ICD-11*; World Health Organization [WHO], 2023) includes categories for specific clinical syndromes that may result from use of 14 classes of psychoactive substances, which comprise illicit substances or "street drugs" as well as prescription and over-the-counter medicines. The *ICD-11* substance classes are alcohol; cannabis; synthetic cannabinoids; opioids; sedative-hypnotics and anxiolytics; cocaine; stimulants, including amphetamines, methamphetamine, and methcathinone; synthetic cathinones; caffeine; hallucinogens; nicotine; volatile inhalants; MDMA and related drugs, including MDA; and dissociative drugs including ketamine and phencyclidine (PCP).

The *ICD-11* also includes categories for "other specified substances," which is important given global variations in use as well as the increasing spread of new psychoactive substances or "designer drugs." These new substances are often drug analogues with subtle molecular variations from known drugs, which have been designed to mimic the effects of existing substances. The global use of two such types of substances—synthetic cannabinoids and synthetic cathinones—has become sufficiently important that these have been given their own categories in the *ICD-11*.

Within each substance class, the *ICD-11* provides categories to capture different harmful patterns of substance use that have an impact on health. This provides a valuable structure to guide health professionals in making important clinical assessments and decisions related to disorders due to substance use. The *ICD-11* Clinical Descriptions and Diagnostic Requirements facilitate a more person-centered approach to assessment, recognizing natural variation in cultural and individual influences. An understanding of the core psychobiological processes underpinning substance use disorders, combined with comprehensive and structured clinical assessment, assist in determining a reliable *ICD-11* substance use disorder diagnosis and, if required, treatment planning. This chapter covers the main antecedents and patterns of disorders due to substance use, core psychological processes that lead to hazardous or repetitive use, mechanisms that result in substance dependence, and key psychological assessment approaches that can be integrated with the *ICD-11* to provide comprehensive assessment and treatment planning for patients with disorders due to substance use.

PRESENTATIONS AND SYMPTOM PATTERNS

The core categories in the *ICD-11* that correspond to the spectrum of substance use that may be a focus of clinical attention range from hazardous use to harmful pattern of substance use to substance dependence, the most severe form of problematic substance use (Figure 15.1). Additional categories are also provided for specific clinical presentations, including episode of harmful substance use, substance intoxication, substance withdrawal, and substance-induced mental disorders. In the *Clinical Descriptions and Diagnostic Requirements for ICD-11 Mental, Behavioural and Neurodevelopmental Disorders* (*CDDR*; WHO, 2024), these syndromes

FIGURE 15.1. The Spectrum of Substance Use and Disorder

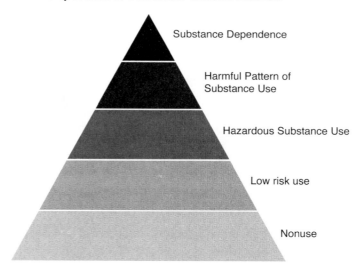

Substance Dependence

Harmful Pattern of Substance Use

Hazardous Substance Use

Low risk use

Nonuse

Note. From "Diagnostic Definitions and Classification of Substance Use Disorders," by J. B. Saunders and N. C. Latt, in N. el-Guebaly, G. Carrà, M. Galanter, and A. M. Baldacchino (Eds.), *Textbook of Addiction Treatment: International Perspectives* (2nd ed., p. 99), 2021, Springer Nature (https://doi.org/10.1007/978-3-030-36391-8_8). Copyright 2021 by Springer Nature. Reprinted with permission.

are described cross-sectionally, with tables describing the specific features of their manifestations due to different substances.

Hazardous Substance Use

Hazardous substance use is characterized by a pattern of substance use that is sufficient in frequency or quantity to increase appreciably the future risk of harmful physical or mental health consequences to the user or to others to an extent that warrants attention and advice from health professionals. The risk may be related to short-term effects of the substance or to longer term cumulative effects on physical or mental health. However, hazardous substance use has not reached the level of having caused specific, concrete harm to the physical or mental health of the user or that of others around the user. For this reason, hazardous substance use is not classified as a mental disorder but rather is listed in the *ICD-11* chapter on "Factors influencing health status or encounters with health services." Hazardous substance use may be a focus of intervention even in the absence of a diagnosable disorder.

The level and pattern of substance use that might be required to be considered hazardous varies across substances, based on evidence linking the quantity, frequency, and pattern of substance use to the development of various disorders. For example, it is known that a mean daily alcohol intake above 100 g per week for both males and females results in a significant increase in the risk of a range of chronic alcohol-related physical disorders (Wood et al., 2018), as well as the risk of various mental disorders including depressive disorders and anxiety and fear-related disorders. Consuming more than 40 g of alcohol on any given day is considered a threshold for significant increased short-term health risk (Connor et al., 2016). As consumption increases over this threshold, so does the risk for unintentional and intentional injuries and trauma to self and others, and medical conditions such as acute pancreatitis. There has been a major emphasis in recent years on health professionals detecting hazardous substance use to assist individuals modify their intake to avoid health consequences. This body of research is most firmly established for hazardous alcohol use (Beyer et al., 2019). Similar intervention approaches have been applied to hazardous use of cannabis, psychostimulants, and opioids, although with mixed results (Humeniuk et al., 2012; Saitz et al., 2014).

Harmful Pattern of Substance Use

Harmful pattern of substance use is diagnosed when recurrent substance use has actually caused harm. In the *ICD-11* it is defined as a pattern of continuous, recurrent, or sporadic use of a psychoactive substance that has caused clinically significant damage to a person's physical or mental health or has resulted in behaviour leading to harm to the health of others (WHO, 2023).

The harm must be accounted for by an identifiable pattern of substance use that is evident over a period of at least 12 months if substance use is episodic or at least 1 month if use is continuous (i.e., daily or almost daily). The harm to the person may occur from (a) intoxication, (b) toxic effects on body organs and systems or exacerbation of preexisting disorders, or (c) a harmful route of administration (e.g., injecting drug use). Harm to health of others includes any form of physical harm, including assault or a mental disorder, that is directly attributable to behavior on the part of the person to whom the diagnosis applies. Importantly, although there is a repetitive pattern of use, the diagnostic features of substance dependence—including impaired ability to control use, continued or escalated use despite harm or negative consequences, and physiological features such as tolerance and withdrawal—are not present. Harmful pattern of substance use is therefore a subdependence diagnosis that occupies the spectrum between hazardous or "at risk" use and "dependent" use, capturing various patterns of substance use—including repeated regular consumption or periodic excessive consumption—that have caused identifiable physical or mental harm.

SUBSTANCE DEPENDENCE

Substance dependence is defined in the *ICD-11* as a disorder of regulation of substance use, characterized by a strong internal drive to use a substance (WHO, 2023). A diagnosis of substance dependence requires the presence of two or more of the following:

- impaired control over substance use (i.e., onset, frequency, intensity, duration, termination, context);

- increasing priority or precedence of substance use over other aspects of life, including maintenance of health, and daily activities and responsibilities, continuation, or escalation of use despite harm or negative consequences; and

- physiological features including (a) tolerance to the effects of the substance, (b) withdrawal symptoms following cessation or reduction in use, or (c) repeated use of the substance or pharmacologically similar substances to prevent or alleviate withdrawal symptoms.

These features are usually evident over a period of at least 12 months, but the diagnosis may be made if use is continuous (daily or almost daily) for at least 3 months.

Physiological features are not a requirement for a diagnosis of substance dependence because they do not appear to occur for certain substances (e.g., hallucinogens, dissociative drugs including ketamine and PCP) even though the other features of substance dependence are present. For most substances, the two classic, predominately physiological features of substance dependence are tolerance and withdrawal, neither of which is present in hazardous substance use or harmful pattern of substance use. Tolerance occurs when a person gradually becomes less responsive to a drug with repeated use. The person consuming the drug requires a larger dose to obtain the same effect. This occurs through two primary mechanisms. First, enzymes that metabolize the drug, usually in the liver, become more effective at eliminating the substance. Second, the brain adapts to regular use and becomes less sensitive to the effects of the substance. Abrupt discontinuation or significant reductions in use can result in substance withdrawal in persons with substance dependence. Withdrawal is time-limited, drug-specific, and influenced by the lifetime and recent dose of the substance.

An often-intense desire or subjective sensation or urge or craving to use a substance is often a key aspect of substance dependence, although it is not required for the diagnosis and is not present invariably for all dependence-producing substances. Repeated use of most psychoactive substances excessively engages brain reward systems. To encourage the brain to return to homeostasis, opponent processes downregulate reward circuitry. As a consequence of these neuroadaptive processes, abstinence from substances can result in altered physiological functions and exaggerated negative emotional states. These states drive a need to relieve distress, described colloquially as craving. Craving assessments and interventions feature prominently in psychological approaches to substance use disorders.

OTHER DIAGNOSTIC CATEGORIES RELATED TO SUBSTANCE USE

The *ICD-11* provides additional diagnostic categories related to substance use for specific clinical situations. Harmful episode of substance use, substance intoxication, and substance withdrawal are particularly likely to be used in the acute management of patients in emergency or other medical settings. Substance-induced mental disorders are provided for situations in which presenting disturbances of perception, cognition, or behavior are substantially excess of those typical of substance intoxication or substance withdrawal and are not accounted for by another mental disorder.

Episode of Harmful Substance Use

This is a new diagnosis in the *ICD-11*. It is defined as an episode of substance use that has caused clinically significant damage to a person's physical or mental health or has resulted in behavior leading to harm to the health of others (WHO, 2023). As with harmful pattern of substance use, the harm to the person may occur from intoxication, toxic effects on body organs and systems, or a harmful route of administration. Harm to the health of others may also be considered in assigning a diagnosis of harmful episode of substance use.

   This category is intended for use in a wide range of health service settings and may be particularly important in primary care and emergency settings, where detailed information on substance use history may not be available, in contrast to specialized mental health and substance abuse treatment centers. Episodes in which substance use has led to harm, either to the self or others, provide important opportunities for brief and low-intensity interventions such as motivational interviewing (Frost et al., 2018) that can be feasibly administered in nonspecialist settings even in the absence of detailed information about the longitudinal pattern of use. If more information becomes available on the person's substance use indicating that the episode is part of a continuous or recurrent pattern of substance use, this diagnosis may be changed to harmful pattern of substance use or substance dependence, as appropriate.

Substance Intoxication

Substance intoxication is a group of disorders in the *ICD-11* that reflect the acute and typically time-limited effects of psychoactive substances, including certain prescribed medications. These conditions mostly refer to discreet episodes of substance use. The diagnosis may be made together with diagnoses that reflect repeated use of the substance, such as substance dependence or harmful pattern of substance use. The essential features of substance intoxication are as follows:

- transient and clinically significant disturbance in consciousness, cognition, perception, affect, behavior, or coordination that develop during or shortly after consumption of a substance;

- the presenting features are compatible with the known pharmacological effects of the substance, and their intensity is closely related to the amount of the substance consumed; and

- the symptoms of intoxication are time-limited and abate as the substance is cleared from the body.

Specific features of intoxication from each class of substance are set out in the *ICD-11*. Substance intoxication may further be specified as mild, moderate, or severe. The diagnosis of substance intoxication is often supported by detecting the substance or a metabolite in blood, urine, or another body fluid, but first and foremost, the diagnosis requires the presence of clinical features that are compatible with the relevant substance.

Substance Withdrawal

Substance withdrawal is also a time-limited syndrome. It may occur when a person who has substance dependence or otherwise a history of prolonged and/or substantial substance use ceases or reduces their level of use. It is defined in the *ICD-11* as follows:

- the occurrence of a clinically significant cluster of symptoms, behaviors, and/or physiological features that occur upon cessation or reduction in use in individuals with substance dependence or use of the substance for a prolonged period or in large amounts; and

- the features are consistent with those known to occur upon cessation or reduction of the particular substance or others in the same pharmacological group. The symptoms vary in degree of severity and duration depending on the substance and the amount and pattern of prior use.

Substance withdrawal can occur in people who take prescribed psychoactive medications (e.g., opioids, anxiolytics, and stimulants), even in standard therapeutic doses. Again, the symptoms of withdrawal differ according to the particular substance or substance group and specific descriptions of the individual syndromes are provided in the *ICD-11*. The features of a withdrawal syndrome are typically the opposite of those of acute intoxication with that substance. For example, alcohol is a central nervous system (CNS) depressant. In withdrawal, agitation and anxiety are key features. On the other hand, amphetamine is a CNS stimulant, and characteristic features of withdrawal often include depressed mood and lethargy. The *ICD-11* provides specifiers for certain withdrawal syndromes (e.g., "with seizures," "with perceptual disturbances").

Substance-Induced Mental Disorders

The *ICD-11* provides for the diagnosis of a series of mental disorders the clinician considers to have been induced by the use of a psychoactive substance and typically have their onset during intoxication or withdrawal or shortly afterward. There are several substance-induced mental disorders which apply to a range of substances. These include the following:

- substance-induced delirium;
- substance-induced psychotic disorder;
- substance-induced mood disorder; and
- substance-induced anxiety disorder.

Two substance-induced mental disorders apply only to psychostimulants:

- substance-induced obsessive-compulsive disorder and
- substance-induced impulse control disorder.

The key features of substance-induced mental disorders are the following:

- significant psychological, cognitive, or behavioral symptoms that develop during or soon after intoxication with or withdrawal from a specified substance or the use of a psychoactive medication;

- the specified substance, in the amount and duration of use, is capable of producing the symptoms;

- the duration or severity of the symptoms is substantially in excess of the disturbances characteristic of intoxication or withdrawal; and

- the symptoms cause significant distress or significant impairment in personal, family, social, educational, occupational, or other important areas of functioning.

There is also the requirement that features are not better explained by another medical or mental disorder.

Substance-induced mental disorders need to be distinguished from co-occurring independent or underlying mental disorders. The difference is that the features of substance-induced mental disorder usually resolve or improve after sustained cessation of substance use. This may take several weeks, and in certain cases, substance-induced mental disorders may run a course of some months before remitting. Certain substance withdrawal syndromes may also have a prolonged course, and the distinction between prolonged withdrawal and the substance-induced mental disorder (e.g., for benzodiazepines) may be difficult.

Other substance-induced mental disorders include substance-induced amnestic disorder, substance-induced dementia, and substance-induced catatonia, which are classified elsewhere in the *ICD*.

A PSYCHOLOGICAL APPROACH TO DISORDERS DUE TO SUBSTANCE USE

There is a large body of psychologically based research that describes the etiology of disorders due to substance use. The development and maintenance of a repetitive pattern of substance use is influenced by specific psychological processes—in particular, the effect of associating the actions of a substance with desired consequences. The pattern and intensity of substance use is further influenced by social mores, informal constraints, and a range of local laws and regulations. Consequently, first-line, evidence-based interventions for disorders due to substance use are primarily behavioral in nature. The main exceptions to this are management of the acute effects of substance intoxication and substance withdrawal, and pharmacological interventions for opioid dependence and nicotine dependence (i.e., opioid substitution therapy and nicotine replacement therapy). Depending on the specific substance, behavioral treatments may be combined with adjunctive pharmacotherapy for relapse prevention and management of craving, particularly for the more severe forms of disorder. Examples of adjunctive treatments include naltrexone and acamprosate for alleviation of craving and promotion of abstinence from alcohol.

Substance use develops in relation to the experience of its effects and the expectations developed as a result, often described as "outcome expectancies."

For example, if a patient consumes a substance, there is often the expectation they will feel more happy, relaxed, or socially confident (Monk & Heim, 2013). These expectations are modified by the individual's psychological state and the prevailing environment. The repeated pairing of environmental cues and perceived social and other benefits enhances the substance's subjective and physiological effects via conditioning and social and cognitive learning (Bandura, 1999). Higher levels of outcome expectancies are associated with a higher risk of alcohol-related problems (Monk & Heim, 2013). In some individuals, substance use becomes more stereotyped over time, less flexible, less responsive to the external environment, and more internally driven, and the individual's capacity to maintain control of consumption diminishes. This sets the stage for substance dependence, in which profound neurobiological changes occur in several neurocircuits in the brain, many clustered within the brain's reward systems (Koob & Volkow, 2016; Volkow et al., 2016).

A complex set of inherited and learned behaviors contribute to psychological vulnerability and risk of developing disorders due to substance use. Genetics plays a significant role, representing approximately 50% of the risk (Yu & McClellan, 2016). The two main mechanisms for genetic effects are variations in brain neurotransmitter activity and drug metabolism in the body. Other strong risk factors include a family history of disorders due to substance use disorders; co-occurring psychopathology; childhood mood, conduct, and dissocial disorders; low self-control; and high impulsivity (Chartier et al., 2010). For example, increased levels of impulsiveness are associated with earlier age of onset of disorders due to substance use, higher levels of consumption, and poorer treatment outcomes (Sher et al., 2000).

A robust clinical assessment typically triangulates self-reported data from the individual, the *ICD-11* diagnostic requirements as evaluated by the clinician, addiction-specific psychometrically valid instruments, and where applicable, biological consumption and organ functioning markers (see description in the Assessment section later in this chapter). Comprehensive addiction assessments should include instruments that not only map onto the *ICD-11* diagnostic requirements but also assess important behavioral treatment targets. This is particularly relevant for psychologically based treatments.

Important targets of psychological assessment and treatment include urges and craving to use, outcome expectancies, self-efficacy, and motivation (Coates et al., 2018; Moos, 2007). Craving is a multidimensional construct that includes the intensity of the drive to use substances, the presence of associated imagery (e.g., smell, taste), and the intrusiveness of cognitions related to desire to use the substance, which often displace more functional, nonsubstance cognitions. It does not invariably occur in persons with substance dependence, but it is a major risk factor for relapse. It may include physiological discomfort, intrusive substance-related thoughts, and affective distress, all of which are important targets of cognitive and behavioral interventions. Individuals may describe craving in a variety of ways, such as desires, wants, and needs. Desires of moderate and even mild intensities may be important to assess, both as targets for psychological interventions and as indicators of change and treatment prognosis. Many substance treatment services report benefits in treatment outcomes related to craving (Pavlick et al., 2009).

Expectations of substance use develop vicariously, typically before use is initiated, via social modeling, direct observation, and exposure to peer and media influences. Common outcome expectancy domains include being more assertive (e.g., "Using alcohol makes me more assertive"), affect modification (e.g., "Cannabis improves my mood"), sexual enhancement (e.g., "Amphetamines make me more attractive and sexually alluring"), cognitive change (e.g., "I use alcohol to slow down my thinking"), and tension reduction ("I use cannabis to relax"). A nuanced assessment of substance use expectancies can identify the unique cluster of positive or negative expectations of substance use that the individual holds. The next step is to apply well-validated psychological interventions to modify strong and unrealistic expectations of substance use and to develop effective strategies to compensate for skills deficits (e.g., social skills training as an alternative to alcohol use before social interactions; Coates et al., 2018; Moos, 2007).

Self-efficacy refers to a person's belief that they can successfully regulate their behavior. Self-efficacy is regarded as a pivotal pathway to change and a foundation of human agency (Bandura, 1997) and is one of the most consistent predictors of treatment outcomes for disorders due to substance use. Dimensions of self-efficacy relevant to substance use include the ability to resist social pressure to use (e.g., "I find it difficult to resist smoking when my friends are smoking"), the ability to resist opportunities to use (e.g., "When someone offers me a drink, it is hard to say no"), and use of substances for emotional relief (e.g., "When I am stressed, it is hard not to smoke cannabis"). Information about substance use expectancies and patterns of self-efficacy profiles can provide a highly effective basis for treatment planning (Moos, 2007).

However, in addition to belief in their ability to change (self-efficacy), it is important to assess the individual's level of motivation to effect this change. The most widely applied theoretical model of motivation in substance use disorder assessment and treatment is the transtheoretical model of change (Prochaska et al., 2002). This model conceptualizes six stages of change, which have major implications for treatment strategies. These stages include *precontemplation* (individual not considering change and unlikely to accept help or professional advice; therapeutic emphasis is on information giving and feedback, raising awareness, and developing rapport), *contemplation* (individual considering changing substance use; therapeutic emphasis is on exploring and resolving ambivalence), *preparation* (individual has made a decision to instigate change; therapeutic emphasis is on reinforcing commitment to change), *action* (the individual is actually initiating change; therapeutic emphasis is on operationalizing change tasks and goals), *maintenance* (the individual is adhering to modified substance use behavior; therapeutic emphasis is on maintaining self-efficacy and planning for high-risk situations), and *relapse* (the individual returns to previous substance use behavior; therapeutic emphasis is on framing relapse as an opportunity to learn).

CO-OCCURRING DISORDERS

A wide range of mental disorders and medical comorbidities are commonly present in disorders due to substance use and are highlighted in the *CDDR*. Some of the mental disorders are in the category of substance-induced mental disorders. Others are termed "co-occurring" mental disorders. These often reflect shared neurobiological, genetic, psychological, and social factors implicated in the development, maintenance, and exacerbation of multiple disorders. Approximately one in four individuals with mental disorders including schizophrenia, depressive disorders, and bipolar disorders also have a disorder due to substance use (National Institute on Drug Abuse, 2018). Prevalence of co-occurring mental disorders is typically higher among persons seeking treatment for substance disorders (Moss et al., 2010).

In most cases of co-occurring disorders, each exacerbates the other, but it is often unclear which came first. Impact on functioning should be emphasized in determining the priority for treatment. However, continued substance use may detrimentally affect engagement in therapy and compromise the benefits of medication, and many clinicians and treatment services focus on achieving a period of abstinence first. In addition, this allows some substance-induced mental disorders to remit or lessen. Improvement or remission in one disorder typically improves severity of the corresponding disorder. For example, effective treatment of alcohol dependence typically results in improved mood for those with co-occurring depressive disorders. This is not surprising given that treatment approaches and strategies for managing substance dependence (such as relaxation techniques, problem-solving, cognitive restructuring, and social skills development) overlap with those used for many other mental health conditions. Neurochemicals such as dopamine and serotonin implicated in mental disorders also regulate subjective feelings of substance intoxication and well-being in response to substances.

DEVELOPMENTAL COURSE

In most countries, alcohol consumption is most commonly initiated during early adolescence (Connor et al., 2016). Drinking rates then increase in a largely linear fashion until young adulthood, which is the age during which heaviest alcohol consumption occurs. Alcohol consumption generally declines from middle to late adulthood (Jackson & Sartor, 2016). A similar trajectory is evident for illicit drug use, although the age of onset is usually later than alcohol (de Girolamo et al., 2019). Early initiation of alcohol or drug use relative to society norms is a predictor of increased chronicity of adult use and of substance dependence (de Girolamo et al., 2019). Approximately half of those with early-onset disorders remit by their late 20s and achieve normative social and vocational functioning. This often occurs without formal intervention as young adults enter the labor market, marry, and assume responsibility for children.

ASSESSMENT

A comprehensive clinical interview as described in this section is the most effective approach to arrive at a reliable *ICD-11* diagnosis and an effective treatment plan for disorders due to substance use. Central to assessment is examination of psychological and behavioral processes pivotal in development and maintenance of a repetitive pattern of substance use and determination if this pattern conforms to the *ICD-11* (a) hazardous use, (b) harmful use, or (c) substance dependence. Obtaining an individual's narrative history is essential in making a diagnosis (Dore et al., 2016), including a consideration of whether time duration requirements are met for different diagnoses.

Depending on the circumstances of the referral, the individual may be forthcoming about their history of substance use, or it may require substantial corroboration and use of ancillary information, such as data from interviews of family members, medical records and tests, and previous interactions with the legal system. For example, a person who has come to the realization that their use of one or more substances is causing them personal or health problems and has booked the appointment and has a goal of working to resolve this issue is more likely to be forthcoming about the various substances they use and their psychological, physical, and personal impact. However, even those who present voluntarily for treatment of disorders due to substance use may exhibit considerable denial about the extent of their substance use and its impact, making accurate assessment difficult.

Assessment requires much sophistication if the patient has reason to understate the level of use or its impact or even to deny certain forms of substance use or its consequences. This is more likely in patients who have been referred by their employers (e.g., through employee assistance programs), for an assessment for fitness for work, for disability assessment (after a previous accident or injury), from the criminal justice system, or have been coerced to seek treatment by family members. If a negative outcome from the diagnosis of a disorder due to substance use is likely, it may be difficult to get reliable diagnostic information. In such cases, corroborating data are more heavily weighted, including biological markers of substance use and organ disease (derived from blood samples) and data from the individual's family, social, and vocational network.

There are three central components of assessing a person's substance use history. These are (a) intake of psychoactive substances, (b) substance dependence, and (c) harms and consequences. These three dimensions are embedded in the WHO Alcohol Use Disorders Identification Test (AUDIT; Saunders et al., 1993), which offers a convenient method of assessing disorders due to alcohol use.

(Available at https://www.who.int/publications/i/item/audit-the-alcohol-use-disorders-identification-test-guidelines-for-use-in-primary-health-care.)

INTAKE OF PSYCHOACTIVE SUBSTANCES

First, for each major substance or class of substances identified as having been used by the patient, either recently or historically, the assessment should consist of the following:

1. An inquiry about the exact *type* of substance. For example, for alcohol, it should include inquiry about when the main drink is beer, wine, spirits, or some other form of alcohol. The purpose is to quantify the concentration of alcohol consumed. For benzodiazepines, the exact compound should be identified—for example, diazepam (Valium is a common brand name), lorazepam (Ativan), or alprazolam (Xanax). Similar to alcohol, there is a dose-dependent relationship with substance harm for other drugs, and the compounds and delivery systems employed are critical in determining exposure.

2. The frequency of use should be identified; typically daily, several times per week, several times per month, or less frequently.

3. The quantity of use should be established and related to a particular time period—that is, per occasion of use, per day, week, month, or year.

4. The pattern or variability of use should be determined. Use may be quite stereotyped from day-to-day, or there may be a recognizable pattern that is relevant to the symptoms or impact the individual may experience. For example, alcohol may be consumed in a binge-like pattern each weekend with little or no consumption during the working week. A particular risk with this pattern of consumption is acute injury. Methamphetamine is often consumed for 3 to 5 days successively (termed the "run"), and because this level of use cannot often be sustained, the person ceases use, may experience a "crash," and may develop stimulant withdrawal syndrome.

5. Mode of administration: Alcohol is almost always consumed orally. Cannabis (marijuana) is typically smoked. Methamphetamine is often snorted or smoked, or it may be injected. Heroin is usually injected but may be smoked or snorted, and cocaine is most commonly snorted. Substances taken orally typically have a slower rate of absorption, more moderate intoxication levels, and longer lasting effects. Inhaling and injecting results in the drug crossing the blood–brain barrier more effectively and quickly and typically results in more immediate intoxication and—depending on the substance— higher levels of intoxication. Injecting drug use comes at elevated risk of bloodborne diseases such as hepatitis C and HIV. Individuals who are being assessed for substance use disorders and are injecting drugs should be offered screening for bloodborne viruses.

6. Duration of the major phases of use: For each major substance used, progression though hazardous substance use to harmful pattern of substance use to substance dependence (if applicable) should be investigated. These different patterns of substance use may coincide with major life events such as the mid- to late teen years, during college, during the first few years of employment, or after retirement from vocational roles.

7. Time and date of last use: This needs to be identified particularly for potentially high risk, time-critical presentations such as substance intoxication, substance withdrawal, and substance-induced mental disorders, including substance-induced delirium.

Standardized psychometric tools can be used as a prompt for patients to recall substance intake. They are particularly useful for patients with cognitive impairment, severe co-occurring mental disorders, or those in substance withdrawal. The most widely used substance intake instrument is the Time-line Follow-Back (Sobell & Sobell, 1992). It has strong psychometric properties and is freely available.

Substance Dependence

The most common publicly available instruments for substance dependence that have strong psychometric properties are the Addiction Severity Index (McLellan et al., 1980) and the Severity of Dependence Scale (Gossop et al., 1995). Both have a recognized threshold for likely substance dependence. The AUDIT questionnaire (Saunders et al., 1993) has three questions (Q 4–6) on alcohol dependence, and an overall score of 15 or higher suggests likely alcohol dependence. Also available are various other substance-specific dependence measures. Use of these instruments assists not only with diagnosis but also in determining appropriate treatment pathways.

Harms and Consequences

On the basis of the interview, the clinician will have identified several areas of concern that are the individual's (or relative's) primary reason for seeking assistance. Inquiry should continue on problems typically associated with the substance in question. These can be grouped in the following domains: (a) mental health consequences/harms (e.g., presence of anxiety, depression, suicidal ideation and attempts, psychotic disorders triggered by the substance use), (b) social consequences (e.g., difficulties in interpersonal relationships; with finances; with work, such as unemployment or engaging in prostitution; legal/forensic trouble, such as drunk driving, assault, or criminal charges), and (c) physical harm/consequences. This may be particularly relevant to psychologists working in general health or medical settings (e.g., acute physical illnesses such as gastritis, pancreatitis, and chronic physical disorders such as liver disease and substance-induced brain damage).

Assessment of Addiction-Specific Psychological Treatment Targets

There are a large range of multifactorial, psychometrically robust substance-specific scales available to measure common psychological targets in addiction treatment. These instruments can also be effectively used to track a patient's progress across treatment. Using alcohol as an example, a widely used craving instrument in research and clinical practice is the Obsessive-Compulsive Drinking Scale for Heavy Drinking (Anton et al., 1995). Outcome expectancies can also be assessed via qualitative interviewing techniques or by using one of several validated and standardized substance-specific expectancy instruments (e.g., Brown et al., 1987). Similar to outcome expectancies, self-efficacy beliefs can also be assessed via qualitative interviewing techniques or by standardized assessments (e.g., Young et al., 1991). Psychometric tools can assist in confirming motivation stages. The most widely used instrument is the Readiness to Change Questionnaire (Heather et al., 1993).

Assessment of Suicide Risk

Consideration of suicide risk should occur in all mental health assessments, even if the individual does not meet the *ICD-11* requirements for a depressive disorder. Substance use significantly increases the risk of death by suicide (Conner et al., 2019). The disinhibition that can occur when a person is intoxicated contributes to these suicide rates. Disinhibition also contributes to self-harming behaviors without suicidal intent. A key strategy for reducing suicide rates is targeting risk factors associated with substance use and substance use disorders. In addition to risk to the individual being assessed, health professionals need to be alert to risk of violence or homicidal intent toward others.

Mental State Examination

This is a vital component of the overall assessment. Emphasis should be placed on identifying common co-occurring mental disorders and neurocognitive impairments. Key components are the person's general appearance, their reaction to the interview, speech, mood, affect, speech, thought form, thought content, perception, presence of hallucinations, cognitive function, attention, concentration, orientation, memory (immediate recall, short- and long-term memory), intelligence, insight, and judgment. As mentioned, risk assessment (of suicidal ideation, and attempts, and of other forms of self-harm and homicidal intent) is mandatory.

Laboratory Investigations

In medical settings, the clinical interview is often complemented by undertaking relevant laboratory tests. These include routine blood tests, urine drug screens (for drugs or metabolites), saliva analysis, breath analysis, and, less commonly, analysis of hair. These samples can be examined for the presence of alcohol, nicotine, prescribed medications, and illicit drugs, and their metabolites. For alcohol, there are several biological markers that reflect a range of pathophysiological effects on blood, the liver, and other organs (e.g., liver cell damage may be assessed by levels of alanine and aspartate aminotransferase [AST, ALT] and γ-glutamyl transferase [GGT] in the blood). It should be noted that none of these tests diagnose substance dependence, harmful substance use, or hazardous substance use. They reflect the presence of the substance that may be affecting organ health.

GENDER-RELATED FEATURES

Males and females may be affected differently by the acute and long-term effects of substances. Gender differences in the biology of brain structure and endocrine and metabolic systems contribute to these differential health risks. For example, females are less effective at metabolizing alcohol than males, resulting in ethanol remaining in the female body for longer periods of time. Females also have lower total body water compared with males, resulting in higher blood alcohol concentrations (and therefore intoxication) from equivalent amounts of alcohol consumed. Gender differences based on biological variation in substances other than alcohol is less well studied. Cultural and social factors relating to women's role in society also contribute to the differential prevalence and health impact of substance use.

CULTURAL AND OTHER CONTEXTUAL CONSIDERATIONS

Culture, religious beliefs, and regional policies and laws influence the use of substances, the development of substance use disorders, and treatment-seeking behavior (McHugh et al., 2018). For example, a number of religions prohibit alcohol consumption. This reduces prevalence of alcohol use disorders in certain geographic areas. Some countries impose legal restrictions to support the upholding of religious belief-based practices; in these countries, alcohol use disorders are rare. There is greater variation based on religious beliefs regarding the use of nonprescribed drugs. Different cultures have their own values, beliefs, customs, and traditions associated with substance use. For example, in some cultures, drug use occurs but is heavily regulated and only used for ceremonial purposes. Prevailing national and local policies relating to substance use contribute to the prevalence of substance use disorders. Some countries have more liberal policies relating to alcohol and drugs, and some are more conservative. However, there is a weak correlation between more restrictive policies and lower consumption and substance use disorder prevalence. Culture as well as gender roles also influence clinical presentation (e.g., the specific expression of priority given to use over other activities in substance dependence). The way in which diagnostics in the *ICD-11* are framed provides scope for consideration of cultural, prevailing normative, and religious factors that may contribute to the diagnosis of disorders due to substance use.

KEY POINTS

- The *ICD-11* includes specific disorder categories related to 14 classes of psychoactive substances, in addition to categories for "other specified substances."

- A central aim of a clinical assessment of disorders due to substance use is to arrive at one of four descriptions of the overall pattern of substance use: (a) no substance use disorder, (b) hazardous substance use, (c) harmful pattern of use of a substance, or (d) substance dependence.

- Additional *ICD-11* categories are provided for substance intoxication, substance withdrawal, episode of harmful substance use, and substance-induced mental disorders, including substance-induced delirium.

- Co-occurrence with other mental disorders is common and is even higher among those who seek mental health treatment.

- The development and maintenance of a repetitive pattern of substance use is influenced by specific psychological processes—in particular, the effect of associating the actions of a substance with desired consequences. Important targets of psychological assessment and treatment include substance craving, outcome expectancies, self-efficacy, and motivation.

- There are three central components of assessing a person's substance use history. These are (a) intake of psychoactive substances, (b) dependence, and (c) harms and consequences.

- Pervading cultural practices, religious beliefs, laws, gender roles, and other societal norms relating to substance use should be considered in substance use disorder assessments.

REFERENCES

Anton, R. F., Moak, D. H., & Latham, P. (1995). The Obsessive Compulsive Drinking Scale: A self-rated instrument for the quantification of thoughts about alcohol and drinking behavior. *Alcoholism, Clinical and Experimental Research, 19*(1), 92–99. https://doi.org/10.1111/j.1530-0277.1995.tb01475.x

Bandura, A. (1997). *Self-efficacy: The exercise of control.* W.H. Freeman & Co.

Bandura, A. (1999). A sociocognitive analysis of substance abuse: An agentic perspective. *Psychological Science, 10*(3), 214–217. https://doi.org/10.1111/1467-9280.00138

Beyer, F. R., Campbell, F., Bertholet, N., Daeppen, J. B., Saunders, J. B., Pienaar, E. D., Muirhead, C. R., & Kaner, E. F. S. (2019). The Cochrane 2018 review on brief interventions in primary care for hazardous and harmful alcohol consumption: A distillation for clinicians and policy makers. *Alcohol and Alcoholism, 54*(4), 417–427. https://doi.org/10.1093/alcalc/agz035

Brown, S. A., Christiansen, B. A., & Goldman, M. S. (1987). The Alcohol Expectancy Questionnaire: An instrument for the assessment of adolescent and adult alcohol expectancies. *Journal of Studies on Alcohol, 48*(5), 483–491. https://doi.org/10.15288/jsa.1987.48.483

Chartier, K. G., Hesselbrock, M. N., & Hesselbrock, V. M. (2010). Development and vulnerability factors in adolescent alcohol use. *Child and Adolescent Psychiatric Clinics of North America, 19*(3), 493–504. https://doi.org/10.1016/j.chc.2010.03.004

Coates, J. M., Gullo, M. J., Feeney, G. F. X., Young, R. M., & Connor, J. P. (2018). A randomized trial of personalized cognitive-behavior therapy for alcohol use disorder in a public health clinic. *Frontiers in Psychiatry, 9*, Article 297. https://doi.org/10.3389/fpsyt.2018.00297

Conner, K. R., Bridge, J. A., Davidson, D. J., Pilcher, C., & Brent, D. A. (2019). Meta-analysis of mood and substance use disorders in proximal risk for suicide deaths. *Suicide & Life-Threatening Behavior, 49*(1), 278–292. https://doi.org/10.1111/sltb.12422

Connor, J. P., Haber, P. S., & Hall, W. D. (2016). Alcohol use disorders. *The Lancet, 387*(10022), 988–998. https://doi.org/10.1016/S0140-6736(15)00122-1

de Girolamo, G., McGorry, P., & Sartorius, N. (Eds.). (2019). *The age of onset of mental disorders: Ethiopathogenetic and treatment implications*. Springer. https://doi.org/10.1007/978-3-319-72619-9

Dore, G. M., Latt, N. C., & Saunders, J. B. (2016). Establishing the diagnosis. In J. B. Saunders, K. M. Conigrave, N. C. Latt, D. J. Nutt, E. J. Marshall, W. Ling, & S. Higuchi (Eds.), *Addiction medicine* (2nd ed., pp. 67–84). Oxford University Press.

Frost, H., Campbell, P., Maxwell, M., O'Carroll, R. E., Dombrowski, S. U., Williams, B., Cheyne, H., Coles, E., & Pollock, A. (2018). Effectiveness of motivational interviewing on adult behaviour change in health and social care settings: A systematic review of reviews. *PLoS One, 13*(10), e0204890. https://doi.org/10.1371/journal.pone.0204890

Gossop, M., Darke, S., Griffiths, P., Hando, J., Powis, B., Hall, W., & Strang, J. (1995). The Severity of Dependence Scale (SDS): Psychometric properties of the SDS in English and Australian samples of heroin, cocaine and amphetamine users. *Addiction, 90*(5), 607–614. https://doi.org/10.1046/j.1360-0443.1995.9056072.x

Heather, N., Rollnick, S., & Bell, A. (1993). Predictive validity of the Readiness to Change Questionnaire. *Addiction, 88*(12), 1667–1677. https://doi.org/10.1111/j.1360-0443.1993.tb02042.x

Humeniuk, R., Ali, R., Babor, T., Souza-Formigoni, M. L., de Lacerda, R. B., Ling, W., McRee, B., Newcombe, D., Pal, H., Poznyak, V., Simon, S., & Vendetti, J. (2012). A randomized controlled trial of a brief intervention for illicit drugs linked to the Alcohol, Smoking and Substance Involvement Screening Test (ASSIST) in clients recruited from primary health-care settings in four countries. *Addiction, 107*(5), 957–966. https://doi.org/10.1111/j.1360-0443.2011.03740.x

Jackson, K. M., & Sartor, C. E. (2016). The natural course of substance use and dependence. In K. J. Sher (Ed.), *The Oxford handbook of substance use and substance use disorders* (Vol. 1, pp. 67–131). Oxford University Press.

Koob, G. F., & Volkow, N. D. (2016). Neurobiology of addiction: A neurocircuitry analysis. *The Lancet Psychiatry, 3*(8), 760–773. https://doi.org/10.1016/S2215-0366(16)00104-8

McHugh, R. K., Votaw, V. R., Sugarman, D. E., & Greenfield, S. F. (2018). Sex and gender differences in substance use disorders. *Clinical Psychology Review, 66*, 12–23. https://doi.org/10.1016/j.cpr.2017.10.012

McLellan, A. T., Luborsky, L., Woody, G. E., & O'Brien, C. P. (1980). An improved diagnostic evaluation instrument for substance abuse patients: The Addiction Severity Index. *Journal of Nervous and Mental Disease, 168*(1), 26–33. https://doi.org/10.1097/00005053-198001000-00006

Monk, R. L., & Heim, D. (2013). A critical systematic review of alcohol-related outcome expectancies. *Substance Use & Misuse, 48*(7), 539–557. https://doi.org/10.3109/10826084.2013.787097

Moos, R. H. (2007). Theory-based active ingredients of effective treatments for substance use disorders. *Drug and Alcohol Dependence, 88*(2–3), 109–121. https://doi.org/10.1016/j.drugalcdep.2006.10.010

Moss, H. B., Chen, C. M., & Yi, H. Y. (2010). Prospective follow-up of empirically derived alcohol dependence subtypes in wave 2 of the National Epidemiologic Survey on Alcohol And Related Conditions (NESARC): Recovery status, alcohol use disorders and diagnostic criteria, alcohol consumption behavior, health status, and treatment seeking. *Alcoholism, Clinical and Experimental Research, 34*(6), 1073–1083. https://doi.org/10.1111/j.1530-0277.2010.01183.x

National Institute on Drug Abuse. (2018). *Common comorbidities with substance use disorders.* https://www.drugabuse.gov/publications/research-reports/common-comorbidities-substance-use-disorders/introduction

Pavlick, M., Hoffmann, E., & Rosenberg, H. (2009). A nationwide survey of American alcohol and drug craving assessment and treatment practices. *Addiction Research and Theory, 17*(6), 591–600. https://doi.org/10.3109/16066350802262630

Prochaska, J. O., Redding, C. A., & Evers, K. (2002). The transtheoretical model and stages of change. In K. Glanz, B. K. Rimer, & F. M. Lewis (Eds.), *Health behavior and health education: Theory, research, and practice* (3rd ed., pp. 99–120). Jossey-Bass.

Rehm, J., & Shield, K. D. (2019). Global burden of disease and the impact of mental and addictive disorders. *Current Psychiatry Reports, 21*(2), Article 10. https://doi.org/10.1007/s11920-019-0997-0

Saitz, R., Palfai, T. P., Cheng, D. M., Alford, D. P., Bernstein, J. A., Lloyd-Travaglini, C. A., Meli, S. M., Chaisson, C. E., & Samet, J. H. (2014). Screening and brief intervention for drug use in primary care: The ASPIRE randomized clinical trial. *JAMA, 312*(5), 502–513. https://doi.org/10.1001/jama.2014.7862

Saunders, J. B. (2016). The nature of addictive disorders. In J. B. Saunders, K. M. Conigrave, N. C. Latt, D. J. Nutt, E. J. Marshall, W. Ling, & S. Higuchi (Eds.), *Addiction medicine* (2nd ed., pp. 449–460). Oxford University Press. https://doi.org/10.1093/med/9780198714750.003.0021

Saunders, J. B., Aasland, O. G., Babor, T. F., de la Fuente, J. R., & Grant, M. (1993). Development of the Alcohol Use Disorders Identification Test (AUDIT): WHO Collaborative Project on Early Detection of Persons with Harmful Alcohol Consumption—II. *Addiction, 88*(6), 791–804. https://doi.org/10.1111/j.1360-0443.1993.tb02093.x

Saunders, J. B., & Latt, N. C. (2021). Diagnostic definitions and classification of substance use disorders. In N. el-Guebaly, G. Carrà, M. Galanter, & A. M. Baldacchino (Eds.), *Textbook of addiction treatment: International perspectives* (2nd ed., pp. 91–113). Springer Nature. https://doi.org/10.1007/978-3-030-36391-8_8

Sher, K. J., Bartholow, B. D., & Wood, M. D. (2000). Personality and substance use disorders: A prospective study. *Journal of Consulting and Clinical Psychology, 68*(5), 818–829. https://doi.org/10.1037/0022-006X.68.5.818

Sobell, L. C., & Sobell, M. B. (1992). Timeline follow-back: A technique for assessing self-reported ethanol consumption. In J. Allen & R. Z. Litten (Eds.), *Measuring alcohol consumption: Psychosocial and biological methods* (pp. 41–72). Humana Press. https://doi.org/10.1007/978-1-4612-0357-5_3

Volkow, N. D., Koob, G. F., & McLellan, A. T. (2016). Neurobiologic advances from the brain disease model of addiction. *The New England Journal of Medicine, 374*(4), 363–371. https://doi.org/10.1056/NEJMra1511480

Wood, A. M., Kaptoge, S., Butterworth, A. S., Willeit, P., Warnakula, S., Bolton, T., Paige, E., Paul, D. S., Sweeting, M., Burgess, S., Bell, S., Astle, W., Stevens, D., Koulman, A., Selmer, R. M., Verschuren, W. M. M., Sato, S., Njølstad, I., Woodward, M., . . . the Emerging Risk Factors Collaboration/EPIC-CVD/UK Biobank Alcohol Study Group. (2018). Risk thresholds for alcohol consumption: Combined analysis of individual-participant data for 599 912 current drinkers in 83 prospective studies. *The Lancet, 391*(10129), 1513–1523. https://doi.org/10.1016/S0140-6736(18)30134-X

World Health Organization. (2023). *ICD-11 for mortality and morbidity statistics* (Version: 01/2023). https://icd.who.int/browse11/l-m/en#/

World Health Organization. (2024). *Clinical descriptions and diagnostic requirements for ICD-11 mental, behavioural and neurodevelopmental disorders.* https://www.who.int/publications/i/item/9789240077263

Young, R. M., Oei, T. P. S., & Crook, G. M. (1991). Development of a drinking self-efficacy questionnaire. *Journal of Psychopathology and Behavioral Assessment, 13*(1), 1–15. https://doi.org/10.1007/BF00960735

Yu, C., & McClellan, J. (2016). Genetics of substance use disorders. *Child and Adolescent Psychiatric Clinics of North America, 25*(3), 377–385. https://doi.org/10.1016/j.chc.2016.02.002

16

Disorders Due to Addictive Behaviors and Impulse Control Disorders

Joël Billieux, Naomi A. Fineberg, Daniel L. King, and Hans-Jürgen Rumpf

OVERARCHING LOGIC

This chapter focuses on two groupings of disorders in the 11th revision of the *International Classification of Diseases* (*ICD-11*; World Health Organization [WHO], 2023): disorders due to addictive behaviors—namely, gambling disorder and gaming disorder—and impulse control disorders, which include pyromania, kleptomania, compulsive sexual behavior disorder, and intermittent explosive disorder. As described in the *Clinical Descriptions and Diagnostic Requirements for ICD-11 Mental, Behavioural and Neurodevelopmental Disorders* (*CDDR*; WHO, 2024), disorders due to addictive behaviors and impulse control disorders are disabling conditions sharing impulsivity and loss of control as core features. A common characteristic of these disorders is that they lie at the extreme pole of an impulsivity continuum linking normal behavior to dysregulated, pathological behavior (Padhi et al., 2012). At the symptomatic level, these disorders may also share common experiences of an overwhelming urge (or craving) before engaging in the behavior and a feeling of relief or pleasure afterwards. A vicious circle involving a dynamic interaction between positive and negative reinforcement therefore can contribute to the maintenance of these conditions (Dell'Osso et al., 2006). Positive reinforcement in the context of these conditions typically relates to feelings of gratification, pleasure, excitement, or euphoria, whereas negative reinforcement typically relates to the relief or reduction of aversive emotional states (e.g., dysphoria, boredom,

https://doi.org/10.1037/0000392-016
A Psychological Approach to Diagnosis: Using the ICD-11 as a Framework, G. M. Reed,
P. L.-J. Ritchie, and A. Maercker (Editors)

anxiety) by the relevant behavior. In terms of neurocognitive underpinnings, both disorders due to addictive behaviors and impulse control disorders are related to impairments in neural circuits involved in reward-processing and top-down executive control (Brand et al., 2019; Grant et al., 2014).

A PSYCHOLOGICAL APPROACH TO DISORDERS DUE TO ADDICTIVE BEHAVIORS AND IMPULSE CONTROL DISORDERS

There are two other important reasons for addressing these two groupings of disorders in the same chapter and for separating them from disorders due to substance use. First, central features of disorders due to substance use such as tolerance or preoccupation are not necessarily indicative of pathological or problematic behavior when they occur in relation to activities such as gaming or gambling (e.g., Billieux et al., 2019; Castro-Calvo et al., 2021). Given that some gamblers or gamers may become highly involved in these activities without necessarily experiencing adverse effects such as impaired control or functional impairment, applying diagnostic requirements from disorders due to substance use to other types of behaviors risks pathologizing normal behavior and promoting unnecessary or inappropriate interventions. Second, the psychological assessment and treatment of both disorders due to addictive behaviors and impulse control disorders should systematically target impulsivity traits and processes related to self-control, factors known to play a pivotal role in the onset, persistence, and recurrence of these disorders (Padhi et al., 2012).

Impulsivity generally refers to a tendency to engage in swift or uncontrolled behavior without forethought or conscious and adaptive judgment. Heightened impulsivity is understood as a transdiagnostic etiological factor (Berg et al., 2015; Slutske et al., 2005) that has been linked to a wide range of behavioral problems and mental health conditions and plays a particular role in the disorders discussed in this chapter. At the same time, impulsivity is an "umbrella" construct, reflecting a combination of separable personality traits. Accordingly, when assessing a patient, a sound and clinically relevant assessment of impulsivity that takes into account its multidimensional nature is important as a basis for formulating treatment needs and selecting appropriately targeted psychological interventions.

A particularly useful framework for conceptualizing impulsivity is the urgency–premeditation–perseverance–sensation seeking (UPPS) impulsivity model (Whiteside & Lynam, 2001). The main advantage of the UPPS framework is that it allows for consideration of the various facets of impulsivity, while other existing frameworks focus on only one or another aspect and therefore do not allow for sufficiently comprehensive impulsivity assessment and profiling. Numerous studies have been conducted based on the UPPS model over the past 2 decades, showing that its various components predict specific psychopathological symptoms and problematic behaviors and are related to distinct (neuro)cognitive mechanisms (e.g., inhibitory control, attentional capacities, decision making) and neuroanatomical underpinnings (Berg et al., 2015; Rochat et al., 2018).

In the UPPS model, *urgency* refers to emotion-related impulsivity, which is generally defined as the tendency to act rashly in intense emotional contexts. Individuals with high urgency tend to overreact when, for example, they are distressed or angry and are at increased risk for displaying maladaptive coping strategies and addictive or compulsive behaviors (Berg et al., 2015). Individuals with elevated urgency also present with reduced inhibitory control (i.e., the ability to refrain from automatic and habitual motor behaviors), which is a central feature of disorders due to addictive behaviors and impulse control disorders. Lack of *premeditation* refers to the tendency not to consider the consequences of an action before engaging in it. Individuals who exhibit lack of premeditation tend to favor short-term considerations, are not good at delaying rewards, and tend to have poorer decision-making and problem-solving abilities, all of which are also features of these disorders. Lack of *perseverance* is defined as difficulty remaining focused on tasks that are boring or cognitively demanding. This attentional component of impulsivity has been linked with difficulties in resisting the intrusion of irrelevant information that interferes with ongoing tasks. People with low perseverance are thus at increased risk for experiencing memory intrusions that promote subjective states of urge or craving (e.g., occurrence of thoughts related to sexual or gaming-related activities). Finally, *sensation seeking* refers to the tendency to enjoy and pursue activities that are exciting and an openness to trying new experiences. This component of impulsivity has been shown to constitute a risk factor for the initiation of various problematic behaviors (e.g., drug use, delinquent acts, gambling, risky sexual behaviors). Importantly, however, sensation seeking does not necessarily predict pathological involvement in these activities, which is more consistently related to other components of the UPPS model (e.g., urgency).

In addition to impulsivity traits, a range of other (neuro)psychological factors have been identified as key features of disorders due to addictive behaviors and impulse control disorders and are therefore relevant in their assessment and treatment (for a review, see Rochat et al., 2019). First, *motivational* processes include individual differences in reinforcement sensitivity (i.e., the extent to which individuals behave to pursue rewards or avoid punishment), attentional bias (i.e., a preferential attentional allocation toward a specific type of stimuli), and implicit association (i.e., automatic approach behavior toward specific types of stimuli). Second, *emotional* processes include adaptive and maladaptive strategies that individuals use to regulate negative emotions. Examples of maladaptive strategies include active suppression (i.e., trying to ignore the negative emotions and to suppress related thoughts) and nonconstructive rumination (i.e., abstract, negative and repetitive patterns of ruminative thinking), which can perpetuate and even increase negative affect and negative emotions (Watkins, 2008). Examples of adaptive strategies that may constitute protective factors include reappraisal of the situation that triggered the adverse emotions (i.e., trying to think about it in a different way) and the use of constructive rumination (i.e., concrete and solution-oriented patterns of thinking).

Consideration of these psychological processes will improve case conceptualization (e.g., by elucidating the functions of the pathological behaviors) and support the implementation of psychological interventions that are tailored to the individual through the identification of specific targets for treatment and individual risk and protective factors. At the same time, assessment and treatment of these disorders should consider the potential unique factors involved in each disorder. Specific motives are linked to activities such as gaming, gambling, or pornography consumption. For example, gaming disorder is frequently associated with motives related to in-game achievement or immersion in virtual worlds, whereas compulsive pornography consumption is frequently motivated by the desire to satisfy fantasies not fulfilled in offline sexual life. Specific dysfunctional cognitions may also be linked to each disorder. For example, the illusion of control, which refers to fallacious beliefs about one's ability to exert control over uncontrollable events, may be important in gambling disorder but not for the other conditions discussed in this chapter.

GAMBLING DISORDER

Presentations and Symptom Patterns

As described in the *CDDR*, individuals with gambling disorder suffer from the inability to control their gambling in terms of context (inappropriate situation), frequency (more often than intended), intensity (e.g., quantity of money spent), or duration (longer than intended). Increasing priority is given to gambling compared with other areas of life (e.g., hobbies, friends, sports, daily activities or duties like going to school or work). The individual persists in gambling despite negative consequences that derive from gambling, such as repeated relationship problems, substantial financial losses, problems at work or school, or negative impact on health. The pattern of gambling behavior manifests over an extended period of time, such as 12 months, and is continuous or episodic and recurrent. The behavior results in significant distress or impairment in life areas related to personal, family, social, educational, or occupational functioning. Additional characteristics may include unsuccessful attempts to reduce or control gambling behavior, increasing amounts of money spent on gambling to achieve the desired excitement, trying to compensate for losses by increasing subsequent bets ("chasing"), the occurrence of urges or cravings to engage in gambling, attempts to deceive others about losses or conceal spending on gambling, gambling to alleviate negative emotions, and the occurrence of detrimental physical and mental health consequences due to disruptions in diet, sleep, or physical exercise. Individuals with gambling disorder can be differentiated according to whether they engage in primarily online gambling versus those who tend to go into gambling venues such as casinos or racetracks to gamble in person, using a "predominantly online" or "predominantly offline" specifier.

Gambling behavior may occur in the absence of co-occurring mental disorders and may develop, for example, from distorted and dysfunctional cognitions, such as false expectations about the probability of winning or mis-beliefs about their own ability to influence gambling outcomes. This is the most common pattern in the disorder and is associated with better treatment outcomes. Alternatively, gambling behavior may occur in the context of preexisting mood disorders and poor emotional regulation, or in relation to substance misuse, personality disorder, attention deficits, or impulsivity.

Gambling disorder—like most other addictive disorders—occurs more often in males than in females and typically develops during adolescence or early adulthood. Available data show that prevalence in adolescents is at least as high as in adults and sometimes even higher (Calado et al., 2017), despite the fact that minors are not legally permitted to gamble in most countries. A chronic progressive course is frequently observed. Nevertheless, studies show that a substantial proportion (about 80%) remit for periods of 12 months or longer without formal treatment. Specific environmental factors such as being unemployed, being an immigrant and the related acculturation process, and being a child of a gambler can predict a worse course of the disorder (Donati et al., 2020; Dowling et al., 2017). The prevalence of past-year gambling disorder in adults ranges from 0.1% and 5.8% in available studies (Calado & Griffiths, 2016), though most population-based representative studies find prevalence estimations below 2%. Variability in prevalence estimates is partly due to methodological differences but may also reflect differences among countries or jurisdictions, such as in accessibility or other legal and cultural differences (Hodgins et al., 2011).

Differential Diagnosis

Gambling disorder must be differentiated from leisure or professional gambling that does not lead to significant distress or functional impairment and is not characterized by the three core features. The *ICD-11* also offers a category of hazardous gambling, which is not considered a disorder but rather is included in the chapter "Factors influencing health status and encounters with health services." This category can be assigned when, in the judgment of the clinician, the individual's gambling behavior appreciably increases the risk of harmful physical or mental health consequences, but the presentation does not fulfill the diagnostic requirements for gambling disorder.

Gambling disorder also should not be confused with gaming disorder. The essential difference between gaming and gambling is that gambling centrally involves the betting of money on an uncertain outcome. However, the boundary between gambling and gaming becomes blurry at times, with, for example, some gaming activities involving financial elements and random rewards such as loot boxes (monetization of games via consumable virtual items). Therefore, the predominant elements characterizing and maintaining the behavior must be considered in making this distinction.

The diagnosis of gambling disorder should only be assigned if the relevant pattern of gambling behavior occurs outside of manic, mixed, or hypomanic mood episodes. In addition, gambling disorder should not be diagnosed if the behavior pattern is induced by specific psychoactive drugs such as dopamine agonists including medications that may be prescribed in Parkinson disease or restless leg syndrome. The co-occurrence of other mental disorders with gambling disorder is frequent and is not an exclusion criterion for gambling disorder. Common co-occurring conditions include disorders due to substance use, mood disorders, anxiety and fear-related disorders, attention deficit hyperactivity disorder (ADHD), and personality disorder (Petry et al., 2005).

GAMING DISORDER

Presentations and Symptom Patterns

There is substantial clinical and public health evidence that video gaming can become dysfunctional and generate psychological distress and functional impairment (Rumpf et al., 2018). As a result, gaming disorder was included as an officially recognized mental health condition for the first time in the *ICD-11*. The diagnostic requirements detailed in the *CDDR* for gaming disorder are analogous to those of gambling disorder, focusing on impaired control over gaming behavior; increasing priority given to gaming over other life interests and daily activities; and continuation of gaming despite the occurrence of negative consequences. The gaming pattern occurs over an extended period, typically 12 months, and must be associated with distress or significant impairment in personal, family, social, or other important areas of functioning (Billieux et al., 2017). Additional features may include unsuccessful efforts to control or reduce gaming, the experience of urges or cravings to engage in gaming, the use of gaming to alleviate negative emotions, as well as the occurrence of detrimental physical and mental health consequences due to disruptions in diet, sleep, or physical exercise. Gaming disorder can be qualified as "predominantly online" (when the gamer favors video games involving other players) or "predominantly offline" (when the gamer favors single-player, often story-driven games). Predominantly online gaming disorder is more common than predominantly offline (Saunders et al., 2017).

Gaming disorder should not be diagnosed merely on high involvement in gaming in the absence of the other characteristic features of the disorder. High rates and long durations of nonproblematic gaming occur more commonly among specific age and social groups (e.g., adolescent males) and in particular contexts such as during the holidays or as a part of organized gaming activities for entertainment. Daily gaming behavior as a part of a routine or the use of gaming for purposes such as developing skills and proficiency in gaming, changing mood, alleviating boredom, or facilitating social interaction does not per se indicate the presence of gaming disorder.

A recent meta-analysis estimated the prevalence of problematic gaming to be 1% to 2% (Stevens et al., 2021). Generally, the age of onset is during puberty or late adolescence, although the disorder may begin in childhood, young adulthood, or adulthood (Saunders et al., 2017). Studies on the course of the disorder over follow-up periods of about 2 years indicate that approximately half of diagnosable individuals have a persistent disorder. Studies on the long-term course of gaming disorder are not available. Gaming disorder is more frequent in males, yet the market for video gaming is evolving, and an increasing number of females are playing video games, which may influence the gender ratio in the future.

Differential Diagnosis

Video games have become one of the most popular leisure activities worldwide and recognizing the distinction between elevated but non-problematic patterns of gaming behavior and gaming disorder is crucial to avoid over-pathologization and stigmatization of recreational gamers (Billieux et al., 2019). It is also important as a part of clinical assessment to consider that gaming behavior may be a maladaptive strategy for coping with emotional distress or other types of symptoms. For example, in social anxiety disorder, excessive gaming can reflect a preference for online interactions and avoidance of real-life interactions. In depressive disorders, excessive gaming may be used to regulate dysphoric mood or negative emotions. In posttraumatic stress disorder, excessive gaming may serve as a way to distance oneself from an unbearable reality. It is important that assessment and intervention focus on the psychological function of the gaming behavior and not only on the behavior itself, although the diagnosis of gaming disorder may still be assigned if all diagnostic requirements are met, together with other applicable diagnoses. Gaming disorder is commonly associated with mood disorders, anxiety and fear-related disorders, disorders due to substance use, ADHD, obsessive-compulsive disorder, and sleep–wake disorders (Saunders et al., 2017).

PYROMANIA

Presentations and Symptom Patterns

Pyromania is defined as a recurrent failure to control strong impulses to set fires, resulting in multiple episodes of deliberate and purposeful acts of, or attempts at, setting fire to property or other objects. The fire setting can occur opportunistically or be carefully planned. In either case, the lack of control over urges or impulses is the central component. Pyromania is associated with an increase in feelings of tension ("hyped up," excited) or emotional arousal before the fire setting, contrasted with pleasure (a "rush"), gratification, or relief when setting fires or when witnessing or participating in their aftermath, as well as a fascination or attraction to fire and the activities and equipment associated with fire-fighting. The disorder is understudied from a neurobiological perspective. It is hypothesized that pyromania may share pathophysiology associated with cognitive impulsivity and poor decision-making with other impulse control disorders.

Individuals with pyromania may show cognitive features of compulsivity as well. Fire setting may occur in response to feelings of depression, anxiety, boredom, loneliness, or other negative emotional states. Many individuals with pyromania exhibit impairments in social communication skills and a history of learning difficulties (Lindberg et al., 2005). Furthermore, individuals with pyromania, particularly women, often report histories of exposure to trauma, self-harm, and sexual abuse (Ducat et al., 2017).

Most research on pyromania focuses on fire setting in children and adolescents; the long-term course of pyromania is poorly understood. The population prevalence is not well established, although it is thought to be rare (lifetime prevalence around 1%; see Odlaug & Grant, 2010); it is uncommon even among those reaching the criminal system with repeated fire setting. However, in a study of hospitalized patients with mental disorders, approximately 3% presented with current symptoms of pyromania and approximately 6% with symptoms consistent with a lifetime diagnosis, suggesting pyromania may be more common in clinical samples than traditionally recognized (Grant et al., 2005). The mean age of onset is 18 ± 5 years (Grant & Kim, 2007).

The majority of convicted fire-setters are male (Ducat et al., 2017), and pyromania is generally considered to be more common among males, particularly young adults with poor social skills or learning difficulties (American Psychiatric Association, 2013). However, robust epidemiological data for pyromania are scarce, and the disorder may not be as gender-specific as traditionally assumed: A study conducted in college students found no gender-based difference in the rate of pyromania (Odlaug & Grant, 2010).

Differential Diagnosis

Acts of fire setting in pyromania lack an apparent motive and are therefore differentiated from intentional fire setting perpetrated for financial or sociopolitical gain, revenge, attention or recognition (e.g., deliberately setting a fire, and then being the first one to discover it and put it out), or another advantage that is planned beforehand. Some intentional forms of fire setting may also represent a manifestation of conduct-dissocial disorder or personality disorder with dissociality and/or disinhibition.

Interest in fires is common during early childhood, and children may accidentally or intentionally set fires as a part of developmental experimentation (e.g., playing with matches). A diagnosis of pyromania is not appropriate in such cases or when the behavior can be accounted for by a disorder of intellectual development or substance intoxication. Individuals with ADHD, particularly children and youth, may also impulsively set fires, but in such cases reckless disregard for consequences is typically seen across multiple contexts. Pyromania should also be differentiated from fire setting as a manifestation of impulsive or disorganized behavior associated with bipolar type I disorder during manic or mixed episodes, as well as fire setting in response to a delusion or a command hallucination associated with schizophrenia or other primary psychotic disorders.

Co-occurrence with other impulse control disorders and other mental disorders is high. For instance, in a relatively small sample of individuals with pyromania (Grant & Kim, 2007), 47.6% met criteria for another disorder characterized by difficulties controlling impulses, with lifetime co-occurrence of 23.8% for kleptomania, 9.5% each for gambling disorder and intermittent explosive disorder, and 4.8% for trichotillomania. There were also significant rates of co-occurrence with disorders due to substance use (33.3%), mood disorders (61.9%), anxiety and fear-related disorder (19%), and personality disorder with borderline pattern (9.5%).

KLEPTOMANIA

Presentations and Symptom Patterns

Kleptomania is defined as a recurrent failure to resist impulses to steal items not needed for personal use. Parallel to other impulse control disorders, the disorder is characterized by an urge to perform an act of stealing that may be pleasurable in the moment but later causes significant distress and dysfunction (e.g., shame, legal issues). There is characteristically a rising sense of tension or emotional arousal before stealing, followed by a sense of pleasure, excitement, relief, or gratification during and immediately after the act. In some cases, arousal before stealing diminishes over the course of the disorder. Although individuals with kleptomania may desire or have use for the stolen items, they do not need them, usually have the financial resources to pay for them, and often end up with multiples of the same unused items. Some individuals end up hoarding the stolen objects or surreptitiously return them.

Episodes of stealing in kleptomania may occur in response to feelings of depression, anxiety, boredom, loneliness, or other negative affective states. Individuals with kleptomania frequently try to resist their impulses to steal and acknowledge their actions are wrong or irrational. Afterward, they may fear being apprehended and experience guilt or shame, but this does not prevent recurrence of the stealing. Some individuals with kleptomania report amnesia or other dissociative symptoms (feelings of being disconnected from own body or environment) during stealing.

The prevalence of kleptomania in the general population has been estimated at just 3–6 per 1,000. Females outnumber males at a ratio of 3:1. However, kleptomania occurs in up to a quarter of individuals arrested for shoplifting and in one study was found to be a commonly co-occurring disorder (approximately 9%) in a sample of hospitalized patients with multiple mental disorders (Grant et al., 2005). The mean age of onset is during adolescence, although the disorder may begin in childhood or any subsequent stage of life. The course is usually chronic and may continue despite multiple shoplifting convictions. In clinical samples, females with kleptomania outnumber males (Lejoyeux et al., 2002), although males may be more likely to be subject to criminal penalties rather than being referred for treatment.

Differential Diagnosis

Stealing is common and most individuals who steal do so because they need or want something they cannot afford or as an act of mischief, anger, or vengeance. To diagnose kleptomania, there should be a lack of an apparent motive for stealing. Kleptomania can be distinguished from conduct-dissocial disorder or personality disorder with dissociality and/or disinhibition based on this lack of motive as well as on the presence of guilt or remorse. To diagnose klepto-mania, the stealing behavior should not be accounted for by a disorder of intel-lectual development or substance intoxication.

Kleptomania has high rates of co-occurrence with other mental disorders including disorders due to substance use, obsessive compulsive or related dis-orders, disorders due to addictive behaviors, other impulse control disorders, mood disorders, particularly bipolar type I disorder, and personality disorders (Padhi et al., 2012). It is also associated with reduced quality of life and increased suicidality (Kim et al., 2017). These findings indicate a need to assess a wide array of potential symptoms in individuals presenting with kleptomania. High rates of arrest, conviction, and incarceration are also common (Grant et al., 2009).

COMPULSIVE SEXUAL BEHAVIOR DISORDER

Presentations and Symptom Patterns

Compulsive sexual behavior disorder is characterized by the failure to control intense, repetitive sexual impulses or urges to engage in sexual activities, leading to repetitive sexual behavior that results in marked distress or signifi-cant impairment in important areas of functioning. The inability to control sexual urges or impulses is manifested in at least one of the following: (a) repet-itive sexual behavior that has become the central part of life to the extent that health, personal care, and other activities, interests, or responsibilities are neglected; (b) frequent but unsuccessful attempts to reduce or control repeti-tive sexual behavior in a significant manner; (c) engagement in repetitive sexual behavior that is continued despite negative consequences, such as marital conflict, financial or legal consequences, or negative impact on health; and (d) continued repetitive sexual behavior even when the person derives no or little satisfaction from it. To make a diagnosis, the behavior pattern involving the failure to control sexual urges and engaging in repetitive sexual behavior must be present over an extended period of time, such as 6 months or longer.

As with other disorders discussed in this chapter, impulsivity and positive reinforcement (pleasure) tend to be the most important elements early in the development of the behavior pattern. Later in the course of the disorder, com-pulsive aspects and negative reinforcement (e.g., alleviation of negative mood) are likely to become increasingly important in sustaining the behaviors (Briken & Basdekis-Jozsa, 2010). In addition, presentations of compulsive sexual behavior disorder involving primarily interpersonal sexual behavior (e.g., casual sex or sex for money) are more likely to be associated with impulsivity, particularly sensation seeking, while presentations involving primarily solitary sexual activities (e.g., masturbation and pornography viewing) are more likely to represent attempts to regulate negative emotions (Gola & Potenza, 2018). Compulsive sexual behavior disorder typically develops in late adolescence or early adulthood. It is more common among men than women, although recent studies have found that prevalence is higher among women than previously thought (Klein et al., 2014). Treatment of compulsive sexual behavior disorder focuses on improving sexual self-control as well as addressing the underlying emotional states and motivations (Briken, 2020; Stein et al., 2020). There is also evidence that certain pharmacological treatments can be helpful in reducing compulsive sexual behavior disorder symptoms (Lew-Starowicz et al., 2022).

Available epidemiological data indicate that subjective difficulty in controlling sexual impulses is common (Dickenson et al., 2018), although this is not sufficient for a diagnosis of compulsive sexual behavior disorder. The *ICD-11* diagnostic requirements for compulsive sexual behavior disorder are beginning to be used in epidemiological studies. A very large study in 42 countries using data from the International Sex Survey found that 4.8% of participants were considered to be at high risk for developing compulsive sexual behavior disorder (Böthe et al., 2023). Country- and gender-based differences were observed, but there was no effect of sexual orientation. The results of a large study in Germany based on a probability-based national sample found that 3.2% of men and 1.8% of women reported experiences consistent with the diagnostic requirements for compulsive sexual behaviour disorder during the previous 12 months (Briken et al., 2022). The researchers attempted to control for the possibility that people with nonpathological patterns of sexual behavior would describe themselves as lacking control over their sexual behavior because of their own moral judgments about it, a phenomenon referred to as moral incongruence (Grubbs et al., 2020). When participants who reported either a strict religious upbringing or conservative attitudes toward sexuality were excluded, the estimated 12-month prevalence rate was approximately half that of the uncorrected rate (1.6% of men and 0.9% of women). This finding illustrates that due to the greater restrictiveness of the *ICD-11* diagnostic requirements for compulsive sexual behavior disorder compared with previous constructs such as "hypersexuality" or "excessive sexual drive," prevalence rates will be correspondingly lower (Kraus et al., 2018).

Differential Diagnosis

It is of particular importance to distinguish high engagement in sexual activities from sexual behavior that is experienced as uncontrollable and leads to significant distress or functional impairment. The 19-item Compulsive Sexual Behavior Disorder Scale (Böthe et al., 2020) is freely available in multiple languages and can be helpful in making this determination. A seven-item version is also available. In individuals with compulsive sexual behaviour disorder, engagement in repetitive sexual behavior is often no longer experienced as pleasurable, but they find they are unable to stop engaging in it. In some cases, religious or moral concerns may lead individuals to believe that their behavior is wrong or abnormal. It is important to differentiate these kinds of attitudes toward sexuality from having compulsive sexual behavior disorder. Although individuals may suffer from a discrepancy between their moral or religious views and their actual behavior, the diagnosis requires the presence of the core features described. Furthermore, it is important to consider the wide variation that exists in sexual activity and related attitudes as well as cognitions such as sexual fantasies. Specific sexual interests or a high sex drive or high frequency of sexual behavior does not indicate the presence of compulsive sexual behavior disorder. Frequent sexual activity and urges can also be related to developmental phases such as adolescence or specific life circumstances like changes in partnership status.

As with other disorders discussed in this chapter, increased sexual behavior may sometimes be a symptom of other disorders such as personality disorder, dementia, or disorders due to substance use. Compulsive sexual behavior disorder should only be assigned if it occurs outside of manic, mixed or hypomanic mood episodes. Several mental disorders co-occur with compulsive sexual behavior disorder in clinical samples, including depressive disorders, anxiety or fear-related disorders, disorders due to substance use, ADHD, and posttraumatic stress disorder (Campbell & Stein, 2016). Among individuals with personality disorder, co-occurring compulsive sexual behavior disorder is related to the trait domains of dissociality and disinhibition as well as to borderline pattern.

INTERMITTENT EXPLOSIVE DISORDER

Presentations and Symptom Patterns

Intermittent explosive disorder is characterized by recurrent, brief, explosive episodes involving verbal aggression (e.g., verbally attacking another person, temper outbursts, yelling) or physical aggression (e.g., hitting another person, assault involving personal injury, destruction of property) in an individual who is at least 6 years old or an equivalent developmental age. The intensity of the outbursts or the degree of aggression is grossly out of proportion to any provocation or precipitating event or situation, and the behavior is not better accounted for by other mental disorders or the effects of a substance or medication. The violent outbursts are typically brief (e.g., less than an hour). They are not planned or intended to achieve a desired outcome but rather are impulsive or reactive in nature, suggesting failure to control aggressive urges. The outbursts often result in physical harm to self or others, although this is not a diagnostic requirement. However, the pattern of aggressive outbursts must result in significant distress to the individual with the disorder or significant functional impairment in social (loss of friends, marital instability), scholastic or occupational (suspension or expulsion, demotion, loss of employment), or other important domains. Frequently, the disorder also has a profound impact on financial and legal status (civil or criminal charges; Rynar & Coccaro, 2018).

The aggressive outbursts are most commonly triggered by perceived threats in social contexts, even if no real threat exists, or by frustration due to impediments in the course of daily events. There is typically little or no prodromal period (no lead-up to the outburst), although in some cases, outbursts may be preceded by symptoms such as tremor, sweating, chest tightness, or a general sense of tension or arousal. During the episode, the individual may feel a sensation of relief and, in some cases, pleasure. Afterward, the individual usually, but not always, experiences depressed mood, fatigue, or other negative emotions such as remorse, shame, or guilt. The outbursts occur regularly over a period of at least 6 months, with no signs of aggression between episodes. Some individuals with intermittent explosive disorder have a history of exposure to trauma, such as violence or childhood physical abuse, and some show nonspecific neurological signs that do not constitute a diagnosable neurological condition.

Data from the World Mental Health Survey (Scott et al., 2020) indicate that the lifetime prevalence of intermittent explosive disorder in 17 countries was 0.8%. Data from U.S. studies have shown a higher prevalence (Coccaro, 2012). The World Mental Health Survey study also found subtypes involving anger attacks that harmed people, comprising 73% of those with intermittent explosive disorder; these individuals had high rates of co-occurring externalizing disorders. Subtypes involving threatening people or destroying property without harming others were associated with higher rates of internalizing than externalizing co-occurring disorders. Suicidal behavior was higher among those with co-occurring disorders and those who perpetrated more violent assaults. The prevalence of suicide attempts and nonlethal self-injurious behaviors among individuals with intermittent explosive disorder has been estimated as 12.5% and 7.4% respectively (McCloskey et al., 2008). In a survey of individuals on probation following a criminal conviction, 7.4% were found to have intermittent explosive disorder, with even higher rates among those with ADHD (18%; Padhi et al., 2012).

Intermittent explosive disorder occurs among prepubertal children, but the mean age of onset is between 13 and 21 years of age. Early in the course of the disorder, children typically display temper tantrums associated with verbal outbursts and aggression against objects, although typically without serious destruction or assault. During adolescence, explosive outbursts often escalate. Intermittent explosive disorder usually follows a chronic course, although the prevalence tends to diminish over the life span. Although intermittent explosive disorder was originally believed to be more prevalent in males, community surveys suggest that the male-to-female ratio is likely closer to equal, with serious physical assault being more common in males.

Differential Diagnosis

Aggressive outbursts, particularly verbal outbursts, are extremely common, especially under stress, and do not necessarily indicate a disorder. One or two isolated incidents are insufficient for a diagnosis, regardless of the severity or consequences. Intermittent explosive disorder must also be differentiated from behaviors due to the effects of a psychoactive substance or medication, including intoxication and withdrawal, or due to dementia or a disease of the nervous system. Explosive or impulsive outbursts of aggression may also occur in autism spectrum disorder, where they are usually associated with a specific trigger related to the core autism spectrum disorder symptoms (e.g., a change in routine, aversive sensory stimulation). Intermittent explosive disorder should also be differentiated from regularly occurring and disproportionately severe temper outbursts that occur in the context of oppositional defiant disorder with chronic irritability-anger, particularly in response to demands by authority figures. It should also be differentiated from the broader and often premeditated or instrumental pattern of antisocial behavior characteristic of conduct-dissocial disorder, which generally also includes behavior such as lying or theft in addition to motivated aggression. Co-occurrence with other mental disorders is common in intermittent explosive disorder, particularly with mood disorders, anxiety and fear-related disorders, disorders due to substance use, eating disorders (especially those involving binge eating), and ADHD (Padhi et al., 2012).

GENERAL PRINCIPLES OF ASSESSMENT

As previously indicated, disorders due to addictive behaviors and impulse control disorders share many etiological and symptomatic similarities, which calls for a unified approach to psychological assessment. The assessment of impulsivity is central in patients presenting with these disorders. Assessment tools derived from the UPPS model of impulsivity assess multiple facets of impulsivity, allowing for fine-grained and individualized profiling. Unlike most other instruments assessing impulsivity, UPPS-based assessment tools also include an emotion-related impulsivity trait: the "urgency trait," which has been found to be consistently related to both disorders due to addictive behaviors and impulse control disorders (Berg et al., 2015).

Long and short versions of the UPPS Impulsive Behavior Scales (the long version is 59 items and the short one 20 items) have been developed. Both have excellent psychometric properties, including a robust and theoretically based factor structure, high internal reliability, and high test–retest stability (long version: Whiteside & Lynam, 2001; short version: Billieux, Rochat, et al., 2012). Both versions of the UPPS Impulsive Behavior Scale have been adapted and validated in many languages, including English, French, Spanish, Italian, German, Arabic, or Chinese. The scale has also been adapted for assessment in children and adolescents (Geurten et al., 2021). All versions are freely available.

Figure 16.1 illustrates how UPPS-based individualized impulsivity profiles can be used to inform case conceptualization and treatment planning (e.g., see Billieux, Lagrange, et al., 2012, for a study showing the heterogeneity of impulsivity profiles assessed by the UPPS scale in a sample of gambling disorder patients). Patient 1 displays a "multi-impulsive" impulsivity profile, which is

FIGURE 16.1. UPPS-Based Impulsivity Profiles

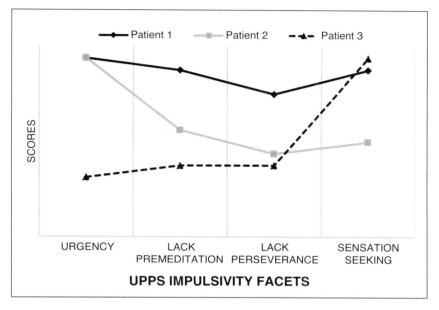

Note. UPPS = urgency–premeditation–perseverance–sensation seeking impulsivity model.

typical of severe disorders due to addictive behaviors or impulse control disorders. In contrast, Patient 2 presents with an impulsivity profile that is especially characterized by an elevated urgency—that is, a tendency to act impulsively in emotional contexts. Such a profile would call for further exploration of emotion regulation skills and consideration of whether the target pathological behavior (e.g., gaming, gambling, sexual behavior) is the consequence of maladaptive coping rather than a primary disorder per se. Finally, Patient 3 presents only with elevated sensation seeking, suggesting that the behavior in question does not necessarily reflect problematic impulsivity. Indeed, individuals with high sensation seeking but low scores in other impulsivity components are more likely to take controlled risks, such as in the case of a skilled poker player who likes the excitement of the game but does not lose control over the game or "chase" losses with additional uncontrolled bets.

Clinicians assessing disorders due to addictive behaviors and impulse control disorders should also be able to evaluate functional impairment rigorously. This is especially crucial in relation to behavior patterns that involve common activities, such as gaming, gambling, or sexual behaviors, which are at risk for over-pathologization (Billieux et al., 2015). Currently, this primarily relies on a clinical assessment because no specific assessment tool for functional impairment in disorders due to addictive behaviors and impulse control disorders exists. Available scales mainly focus on items related to physical functioning, which is rather rarely affected in disorders due to addictive behaviors and impulse control disorders. The Sheehan Disability Scale is a better fit in terms of content; however, it is not free of charge. The International Consortium for Health Outcome Measures (ICHOM) recently developed a set of scales for disorders due to substance use and disorders due to addictive behaviours (https://www.ichom.org/portfolio/addiction/).

Because of symptomatic overlap and co-occurrence of disorders due to addictive behaviors and impulse control disorders with a variety of other mental disorders, their assessment needs to be grounded in a broad assessment of psychopathology, particularly mood disorders, anxiety and fear-related disorders, disorders due to substance use, and personality disorder. Behaviors such as excessive gambling, gaming, sexual behavior, fire setting, stealing, or temper outbursts can sometimes be presenting features of other disorders (e.g., they occur in response to negative emotional states related to the other disorder). It is important to evaluate carefully the factors that precipitate and maintain the behaviors to arrive at the most accurate diagnosis and most helpful case formulation. Treatment of the other disorder may stand in the foreground initially even if a co-occurring diagnosis of a disorder due to addictive behavior or impulse control disorder is also assigned.

Finally, the comprehensive psychological assessment of disorders due to addictive behaviors and impulse control disorders often requires consideration of disorder-specific symptoms or psychological factors. This type of assessment is particularly useful to determine the severity of a disorder (when normative data are available) or to measure the effect of a therapeutic intervention objectively. Multiple instruments assessing symptom severity for gambling disorder, gaming disorder, and compulsive sexual behavior disorder have been developed; most are freely available. Specific items have also been developed to assess symptom severity in pyromania and kleptomania (e.g., Chamberlain & Grant, 2018).

KEY VALIDITY ISSUES

Given the commonalities discussed in this chapter, the boundary between disorders due to addictive behaviors and impulse control disorders is in some ways arbitrary (Grant et al., 2014; Kraus et al., 2016). With regard to disorders due to addictive behaviors, legitimate concerns have been raised about opening the door to the creation of controversial new conditions of questionable validity, such as love addiction, shopping addiction, exercise addiction, or work addiction (Billieux et al., 2015). However, evidence that these behavior patterns constitute addictions is generally of low quality and fails to consider the critical distinction between high involvement (not associated with loss of control and functional impairment) and pathological involvement. Moreover, apart from anecdotal single case descriptions, such potentially new disorders have not been demonstrated to be associated with demands for clinical services.

KEY POINTS

- Disorders due to addictive behaviors and impulse control disorders share commonalities—namely, impulsivity and loss of control as core features. The behavior patterns that characterize these disorders are perpetuated through a dynamic interaction between positive and negative cycles of reinforcement.

- Functional impairment is a central feature in the diagnosis of disorders due to addictive behaviors and impulse control disorders. Elevated involvement in activities such as gaming, gambling, or sexual behavior that is not associated with functional impairment should not be viewed as inherently pathological.

- In the clinical context, a detailed assessment of impulsivity and related psychological dimensions is central to informing appropriately tailored empirically based interventions.

- Disorders due to addictive behaviors and impulse control disorders have high rates of co-occurrence with other mental disorders, including mood disorders, anxiety and fear-related disorders, disorders due to substance use, and personality disorder.

- At times, behaviors such as excessive gambling, gaming, sexual behavior, fire setting, stealing, or temper outbursts can be presenting features of other disorders (e.g., the behaviors are undertaken in response to negative emotional states). Careful evaluation of the factors that precipitate and maintain the behaviors is important to arrive at the most accurate diagnosis and helpful case formulation.

REFERENCES

American Psychiatric Association. (2013). *Diagnostic and statistical manual of mental disorders* (5th ed.).

Berg, J. M., Latzman, R. D., Bliwise, N. G., & Lilienfeld, S. O. (2015). Parsing the heterogeneity of impulsivity: A meta-analytic review of the behavioral implications of the UPPS for psychopathology. *Psychological Assessment, 27*(4), 1129–1146. https://doi.org/10.1037/pas0000111

Billieux, J., Flayelle, M., Rumpf, H.-J., & Stein, D. J. (2019). High involvement versus pathological involvement in video games: A crucial distinction for ensuring the validity and utility of gaming disorder. *Current Addiction Reports, 6*(3), 323–330. https://doi.org/10.1007/s40429-019-00259-x

Billieux, J., King, D. L., Higuchi, S., Achab, S., Bowden-Jones, H., Hao, W., Long, J., Lee, H. K., Potenza, M. N., Saunders, J. B., & Poznyak, V. (2017). Functional impairment matters in the screening and diagnosis of gaming disorder. *Journal of Behavioral Addictions, 6*(3), 285–289. https://doi.org/10.1556/2006.6.2017.036

Billieux, J., Lagrange, G., Van der Linden, M., Lançon, C., Adida, M., & Jeanningros, R. (2012). Investigation of impulsivity in a sample of treatment-seeking pathological gamblers: A multidimensional perspective. *Psychiatry Research, 198*(2), 291–296. https://doi.org/10.1016/j.psychres.2012.01.001

Billieux, J., Rochat, L., Ceschi, G., Carré, A., Offerlin-Meyer, I., Defeldre, A.-C., Khazaal, Y., Besche-Richard, C., & Van der Linden, M. (2012). Validation of a short French version of the UPPS-P Impulsive Behavior Scale. *Comprehensive Psychiatry*, *53*(5), 609–615. https://doi.org/10.1016/j.comppsych.2011.09.001

Billieux, J., Schimmenti, A., Khazaal, Y., Maurage, P., & Heeren, A. (2015). Are we over-pathologizing everyday life? A tenable blueprint for behavioral addiction research. *Journal of Behavioral Addictions*, *4*(3), 119–123. https://doi.org/10.1556/2006.4.2015.009

Böthe, B., Koós, M., Nagy, L., Kraus, S. W., Demetrovics, Z., Potenza, M. N., Michaud, A., Ballester-Arnal, R., Batthyány, D., Bergeron, S., Billieux, J., Briken, P., Burkauskas, J., Cárdenas-López, G., Carvalho, J., Castro-Calvo, J., Chen, L., Ciocca, G., Corazza, O., . . . Vaillancourt-Morel, M. P. (2023). Compulsive sexual behavior disorder in 42 countries: Insights from the International Sex Survey and introduction of standardized assessment tools. *Journal of Behavioral Addictions*, *12*(2), 393–407. https://doi.org/10.1556/2006.2023.00028

Böthe, B., Potenza, M. N., Griffiths, M. D., Kraus, S. W., Klein, V., Fuss, J., & Demetrovics, Z. (2020). The development of the Compulsive Sexual Behavior Disorder Scale (CSBD-19): An *ICD-11* based screening measure across three languages. *Journal of Behavioral Addictions*, *9*(2), 247–258. https://doi.org/10.1556/2006.2020.00034

Brand, M., Wegmann, E., Stark, R., Müller, A., Wölfling, K., Robbins, T. W., & Potenza, M. N. (2019). The Interaction of Person-Affect-Cognition-Execution (I-PACE) model for addictive behaviors: Update, generalization to addictive behaviors beyond internet-use disorders, and specification of the process character of addictive behaviors. *Neuroscience and Biobehavioral Reviews*, *104*, 1–10. https://doi.org/10.1016/j.neubiorev.2019.06.032

Briken, P. (2020). An integrated model to assess and treat compulsive sexual behaviour disorder. *Nature Reviews Urology*, *17*(7), 391–406. https://doi.org/10.1038/s41585-020-0343-7

Briken, P., & Basdekis-Jozsa, R. (2010). Sexuelle sucht? Wenn sexuelles verhalten ausser kontrolle gerät [Sexual addiction? When sexual behavior gets out of control]. *Bundesgesundheitsblatt, Gesundheitsforschung, Gesundheitsschutz*, *53*(4), 313–318. https://doi.org/10.1007/s00103-010-1033-z

Briken, P., Wiessner, C., Štulhofer, A., Klein, V., Fuss, J., Reed, G. M., & Dekker, A. (2022). Who feels affected by "out of control" sexual behavior? Prevalence and correlates of indicators for *ICD-11* compulsive sexual behavior disorder in the German Health and Sexuality Survey (GeSiD). *Journal of Behavioral Addictions*, *11*(3), 900–911. https://doi.org/10.1556/2006.2022.00060

Calado, F., Alexandre, J., & Griffiths, M. D. (2017). Prevalence of adolescent problem gambling: A systematic review of recent research. *Journal of Gambling Studies*, *33*(2), 397–424. https://doi.org/10.1007/s10899-016-9627-5

Calado, F., & Griffiths, M. D. (2016). Problem gambling worldwide: An update and systematic review of empirical research (2000–2015). *Journal of Behavioral Addictions*, *5*(4), 592–613. https://doi.org/10.1556/2006.5.2016.073

Campbell, M. M., & Stein, D. (2016). Hypersexual disorder. In N. M. Petry (Ed.), *Behavioral addictions: DSM-5 and beyond* (pp. 101–123). Oxford University Press.

Castro-Calvo, J., King, D. L., Stein, D. J., Brand, M., Carmi, L., Chamberlain, S. R., Demetrovics, Z., Fineberg, N. A., Rumpf, H. J., Yücel, M., Achab, S., Ambekar, A., Bahar, N., Blaszczynski, A., Bowden-Jones, H., Carbonell, X., Chan, E. M. L., Ko, C. H., de Timary, P., . . . Billieux, J. (2021). Expert appraisal of criteria for assessing gaming disorder: An international Delphi study. *Addiction*, *116*(9), 2463–2475. Advance online publication. https://doi.org/10.1111/add.15411

Chamberlain, S. R., & Grant, J. E. (2018). Minnesota Impulse Disorders Interview (MIDI): Validation of a structured diagnostic clinical interview for impulse control disorders in an enriched community sample. *Psychiatry Research*, *265*, 279–283. https://doi.org/10.1016/j.psychres.2018.05.006

Coccaro, E. F. (2012). Intermittent explosive disorder as a disorder of impulsive aggression for *DSM-5*. *The American Journal of Psychiatry*, *169*(6), 577–588. https://doi.org/10.1176/appi.ajp.2012.11081259

Dell'Osso, B., Altamura, A. C., Allen, A., Marazziti, D., & Hollander, E. (2006). Epidemiologic and clinical updates on impulse control disorders: A critical review. *European Archives of Psychiatry and Clinical Neuroscience, 256*(8), 464–475. https://doi.org/10.1007/s00406-006-0668-0

Dickenson, J. A., Gleason, N., Coleman, E., & Miner, M. H. (2018). Prevalence of distress associated with difficulty controlling sexual urges, feelings, and behaviors in the United States. *JAMA Network Open, 1*(7), e184468. https://doi.org/10.1001/jamanetworkopen.2018.4468

Donati, M. A., Primi, C., Mazzarese, M., Sanson, F., & Leone, L. (2020). Immigrant status and problem-gambling severity in adolescents: Evidence for moderation by sensation seeking. *Addictive Behaviors, 107*, Article 106395. https://doi.org/10.1016/j.addbeh.2020.106395

Dowling, N. A., Merkouris, S. S., Greenwood, C. J., Oldenhof, E., Toumbourou, J. W., & Youssef, G. J. (2017). Early risk and protective factors for problem gambling: A systematic review and meta-analysis of longitudinal studies. *Clinical Psychology Review, 51*, 109–124. https://doi.org/10.1016/j.cpr.2016.10.008

Ducat, L., McEwan, T., & Ogloff, J. R. P. (2017). A comparison of psychopathology and reoffending in female and male convicted firesetters. *Law and Human Behavior, 41*(6), 588–599. https://doi.org/10.1037/lhb0000264

Geurten, M., Catale, C., Gay, P., Deplus, S., & Billieux, J. (2021). Measuring impulsivity in children: Adaptation and validation of a short version of the UPPS-P Impulsive Behaviors Scale in children and investigation of its links with ADHD. *Journal of Attention Disorders, 25*(1), 105–114. https://doi.org/10.1177/1087054718775831

Gola, M., & Potenza, M. N. (2018). Promoting educational, classification, treatment, and policy initiatives. *Journal of Behavioral Addictions, 7*(2), 208–210. https://doi.org/10.1556/2006.7.2018.51

Grant, J. E., Atmaca, M., Fineberg, N. A., Fontenelle, L. F., Matsunaga, H., Janardhan Reddy, Y. C., Simpson, H. B., Thomsen, P. H., van den Heuvel, O. A., Veale, D., Woods, D. W., & Stein, D. J. (2014). Impulse control disorders and "behavioural addictions" in the *ICD-11. World Psychiatry, 13*(2), 125–127. https://doi.org/10.1002/wps.20115

Grant, J. E., & Kim, S. W. (2007). Clinical characteristics and psychiatric comorbidity of pyromania. *The Journal of Clinical Psychiatry, 68*(11), 1717–1722. https://doi.org/10.4088/JCP.v68n1111

Grant, J. E., Levine, L., Kim, D., & Potenza, M. N. (2005). Impulse control disorders in adult psychiatric inpatients. *The American Journal of Psychiatry, 162*(11), 2184–2188. https://doi.org/10.1176/appi.ajp.162.11.2184

Grant, J. E., Odlaug, B. L., Davis, A. A., & Kim, S. W. (2009). Legal consequences of kleptomania. *Psychiatric Quarterly, 80*(4), 251–259. https://doi.org/10.1007/s11126-009-9112-8

Grubbs, J. B., Kraus, S. W., Perry, S. L., Lewczuk, K., & Gola, M. (2020). Moral incongruence and compulsive sexual behavior: Results from cross-sectional interactions and parallel growth curve analyses. *Journal of Abnormal Psychology, 129*(3), 266–278. https://doi.org/10.1037/abn0000501

Hodgins, D. C., Stea, J. N., & Grant, J. E. (2011). Gambling disorders. *The Lancet, 378*(9806), 1874–1884. https://doi.org/10.1016/S0140-6736(10)62185-X

Kim, H. S., Christianini, A. R., Bertoni, D., de Oliveira, M. D. C. M., Hodgins, D. C., & Tavares, H. (2017). Kleptomania and co-morbid addictive disorders. *Psychiatry Research, 250*, 35–37. https://doi.org/10.1016/j.psychres.2017.01.048

Klein, V., Rettenberger, M., & Briken, P. (2014). Self-reported indicators of hypersexuality and its correlates in a female online sample. *The Journal of Sexual Medicine, 11*(8), 1974–1981. https://doi.org/10.1111/jsm.12602

Kraus, S. W., Krueger, R. B., Briken, P., First, M. B., Stein, D. J., Kaplan, M. S., Voon, V., Abdo, C. H. N., Grant, J. E., Atalla, E., & Reed, G. M. (2018). Compulsive sexual behaviour disorder in the *ICD-11*. *World Psychiatry*, *17*(1), 109–110. https://doi.org/10.1002/wps.20499

Kraus, S. W., Voon, V., & Potenza, M. N. (2016). Should compulsive sexual behavior be considered an addiction? *Addiction*, *111*(12), 2097–2106. https://doi.org/10.1111/add.13297

Lejoyeux, M., Arbaretaz, M., McLoughlin, M., & Adès, J. (2002). Impulse control disorders and depression. *Journal of Nervous and Mental Disease*, *190*(5), 310–314. https://doi.org/10.1097/00005053-200205000-00007

Lew-Starowicz, M., Draps, M., Kowalewska, E., Obarska, K., Kraus, S. W., & Gola, M. (2022). Tolerability and efficacy of paroxetine and naltrexone for treatment of compulsive sexual behaviour disorder. *World Psychiatry*, *21*(3), 468–469. https://doi.org/10.1002/wps.21026

Lindberg, N., Holi, M. M., Tani, P., & Virkkunen, M. (2005). Looking for pyromania: Characteristics of a consecutive sample of Finnish male criminals with histories of recidivist fire-setting between 1973 and 1993. *BMC Psychiatry*, *5*(1), 47. https://doi.org/10.1186/1471-244X-5-47

McCloskey, M. S., Ben-Zeev, D., Lee, R., & Coccaro, E. F. (2008). Prevalence of suicidal and self-injurious behavior among subjects with intermittent explosive disorder. *Psychiatry Research*, *158*(2), 248–250. https://doi.org/10.1016/j.psychres.2007.09.011

Odlaug, B. L., & Grant, J. E. (2010). Impulse-control disorders in a college sample: Results from the self-administered Minnesota Impulse Disorders Interview (MIDI). *The Primary Care Companion to the Journal of Clinical Psychiatry*, *12*, Article PCC.09m00842. https://doi.org/10.4088/PCC.09m00842whi

Padhi, A. K., Mehdi, A. M., Craig, K. J., & Fineberg, N. A. (2012). Current classification of impulse control disorders: Neurocognitive and behavioral models of impulsivity and the role of personality. In J. E. Grant & M. N. Potenza (Eds.), *The Oxford handbook of impulse control disorders* (pp. 26–46). Oxford University Press.

Petry, N. M., Stinson, F. S., & Grant, B. F. (2005). Comorbidity of *DSM-IV* pathological gambling and other psychiatric disorders: Results from the National Epidemiologic Survey on Alcohol and Related Conditions. *The Journal of Clinical Psychiatry*, *66*(5), 564–574. https://doi.org/10.4088/JCP.v66n0504

Rochat, L., Billieux, J., Gagnon, J., & Van der Linden, M. (2018). A multifactorial and integrative approach to impulsivity in neuropsychology: Insights from the UPPS model of impulsivity. *Journal of Clinical and Experimental Neuropsychology*, *40*(1), 45–61. https://doi.org/10.1080/13803395.2017.1313393

Rochat, L., Maurage, P., Heeren, A., & Billieux, J. (2019). Let's open the decision-making umbrella: A framework for conceptualizing and assessing features of impaired decision making in addiction. *Neuropsychology Review*, *29*(1), 27–51. https://doi.org/10.1007/s11065-018-9387-3

Rumpf, H.-J., Achab, S., Billieux, J., Bowden-Jones, H., Carragher, N., Demetrovics, Z., Higuchi, S., King, D. L., Mann, K., Potenza, M., Saunders, J. B., Abbott, M., Ambekar, A., Aricak, O. T., Assanangkornchai, S., Bahar, N., Borges, G., Brand, M., Chan, E. M., . . . Poznyak, V. (2018). Including gaming disorder in the *ICD-11*: The need to do so from a clinical and public health perspective. *Journal of Behavioral Addictions*, *7*(3), 556–561. https://doi.org/10.1556/2006.7.2018.59

Rynar, L., & Coccaro, E. F. (2018). Psychosocial impairment in *DSM-5* intermittent explosive disorder. *Psychiatry Research*, *264*, 91–95. https://doi.org/10.1016/j.psychres.2018.03.077

Saunders, J. B., Hao, W., Long, J., King, D. L., Mann, K., Fauth-Bühler, M., Rumpf, H. J., Bowden-Jones, H., Rahimi-Movaghar, A., Chung, T., Chan, E., Bahar, N., Achab, S., Lee, H. K., Potenza, M., Petry, N., Spritzer, D., Ambekar, A., Derevensky, J., . . . Poznyak, V. (2017). Gaming disorder: Its delineation as an important condition for diagnosis, management, and prevention. *Journal of Behavioral Addictions*, *6*(3), 271–279. https://doi.org/10.1556/2006.6.2017.039

Scott, K. M., de Vries, Y. A., Aguilar-Gaxiola, S., Al-Hamzawi, A., Alonso, J., Bromet, E. J., Bunting, B., Caldas-de-Almeida, J. M., Cía, A., Florescu, S., Gureje, O., Hu, C. Y., Karam, E. G., Karam, A., Kawakami, N., Kessler, R. C., Lee, S., McGrath, J., Oladeji, B., . . . de Jonge, P. (2020). Intermittent explosive disorder subtypes in the general population: Association with comorbidity, impairment and suicidality. *Epidemiology and Psychiatric Sciences, 29*, Article 138. https://doi.org/10.1017/S2045796020000517

Slutske, W. S., Caspi, A., Moffitt, T. E., & Poulton, R. (2005). Personality and problem gambling: A prospective study of a birth cohort of young adults. *Archives of General Psychiatry, 62*(7), 769–775. https://doi.org/10.1001/archpsyc.62.7.769

Stein, D. J., Szatmari, P., Gaebel, W., Berk, M., Vieta, E., Maj, M., de Vries, Y. A., Roest, A. M., de Jonge, P., Maercker, A., Brewin, C. R., Pike, K. M., Grilo, C. M., Fineberg, N. A., Briken, P., Cohen-Kettenis, P. T., & Reed, G. M. (2020). Mental, behavioral and neurodevelopmental disorders in the *ICD-11*: An international perspective on key changes and controversies. *BMC Medicine, 18*(1), Article 21. https://doi.org/10.1186/s12916-020-1495-2

Stevens, M. W., Dorstyn, D., Delfabbro, P. H., & King, D. L. (2021). Global prevalence of gaming disorder: A systematic review and meta-analysis. *The Australian and New Zealand Journal of Psychiatry, 55*(6), 553–568. https://doi.org/10.1177/0004867420962851

Watkins, E. R. (2008). Constructive and unconstructive repetitive thought. *Psychological Bulletin, 134*(2), 163–206. https://doi.org/10.1037/0033-2909.134.2.163

Whiteside, S. P., & Lynam, D. R. (2001). The five factor model and impulsivity: Using a structural model of personality to understand impulsivity. *Personality and Individual Differences, 30*(4), 669–689. https://doi.org/10.1016/S0191-8869(00)00064-7

World Health Organization. (2023). *ICD-11 for mortality and morbidity statistics* (Version: 01/2023). https://icd.who.int/browse11/l-m/en#/

World Health Organization. (2024). *Clinical descriptions and diagnostic requirements for ICD-11 mental, behavioural and neurodevelopmental disorders.* https://www.who.int/publications/i/item/9789240077263

17

Personality Disorder

Michaela A. Swales, Lee Anna Clark, and Alireza Farnam

OVERARCHING LOGIC

Personality disorder is fundamentally different from other forms of mental disorder and distress. We all have a personality. Our personality is integral if not synonymous with who we are and who we perceive ourselves to be. Thus, to consider personality as disordered touches closely on our sense of who we are as well as on issues of social norms of acceptable and typical behavior. Diagnosing people with personality disorder has been used as a mechanism of social control and can be a source of state power over individuals. Clinicians are advised to proceed with caution.

Until the advent of the 11th revision of the *International Classification of Diseases* (*ICD-11*; World Health Organization [WHO], 2023), the classification of personality disorder was based largely on outdated, unscientific descriptions of prototypical presentations. These previous systems were lists of criteria for up to 10 "prototype" disorders, which required clinicians to be familiar with more than 70 diagnostic criteria. In practice, clinicians rarely diagnosed personality disorder at all, and when they did, they mostly used only three categories: borderline personality disorder, antisocial personality disorder, and personality disorder not otherwise specified, with the last reflecting that, in many cases, the clinical presentation failed to match any of the designated

Thanks to Jared Keeley for allowing us to adapt the case vignettes he developed for the World Health Organization field testing for use in this chapter.

https://doi.org/10.1037/0000392-017
A Psychological Approach to Diagnosis: Using the ICD-11 as a Framework, G. M. Reed, P. L.-J. Ritchie, and A. Maercker (Editors)

categories. (In the *ICD-10*, these categories were called emotionally unstable personality disorder, borderline type; dissocial personality disorder; and personality disorder, unspecified, respectively.) Because the categories were not based on systematic research, there was no evidence that they were actually discrete entities, so people commonly presented with elements of more than one, leading to high levels of "comorbidity," which indicated a problem with the classification.

These problems and the lack of clinical utility of previous classifications were the drivers for a recent seismic shift in personality disorder classification: *ICD-11* moved decisively away from a categorical classification to base personality disorder diagnosis on current research that links problematic personality presentations to extremes of normal functioning using a trait-descriptor model. The classification emphasizes clinical utility by asking clinicians to assess the severity of the presentation—which is the best-known predictor of outcome— as part of the diagnosis itself. Uniquely, the *ICD-11* classification is more closely akin to the psychological structure of normal personality variation; therefore, it is believed that its assessment and use as part of a psychological formulation of clients' presenting difficulties will prove relatively straightforward for practicing clinicians.

Clinicians considering an *ICD-11* personality disorder diagnosis must first decide whether a person's interpersonal and self-functioning are sufficiently and pervasively enough impaired to warrant a diagnosis at all. If the person's problems are above threshold, the next step is to establish their severity— mild, moderate, or severe—which reliably predicts such clinical outcomes as residual symptoms, long-term functioning, and health service use and cost (Tyrer et al., 2019). Thus, incorporating severity into the diagnostic process itself promotes awareness of likely clinical outcomes from the outset. Following the decision on severity level, clinicians may then apply up to five trait domain specifiers: "negative affectivity," "detachment," "dissociality," "disinhibition," and "anankastia." Dissocial personality traits are sometimes referred to as antisocial, and anankastic traits are sometimes referred to as obsessive-compulsive personality traits, but the terms "dissociality" and "anankastia" are used in the *ICD-11* to avoid conflation with these overlapping concepts. The trait domains are described in detail later this chapter. In addition, to facilitate access to existing treatments, the *ICD-11* includes a borderline pattern specifier.

A PSYCHOLOGICAL APPROACH TO PERSONALITY DISORDER

The origins of personality are found in the crucible of genetics and early environmental experiences. From as young as 3 years, children show personality traits that are approximately 50% heritable, which gradually stabilize across the life span until at least age 60 (Roberts & DelVecchio, 2000). Life experiences across development transact with genetics and temperament to shape personality, in that each of these components reciprocally influence one another. For example, early adverse life experiences such as trauma can shape a child's developing neurobiology, making a child more sensitive and reactive, which in turn may elicit more rejection or harsh responses from caregivers. In essence, personality is a set of repertoires of interpersonal and intrapersonal behaviors that the individual predictably demonstrates, in the case of overt behaviors, or verbally reports, in the case of covert behaviors (thoughts and emotions) across contexts and across time. Over the past 20 years, personality research has explored these behavioral repertoires and reliably observed an organized structure of five major ways in which people differ, known as the "Big 5": neuroticism (or negative affectivity vs. emotional stability), extraversion, agreeableness, conscientiousness, and openness (Markon et al., 2005). As traits emerge early in development, they transact with the person's environment in ways that lead to behavioral repertoires that reflect these traits and are more or less functional for the individual. Environments high in adversity and low on parental care, nurturance, and support are most likely to promote ways of coping that, although they may aid survival in such adverse environments, become less functional in wider society or other relationship contexts.

ICD-11, in using personality trait assessment as its basis, places the understanding of personality disorder in this framework. Practitioners making a personality disorder diagnosis using *ICD-11* should consider patients' developmental histories and how their personality profile has been formed across their life span in response to life experiences. For everyone, the development of personality, whether disordered or not, can be understood from a developmental perspective as an individual's attempt to respond as effectively as possible in the environments that they inhabit given their genetic inheritance. Maintaining this perspective will enable clinicians to adopt a compassionate and nonjudgmental stance toward individuals presenting with these complex and challenging difficulties.

PRESENTATIONS AND SYMPTOM PATTERNS

A personality disorder diagnosis first and foremost requires disturbance in sense of self and/or interpersonal function that is significantly different in quality or frequency from normal personality function. Sense-of-self dysfunction may manifest as persistent difficulties in maintaining a sense of identity, a pervasive sense of impoverished or highly overvalued self-worth, inaccuracies in self-perception, challenges in self-direction and decision-making, or a combination of these. The features of interpersonal dysfunction commonly manifest as inability to make and sustain mutually satisfying relationships, difficulties managing interpersonal conflict, or problems recognizing or understanding others' perspectives. Patterns of cognition, emotional experience and expression, and behavior are often dysregulated or overly rigid and are often mismatched with what is required in given circumstances. That is, individuals with personality disorder struggle to adapt their behavior to changing environmental circumstances. For a diagnosis of personality disorder, these patterns must be present across a range of personal and social situations and contexts and are not be developmentally appropriate or explainable by social or cultural factors, the effects of medication or substance abuse, or any other mental health condition or physical illness. Its features have typically been evident since adolescence or earlier, and problems must have existed for at least the past 2 years.

Clinicians may encounter people in which the extent of disturbance and its impact on functioning is insufficient to warrant a personality disorder diagnosis but whose personality nevertheless presents difficulties for them in circumscribed areas of functioning (e.g., in effectively accessing health care). In these circumstances, clinicians may diagnose "personality difficulty", which is not considered a mental disorder but is found in the chapter "Factors influencing health status or contacts with health services" in *ICD-11*. Personality difficulty may also be considered in circumstances in which adolescents are demonstrating features of personality disorder that are not yet sufficiently persistent over time to warrant the diagnosis.

SEVERITY OF PERSONALITY DISORDER

Once the clinician has determined that personality disorder is present, the next step is to ascertain the severity of the disturbance: mild, moderate, or severe. The *Clinical Descriptions and Diagnostic Requirements for ICD-11 Mental, Behavioural and Neurodevelopmental Disorders* (*CDDR*; WHO, 2024) provide detailed descriptions of each level, alongside examples of common types of disturbances. The general principles underlining the distinctions between levels are the number of areas of the individual's life that are affected (e.g., occupational functioning, family life, social relationships, the extent of the disruption to the individual's life, distress caused to self and other, and, finally, the level of risk of harm to self and/or others). For example, mild personality disorder is not typically associated with threat of harm to self or others, whereas severe personality disorder often is. Mild personality disorder will likely affect only circumscribed areas of life, or, if the disturbance is across many areas, the intensity of the disturbance will be less. Severe personality disorder, in contrast, affects almost all of a person's functioning in many areas and will be clearly evident to those around them.

CLINICAL CASES

This section provides case examples of personality disorder at different levels of severity. These case examples are based on the authors' real experiences, but they are composites that do not represent specific individuals. The identities of any individual patients involved in these examples have been properly disguised to protect their confidentiality.

Case Example: Mild Personality Disorder With Anankastia and Negative Affectivity

Angela is a businesswoman in her mid-40s. Her employer referred her to the current appointment due to decreasing productivity at her job. Angela attended the appointment with her eldest son.

Angela acknowledged that her productivity at work was declining. She was recently put in charge of a major project and her desire to ensure everything is perfect has paralyzed her. Her coworkers say she is impossible to work with because of her exacting standards. In the past, she has always worked on projects for this company by herself, and her attention to detail has served her relatively well. Her coworkers have tolerated her eccentricities, but now several of them have threatened to leave because she belittles them for their mistakes.

Angela married when she was 19 years old, and she and her husband had three children within 3 years of the marriage. She describes the marriage as very strained because she felt she always had to take care of him as if he were her own child. They separated when she was 26 and have lived apart ever since. In a separate interview, Angela's son describes her as a "hard woman." He recounts several stories of the intense pressure she placed on him to perform well in school. When he was participating in sports, she made him practice for long hours. He has come to realize that not everyone has the same high standards and that her harshness negatively affected him growing up.

Angela attends religious services multiple times per week, along with a women's group. In the group, she describes several friends but also has tense relationships with some members. She often "butts heads" with the leader of the group when they disagree about something.

Case Example: Moderate Personality Disorder With Negative Affectivity and Disinhibition (Borderline Pattern Specifier)

Susan, a 24-year-old medical student, referred herself for services after the completed suicide of a classmate. She describes a history of self-harm and suicidal thoughts; these urges and actions have increased in frequency in association with her grief over the death of her friend. She says the pain from cutting helps distract her from the overwhelming emotional pain she is experiencing over this loss. Susan believes she feels things more intensely than other people. Her mood tends to shift dramatically in response to minor things. For example, when negotiating the schedule of clinical rotations with her classmates, she yelled and screamed when she did not get the times she wanted. A few minutes later, she was extremely apologetic and tearful at the realization that she may have threatened her friendship with them. She says outbursts like these are common, and as a result, her peers tend either to avoid her or to treat her very carefully. Similarly, she has had problems taking feedback from her supervisors, alternating between crying when they give her any sort of criticism and becoming very angry that they do not recognize her skills and abilities. She is aware that these problems are approaching a crisis point that may preclude her continuing her training. Susan also describes difficulties maintaining romantic relationships. When she finds herself attracted to a potential partner, she falls in love with him very quickly, idealizing everything about him. The intensity of her attraction tends to scare away boyfriends.

Susan's parents were an international, interracial couple who met when her father was deployed in his country's military. She was very close to her father until his death when she was 16. He suffered from a debilitating chronic illness, and she was his primary caretaker for the last 4 years of his life. She felt that he was always very supportive of her. She describes her mother as hypercritical of everything she does, and Susan feels that in her mother's eyes she could never do anything right. She and her mother would often get into loud verbal arguments. Following the death of her father, she began staying away from home for days at a time, indiscriminately engaging multiple sexual partners and drinking heavily. Despite her behavior, she continued to perform well in school, earning perfect grades.

Case Example: Severe Personality Disorder With Dissociality and Detachment

Peter is a 34-year-old male referred for evaluation pending trial. He has been charged with embezzling money from at least four different victims. Despite the seriousness of his charge, Peter appears to be in a good mood and states that he is confident the charges will be dropped if he can just clear up the misunderstanding. Over the past 12 years, he has developed relationships with four single women. He brags about how he convinced the women to fall in love with him, even though he professed feeling nothing for any of them. Once the relationship had progressed, he would inform them that he had identified a unique investment opportunity. From each he received sizable sums of money, but he never invested any of it, instead using the money to purchase expensive cars for himself or gifts for the other women. When they would confront him about the return on their investment, he would claim he needed more time or more money to make it work. Peter claims that there should not be any problem with his actions because the money he received was all "gifts" and denies that he made any promises about returning the money. He discounts the idea that he has harmed these women in any way, stating that they should be happy he is in their life. At least two of the women claim that he has hit them if they disagreed with him or tried to end the relationship.

Peter currently has no permanent residence, instead alternating staying with each of the women for no more than a few nights at a time. He has never held any form of employment, instead relying on these women to support him financially. Peter has no other substantial relationships in his life, having alienated all family members by constantly asking for money.

Peter had a troubled childhood, frequently fighting with other children, claiming that they disrespected him in some way. He resisted all attempts at discipline from his parents, and his teachers complained that he would make excuses for not completing assignments. His classmates perceived him as a bully and did their best to avoid him. Peter attended a college for 2 years before being expelled for cheating on a test.

Discussion of Case Examples

In these three case studies, the progression of severity is evident in terms of the number of areas of life affected, the presence or absence of harm to self and others, and the level of function of the client in terms of social and occupational roles fulfilled. Angela (in the first case, mild personality disorder) has maintained her occupation relatively successfully until recently and illustrates how some personality traits—in this case, perfectionism and attention to detail—that may be at the extreme can, in some contexts, contribute to functionality. Angela's detail-focused approach, when she worked alone, resulted in projects completed to a high standard that were valued by her employer. When occupational expectations changed, requiring her to work more with others, her approach led to conflict and seems to have precipitated the referral to services. Her characteristic interpersonal habits, comprising excessively high expectations of herself and others, also significantly affect her family life and manifest in her other social relationships. Despite these difficulties, however, Angela does retain her family relationships to a degree and also maintains some social contacts.

In the second case, moderate personality disorder, Susan's disturbance in her interpersonal roles is more extensive, and this is likely linked to her more dysregulated emotional style. Her emotional outbursts affect friendships, work supervisors, and potential romantic partners. She is on the brink of losing her place in medical school as a result of her personality difficulties. She also cuts herself as a means of regulating intensely felt emotions. The self-harm and the more extensive interpersonal aspect of her difficulties leads to a moderate personality disorder diagnosis. In Susan's case, we know a little of her childhood background in which we can see how these patterns of behavior and emotional expression may have been learned and indeed may have functioned as a way of fitting in and coping in her family. Notwithstanding the understandability of their origin, they remain problematic patterns in the present.

In this third case, Peter demonstrates severe personality disorder primarily because of the extent of harm to others. His deliberate exploitation of four women, alongside a callous disregard for their feelings, contribute to the severe personality disorder diagnosis. His skills in persuading the women he exploits to provide for him indicate a degree of functional capacity, but he lacks typical social and occupational roles. He also demonstrates an absence of insight, awareness, and concern for his situation combined with an unrealistic self-view, which is common in severe personality disorder.

Once the clinician has established the presence or absence of personality disorder and determined its severity, there is the option to proceed no further. In some jurisdictions with limited resources and or less training in assessing personality function, this will be common and, given the strong predictive power of severity, will suffice as a tool in treatment. In other circumstances, clinicians may find it helpful to proceed to identify trait specifiers that describe the form the disorder takes in the individual.

TRAIT DOMAIN SPECIFIERS

The Big 5 trait structure of normal personality is essentially replicated in individuals with personality dysfunction; the *ICD-11* trait domain specifiers are continuous with normal personality traits. Identifying them in an individual with personality disorder requires that they are at an extreme end of the distribution of typical functioning. Although traits are continuous in nature, for the purpose of diagnosis, trait domain specifiers are applied dichotomously, as either prominent or not, and clinicians may list as many of the trait domain specifiers as are applicable to the presentation (WHO, 2024). Treatments for personality disorder inevitably focus on the behavioral manifestations of these traits. It is hoped that future treatment research will examine interventions for more specific trait domain patterns.

Negative Affectivity

Negative affectivity is characterized by the experience of a broad range of negative emotions at high intensity and frequency often out of keeping with the circumstances of the situation. Although it may not be immediately apparent to the casual observer, skillful clinicians who understand more about the person's background will recognize that the emotional responses make sense within the individual's context and learning history, as is the case with Susan in the second case example. Individuals with high levels of negative affectivity often have poor emotion regulation skills. The ways in which they cope with their excessive emotionality will be evident in their other traits. For example, some individuals who are also high on disinhibition may act impulsively or recklessly in the face of strong emotion, as we saw in Susan's case in her responses to feedback from others. Under stress, those high on anankastia may rigidly insist on extreme or unattainable standards and perseverate even more than usual or intensify their perfectionistic behaviors. Angela, faced with the increasing pressure of the new assignment at work, found herself in this trap. Those high on detachment may withdraw even further from social contact.

Detachment

The detachment trait specifier comprises both social and emotional detachment, although individuals vary in the extent to which they express these two components. Social detachment essentially refers to the avoidance of social contacts and lack of friendships and intimacy, whereas emotional detachment describes a reserved and aloof interpersonal style often characterized by a lack of emotional expressiveness and, in severe cases, a lack of emotional experience. Individuals may describe feeling dead inside or that they cannot even discern basic bodily sensations (e.g., hunger, thirst, or the need to urinate).

Dissociality

Individuals high on dissociality disregard the feelings and rights of others. This trait domain includes a lack of empathy and extreme focus on the needs of the self at the expense of others, either overtly and directly, or as a consequence of a seeming lack of awareness of the needs of others, as we saw in the case of Peter. Individuals may demonstrate dramatically—and in extreme cases, cruelly—their intense displeasure when their needs are not met or when their skills and attributes are not recognized to the extent that they believe they deserve. Lack of empathy may drive the exploitation and physical or emotional harm to others, and individuals high on this trait may ruthlessly focus on their own desires and goals at the expense of others.

Disinhibition

The disinhibition domain encompasses a range of impulsive and often reckless or irresponsible responses to internal or external stimuli. Emotional and interpersonal cues are the most common prompting events, although internal bodily sensations or thoughts may also prompt problematic acts. Disinhibition may be evident in distractibility, with accompanying sensations of boredom and disinterest and a search for more immediately rewarding stimuli or contexts, alongside an absence of planning and a tendency to focus on short-term over longer term goals and opportunities. This trait will often have a significant impact on employment and educational ability and functioning.

Anankastia

Emotional and behavioral constraint and perfectionism constitute the core features of anankastia. Individuals strong in this trait domain have extreme capacity to deny their own needs in the pursuit of accuracy, detail, and rule-following. They are frequently hyper-organized, neat, and orderly in their approach to life. They are capable of high levels of behavioral control and rarely express emotions, as such displays constitute a lack of control. They may be extremely judgmental of emotional expressiveness in others. These characteristics make interpersonal relationships extremely challenging because they hold others to the same high levels of skill and constraint as themselves, and they can be extremely critical of people who do not live up to their exacting standards. The absence of emotional expression and high levels of constraint can misleadingly give the impression that individuals high on anankastia are unemotional, but often such individuals are high on negative affectivity and devote a lot of energy to controlling their high levels of emotional arousal.

Borderline Pattern

Borderline pattern is not a trait domain but rather a constellation of different personality characteristics. This specifier was included to ensure that patients in jurisdictions that require this diagnosis to get treatment would not be disadvantaged by the new classification. As the specifier aims to retain continuity, it remains essentially the same as the borderline personality disorder diagnosis in previous classifications. As personality disorder becomes more severe, more trait domains are affected. Thus, individuals who receive a borderline pattern specifier typically will have either moderate or severe personality disorder with negative affectivity and often disinhibition or dissociality. *ICD-11* encourages clinicians who use the borderline pattern specifier nevertheless to follow the *ICD-11* process of first diagnosing a personality disorder, then establishing severity, and finally applying relevant trait domains, which will facilitate the transition to the new classification.

ASSESSMENT

Given the risks and potential harms in making a personality disorder diagnosis, careful assessment is required. Assessment typically comprises clinical interviews, observations, and psychometric assessment. High-quality assessment typically takes place over more than one meeting. Several areas require assessment during the clinical interview. The clinician will first ask for individuals' reports of their functioning and its history. Concurrent information from an informant known to the person, with the client's consent, can provide useful additional and/or corroborative information. A developmental history with attention to the experience of early adversity, which may include trauma, will also provide useful background context. Observation of the person during the interview may yield additional information. Throughout, the clinician should seek to establish the breadth of areas in which the person is experiencing difficulty. For example, they should assess functioning in social, family, educational, and occupational roles and not limit their enquiries to single functioning domains. Sufficient duration of difficulties (more than 2 years) must be determined and also whether alternative explanations for difficulties exist (e.g., other diagnoses, such as complex posttraumatic stress disorder, or other contextual factors, such as living in an abusive environment).

Broadly speaking, presentation—and therefore assessment—is affected by whether the person experiences significant difficulties in the control of emotion, thought, and behavior. Individuals with high negative affectivity and disinhibition are more likely to report these difficulties directly and are more likely to present at a younger age. Often self-harm is part of the presentation. In these circumstances, clinicians are more likely to consider personality disorder as a possible diagnosis. Individuals who are high on anankastia and detachment are far less likely to report these as their difficulties and tend to present later and with another primary presenting problem, such as recurring or nonremitting anxiety or depression or noncompliance with recommended health care regimens.

Several measures for both severity and the trait domains are available to augment clinical interviews and observations to support clinicians in the process of diagnosis. The *ICD-11* Personality Disorder Severity Scale (PDS-ICD-11) is a 14-item self-report specifically designed to assess the severity of personality disorder as described in the *ICD-11* CDDR (Bach et al., 2021), with emerging evidence of its validity and utility (Brown & Sellbom, 2023). The Personality Inventory for *ICD-11* (Oltmanns & Widiger, 2018), a 60-item self-report measure designed to assess the five *ICD-11* trait domains of personality disorder, also has accumulating validity evidence (Oltmanns & Widiger, 2021) and is being tested in multiple languages. More comprehensive measures are also being developed (Clark et al., 2021).

Given the potential stigmatizing effect of a personality disorder diagnosis, clinicians should ensure that there are no other diagnoses that reflect the presenting problem more accurately. For example, complex posttraumatic stress disorder may have many of the features of personality disorder, as extensive trauma will almost always affect the developing personality. In a brief interview, clinicians may be reluctant to ask about early trauma, and people presenting for assessment may be reluctant to disclose information about these experiences at a first meeting. Before asking whether clients have experienced traumatic events, reassuring them that they will not be pressed for details of past trauma beyond what they wish to disclose and that the focus will be on the experience of current symptoms may assist in eliciting accurate information. Although a diagnosis of complex posttraumatic stress disorder does not preclude a personality disorder diagnosis, clinicians should be convinced that the personality functioning issues are at least somewhat separable from the sequelae of trauma and that the additional diagnosis provides some benefit. For example, when a personality disorder diagnosis might enable access to a treatment that will assist the person in overcoming their mental health and personality issues, the additional diagnosis should be considered. These two principles—whether the personality disorder clearly presents in distinction to another mental health diagnosis and whether the diagnosis provides added value to the individual—are relevant in all circumstances in which an additional diagnosis is being considered.

Although clinicians must be cautious not to overdiagnose, failing to recognize other mental health diagnoses also may occasionally be a problem. Because individuals with personality disorder frequently present challenges to services, the presence of the diagnosis has been used in some countries to deny access to services or resulted in other aspects of a person's mental health being disregarded or left untreated. The presence of a personality disorder does not mean that an individual may not also experience anxiety or depression or any other condition, and clinicians should ensure that they conduct a broad assessment of issues for treatment and not allow a personality disorder presentation to narrow their focus.

In making a diagnosis of personality disorder, clinicians should be mindful that this diagnosis is one of, if not the most, stigmatizing of diagnoses. For all of us, our personality is central to our sense of self, and to describe or label someone as having a personality disorder is potentially a devastating experience and, when conducted poorly, can be extremely harmful. However, failure to consider personality function in a mental health assessment is also potentially harmful because clinicians may incorrectly advise on clinical interventions or may fail to adjust interventions to address a person's personality style. In giving a diagnosis, clinicians should develop and embody a nonjudgmental and compassionate stance toward clients and assist them in understanding how their own interpersonal patterns and self-functioning have developed. Considering personality function as evolving out of an early interaction between genetics and environmental events can assist in this process. Clinicians can use their understanding of how patterns of behavior have developed to identify and incorporate interventions into the treatment plan that may help the person overcome the difficulties resulting from their personality dysfunction. Current treatments indicate that even individuals with severe disturbance may change; thus, remaining focused on patterns of overt and covert behaviors provides a more direct route into treatment planning and intervention.

CO-OCCURRING DISORDERS

Personality disorder may present in isolation but often co-occurs with other mental health disorders. Common co-occurring presentations are depression, anxiety, posttraumatic stress disorder, and self-harm. Indeed, in assessing for personality disorder, clinicians will want to be sure that the person's presenting problems cannot be described by these other disorders alone. Chronic or unremitting presentations of depression and anxiety may indicate the presence of personality disorder—indeed, experiencing any other mental health disorder that does not respond to treatment will likely affect a person's personality and may lead to a personality disorder diagnosis. Personality disorders also commonly co-occur with long-standing health problems. The direction of causality in both of these circumstances is not clearly understood. Presence of a personality disorder may increase the likelihood of experiencing depression, anxiety, and poorer physical health simply because the origins of personality disorder in early adversity make a person vulnerable to many mental and physical health problems. Equally, experiencing a chronic life-limiting health condition or a mental health disorder that is unresponsive to treatment will likely affect one's personality, which may then affect future responses to treatment.

GENDER-RELATED FEATURES

The scientific literature reveals gender-based rating biases more than actual gender-based differences. Moreover, even when actual gender-based differences are found, they typically are small to moderate. The largest and most consistent differences are in the dissocial domain, with men showing more of such traits (e.g., aggression, self-aggrandizement), followed by negative affectivity, with women showing somewhat more emotionality/emotional lability. These differences tend to be found cross-culturally, although the magnitude of difference varies (Lippa, 2010). Finally, consistent with gender-based rating biases, differences are larger when clinicians are asked to rate men/women in general or men/women with a particular form of personality disorder than when they are asked to rate particular clients with the same form of personality disorder. Thus, clinicians are cautioned against relying on gender stereotypes when considering clients maladaptive personality traits in the context of making a personality disorder diagnosis.

DEVELOPMENTAL COURSE

In typically developing children and average expectable environments, relatively stable personality differences can be assessed by year 3, with the greatest personality changes occurring over the next decade as children venture out of the home into the world and are affected by a wider range of environments. Whether a person is relatively high or low on a specific trait becomes increasingly stable across adolescence into early adulthood. Certain behaviors common in personality disorder (e.g., risk-taking, self-harm, and moodiness) are more common in adolescents. These features tend to peak in the early teenage years and then gradually decline in most individuals. Thus, when assessing adolescents, clinicians must ensure that these features had an earlier onset, are more persistent, or are present to a greater extent than in the typically developing adolescent before considering a personality disorder diagnosis (Newton-Howes et al., 2015). If the clinician is uncertain whether to diagnose personality disorder, the condition personality difficulty may be listed, along with the relevant trait specifiers. This will ensure a period of "watchful waiting" to determine whether the condition abates or develops into a diagnosable personality disorder.

After about 30 years of age, personality differences across individuals continue to stabilize, albeit more slowly, at least until age 60 (Roberts & DelVecchio, 2000). Negative affectivity and detachment tend to decrease considerably across adolescence until the mid-30s to age 40, then continue to decrease slowly until the mid-60s. In contrast, dissociality and disinhibition decrease relatively linearly across adolescence through age 70 to 80. Little information is available on the life course of anankastia.

Evidence suggests that even when personality pathology as traditionally diagnosed is no longer above threshold, considerable psychosocial dysfunction remains (Skodol et al., 2005), which suggests that the *ICD-11* approach to personality diagnosis more accurately reflects the actual course of the disorder. That is, although more flagrant indicators of personality pathology may be manifested less clearly and less frequently over time, long-term maladaptive behavioral patterns remain. That said, less is known about personality disorder later in life, and some research suggests that although maladaptive-range trait manifestations decline when self-reported, informant reports indicate worsening with age (Cooper et al., 2014). Evidence thus provides more optimism regarding treatment of personality pathology while simultaneously indicating that it remains challenging throughout life.

CULTURAL AND CONTEXTUAL CONSIDERATIONS

The diagnostic requirements for personality disorder in the *ICD-11 CDDR* are based on principles that are fundamentally pan-human. Insofar as those individual differences that we call personality underlie socially based human behavior, successful interpersonal functioning is thus a core feature of personality normality. Likewise, work and occupational activities are central functions in successful complex societies and social skills are fundamental to personality functioning. Although these individual differences take on different forms in the complex global array of human societies, the underlying principles are universally acknowledged. Given this perspective, the *ICD-11* system of personality disorder diagnosis ensures that the diagnostic requirements do not reflect any particular set of cultural values. Thus, it was important to emphasize within the trait descriptions that neither nonconformity nor firm adherence to social values is in itself indicative of personality psychopathology.

Nonetheless, the paucity of research outside of Western contexts, and minimal resources in those clinical contexts with few specialist mental health professionals, means that our knowledge of presentations and prevalence of personality disorder outside Western cultures is limited. Specific manifestations of prominent traits may differ from culture to culture. Neuroticism is a universal individual-difference domain, underpinned by the common physiological processes of negative affect; however, the specific way in which negative affect manifests itself behaviorally may vary. For example, negative affect is expressed somatically to different degrees across cultures, and, at the same time, there is within-culture individual variation in somatic expression. Similarly, disinhibition is recognized across cultures, yet its expression and the extent to which it is seen as violating social norms in an individualized Western culture may differ considerably from its expression and interpretation in a collectivist culture, although at the extreme, trait expression may be more similar than different. Of course there are also age and gender differences within cultures, as discussed earlier, that should be considered. Practitioners operating outside the contexts in which personality disorder diagnoses have been studied must exercise caution in making judgments about the presence and severity of personality disorder, ensuring that patterns of behavior and functioning are well outside what is normative and functional for the culture in which the practitioner is operating.

Personality function is strongly interpersonal and contextual, and thus clinicians must take special care to ensure that what they observe in the person is actually a result of personality dysfunction and not a consequence of the person's personal circumstances or the societal context. Situations requiring special caution include younger adolescents for whom presentations that match a personality disorder description are a normal response to an abnormal environmental situation—for example, a young person who demonstrates self-harm and impulsive behavior because they are being sexually abused. Caution is also required in cultural contexts in which oppressive cultural norms and practices are applied to minority groups when defiance of these norms and practices may result in individuals being considered disordered—for example, when they express divergent political or religious views from the society in which they live.

PREVALENCE

Limited development of reliable and valid measures of personality disorder that are easy to use has restricted extensive studies of prevalence across countries, so only broad estimates are available (Tyrer et al., 2015). North American and European studies form the majority of the research base and describe point prevalences in community samples of between 4% and 15%. Prevalence rises significantly in health care settings, with approximately 25% of patients in primary care and 50% in outpatient mental health settings meeting the diagnostic requirements for personality disorder. Figures are even higher in inpatient mental health settings. Given the impact of personality disorder on treatment outcomes for other conditions—both physical and mental—these figures should give pause to all clinicians, as personality disorder is rarely considered and diagnosed even less.

KEY POINTS

- Personality disorder develops as a transaction among genetics, temperament, and life experience.

- Personality disorder reflects disturbances in sense of self and interpersonal functioning that are pervasive across time and context.

- The *ICD-11* departs significantly from previous classifications in its conceptualization of personality disorder. The focus, first and foremost, is on the presence or absence of personality disorder and its severity. *ICD-11* personality disorder has three levels of severity: mild, moderate and severe. Because severity reliably relates to outcome, this initial step guides clinicians to consider the likely level of complexity of intervention in a given case.

- Personality disorder can be described further with five trait domain specifiers: "negative affectivity," "dissociality," "detachment," "disinhibition," and "anankastia." Treatments for personality disorder inevitably focus on the behavioral manifestations of these traits.

- Personality disorder diagnoses are highly stigmatizing, so great care should be given to thoughtful and comprehensive assessment.

REFERENCES

Bach, B., Brown, T. A., Mulder, R. T., Newton-Howes, G., Simonsen, E., & Sellbom, M. (2021). Development and initial evaluation of the *ICD-11* personality disorder severity scale: PDS-ICD-11. *Personality and Mental Health, 15*(3), 223–236. https://doi.org/10.1002/pmh.1510

Brown, T. A., & Sellbom, M. (2023). Further validation of the personality disorder severity for *ICD-11* (PDS-ICD-11) scale in a community mental health sample. *Psychological Assessment, 35*(8), 706–714. https://doi.org/10.1037/pas0001253

Clark, L. A., Corona-Espinosa, A., Khoo, S., Kotelnikova, Y., Levin-Aspenson, H. F., Serapio-García, G., & Watson, D. (2021). Preliminary scales for *ICD-11* personality disorder: Self and interpersonal dysfunction plus five personality disorder trait domains. *Frontiers in Psychology, 12,* Article 668724. https://doi.org/10.3389/fpsyg.2021.668724

Cooper, L. D., Balsis, S., & Oltmanns, T. F. (2014). Aging: Empirical contribution: A longitudinal analysis of personality disorder dimensions and personality traits in a community sample of older adults: Perspectives from selves and informants. *Journal of Personality Disorders, 28*(1), 151–165. https://doi.org/10.1521/pedi.2014.28.1.151

Lippa, R. A. (2010). Gender differences in personality and interests: When, where, and why? *Social and Personality Psychology Compass, 4*(11), 1098–1110. https://doi.org/10.1111/j.1751-9004.2010.00320.x

Markon, K. E., Krueger, R. F., & Watson, D. (2005). Delineating the structure of normal and abnormal personality: An integrative hierarchical approach. *Journal of Personality and Social Psychology, 88*(1), 139–157. https://doi.org/10.1037/0022-3514.88.1.139

Newton-Howes, G., Clark, L. A., & Chanen, A. (2015). Personality disorder across the life course. *The Lancet, 385*(9969), 727–734. https://doi.org/10.1016/S0140-6736(14)61283-6

Oltmanns, J. R., & Widiger, T. A. (2018). A self-report measure for the *ICD-11* dimensional trait model proposal: The Personality Inventory for *ICD-11. Psychological Assessment, 30*(2), 154–169. https://doi.org/10.1037/pas0000459

Oltmanns, J. R., & Widiger, T. A. (2021). The self- and informant-personality inventories for *ICD-11*: Agreement, structure, and relations with health, social, and satisfaction variables in older adults. *Psychological Assessment, 33*(4), 300–310. https://doi.org/10.1037/pas0000982

Roberts, B. W., & DelVecchio, W. F. (2000). The rank-order consistency of personality traits from childhood to old age: A quantitative review of longitudinal studies. *Psychological Bulletin, 126*(1), 3–25. https://doi.org/10.1037/0033-2909.126.1.3

Skodol, A. E., Pagano, M. E., Bender, D. S., Shea, M. T., Gunderson, J. G., Yen, S., Stout, R. L., Morey, L. C., Sanislow, C. A., Grilo, C. M., Zanarini, M. C., & McGlashan, T. H. (2005). Stability of functional impairment in patients with schizotypal, borderline, avoidant, or obsessive-compulsive personality disorder over two years. *Psychological Medicine, 35*(3), 443–451. https://doi.org/10.1017/S003329170400354X

Tyrer, P., Mulder, R., Kim, Y. R., & Crawford, M. J. (2019). The development of the *ICD-11* classification of personality disorders: An amalgam of science, pragmatism, and politics. *Annual Review of Clinical Psychology, 15*(1), 481–502. https://doi.org/10.1146/annurev-clinpsy-050718-095736

Tyrer, P., Reed, G. M., & Crawford, M. J. (2015). Classification, assessment, prevalence, and effect of personality disorder. *The Lancet, 385*(9969), 717–726. https://doi.org/10.1016/S0140-6736(14)61995-4

World Health Organization. (2023). *ICD-11 for mortality and morbidity statistics* (Version: 01/2023). https://icd.who.int/browse11/l-m/en#/

World Health Organization. (2024). *Clinical descriptions and diagnostic requirements for ICD-11 mental, behavioural and neurodevelopmental disorders.* https://www.who.int/publications/i/item/9789240077263

18

Neurocognitive Disorders

Antonio E. Puente, Theophilus Lazarus, Miguel Pérez-García, and Janna Glozman

The prevalence of neurocognitive disorders is increasing rapidly due to the global increase in life span. Delirium affects approximately 30% of hospitalized adults and a more significant percentage of older adults (Ospina et al., 2018). Between 14% and 18% of the population will experience mild neurocognitive disorder by age 70 (Peterson et al., 2009). Globally, there are 55 million people in the world with a diagnosis of dementia. An additional 10 million are diagnosed each year (World Health Organization [WHO], 2022), and there are expected to be 115 million individuals with dementia worldwide by 2050. There is evidence of an increasingly disproportionate impact of these trends on women, both in terms of the greater risk women have for dementia (Artero et al., 2008; Chêne et al., 2015; Niu et al., 2017) and the greater burden of caring for family members with dementia that falls on women (Bamford & Walker 2012). At the same time, the rate of detection of neurocognitive disorders varies greatly because of limited access in many settings to appropriate assessments and adequately trained personnel.

The 11th revision of the *International Classification of Diseases* (*ICD-11*; WHO, 2023) has substantially changed the classification of neurocognitive disorders. The nature of neurocognitive disorders, which embody psychological and neurological components simultaneously, posed conceptual and political challenges for the developers of *ICD-11* related to whether they would be classified in the chapter on mental, behavioral, or neurodevelopmental disorders or the chapter on diseases of the nervous system (Gaebel et al., 2018). After much

https://doi.org/10.1037/0000392-018
A Psychological Approach to Diagnosis: Using the ICD-11 as a Framework, G. M. Reed, P. L.-J. Ritchie, and A. Maercker (Editors)

discussion and negotiation, different aspects of neurocognitive disorders are found in both sections and intended to be used together (Gaebel et al., 2019). Essentially, the mind versus body, functional versus organic split embodied in the classification of these disorders in *ICD-10* has been replaced in *ICD-11* by an integrative model that explicitly recognizes the psychological and syndromal aspects of these disorders as well as their neurological basis (Reed et al., 2019). Although this classification model more accurately reflects the nature of these disorders, it also makes understanding and diagnosing them more complicated. The diagnosis of neurocognitive disorders is also complex because of their heterogeneity, the presence of both somatic and psychological symptoms, and their differential diagnosis and co-occurrence with a host of other disorders. This chapter introduces the interface between the psychological and neurological components of neurocognitive disorders. Neurocognitive disorders are conceptualized in this chapter using psychological principles while integrating information about neurological processes involved in their etiology and associated impairment. Their assessment involves the integration of neuropsychological as well as social, cultural, and historical information.

OVERARCHING LOGIC

The *ICD-11* defines neurocognitive disorders as primary clinical deficits in neurocognitive functioning that are acquired rather than developmental. Neurocognitive functioning specifically refers to neurologically based cognitive skills and abilities believed to be directly related to brain functioning, including but not limited to attention/concentration, memory, language, visual-spatial/perceptual skills, processing speed, and executive functioning (e.g., problem-solving, judgment). Neurocognitive disorders always involve an observable decline from a previous level of functioning in one or more of these areas. They are distinct from neurodevelopmental disorders, which are characterized by deficits in neurocognitive functioning that are present from birth or arise during the developmental period (i.e., before age 18). The term *primary* clinical deficits is meant to indicate that deficits in neurocognitive functioning are the core features of the disorder, in contrast to cognitive symptoms that may be present in many other mental disorders (e.g., schizophrenia, mood disorders).

The four major neurocognitive disorders are

- Delirium
- Mild neurocognitive disorder
- Amnestic disorder
- Dementia

As described in the *Clinical Descriptions and Diagnostic Requirements for ICD-11 Mental, Behavioural and Neurodevelopmental Disorders* (*CDDR*; WHO, 2024), neurocognitive disorders are syndromal diagnoses. They are based on the pattern of cognitive and behavioral deficits, their temporal pattern, and the degree of associated functional impairment. There is a wide range of causes of neurocognitive disorders, and the *ICD-11* provides mechanisms for indicating an established or presumed etiology for each diagnosis. The first significant set of causes comprises diseases or other insults that directly affect the brain. These are often diseases of the nervous system (e.g., Alzheimer disease, cerebrovascular disease), but may also be infectious diseases (e.g., HIV) or be caused by nutritional deficiencies (e.g., pellagra), exposure to environmental toxins, or injury. The second primary set of causes is psychoactive substances or medications. A wide variety of psychoactive substances can cause delirium, and certain specific substances (i.e., alcohol, sedatives, hypnotics or anxiolytics, and volatile inhalants) can also cause amnestic disorder or dementia. If it is known, the etiological disease process (e.g., Parkinson disease, alcohol dependence) should be diagnosed along with the corresponding neurocognitive disorder.

Diagnosis of neurocognitive disorders is challenging because they are not only highly heterogeneous in terms of their etiology but also because various etiologies may interact. Moreover, these disorders' cognitive and behavioral expression is highly variable, and the associated degree of functional impairment can range from relatively benign alterations in cognitive abilities to a complete inability to care for oneself. The onset of symptoms and impairment be sudden or gradual and may be progressive or stable or remit over time.

Conceptualizing and diagnosing neurocognitive disorders requires that we transcend traditional mind–body dualism, in which a disorder is conceptualized as either physical or "organic" (e.g., cancer) on the one hand, or mental, "functional," or "nonorganic" (e.g., generalized anxiety disorder), on the other. Neurocognitive disorders were called "organic mental disorders" in the *ICD-10*, implicitly in comparison to presumably "nonorganic mental disorders," which did not have a readily identifiable physiological substrate. We now understand that this is a false dichotomy in regard to most disorders. Neurocognitive disorders, in particular, are associated with changes in mental processes and brain functioning, producing not just motor and sensory neurological symptoms but also demonstrable and clinically significant changes in cognition and behavior.

A PSYCHOLOGICAL APPROACH TO NEUROCOGNITIVE DISORDERS

A psychological approach to neurocognitive disorders seeks to understand and integrate neurological and cognitive functioning simultaneously using a holistic and comprehensive analysis. Although these disorders have a basis in changes in the brain, the syndrome is psychologically expressed and described, with the assumption that physical changes occurred before the observable cognitive and behavioral symptoms. One principle of this approach is that every patient should be understood within a bio-psycho-socio-cultural system (Puente & McCaffrey, 1992). In other words, neurocognitive deficits exist inside a brain, which lives inside a person who resides within a complex psycho-socio-cultural context. A part of what defines neurocognitive disorders is the interaction between the person and their environment, for example, as expressed in impairment in the execution of tasks in daily living, which is in part a function of the demands of the person's environment and the type and amount of support or assistance available (WHO, 2001). Therefore, although the *Clinical Descriptions and Diagnostic Requirements* (*CDDR*) offer authoritative guidance in diagnosing neurocognitive disorders, it must be applied to each individual in a flexible and customizable manner.

PRESENTATIONS AND SYMPTOM PATTERNS

The core presenting symptoms of the four major neurocognitive disorder diagnoses are described in this section. For each diagnosis, a description is also provided of how the *ICD-11* addresses the characterization of its etiology.

Delirium

Delirium is characterized by a disturbance of attention, orientation, and awareness developing within a short period (e.g., within hours or days), typically presenting as significant confusion or global neurocognitive impairment. Symptoms may be transient or fluctuating depending on the underlying causal condition or etiology. Cognition is commonly impaired in a global manner, with deficits in multiple areas of neurocognitive functioning. For example, delirium may include impaired perception, which can manifest as illusions (e.g., misinterpretations of sensory inputs), delusions, or hallucinations in the absence of other features of schizophrenia and other primary psychotic disorders. Delirium often includes disturbances of emotion, such as anxiety symptoms, depressed mood, irritability, fear, anger, euphoria, or apathy. Behavioral symptoms such as agitation, restlessness, or impulsivity may also be present. Disturbance of the sleep–wake cycle is often present, manifested in diminished ability to sleep, reversal of the sleep–wake cycle, hypersomnia, or reduced arousal. Symptoms should not be better accounted for by a typical syndrome of substance intoxication or substance withdrawal, although delirium can occur as a complication of intoxication or withdrawal states.

Identifying and treating delirium rapidly is highly important. Depending on the etiology, treatment delay is associated with a longer course of delirium (e.g., in cancer, HIV, and postsurgical patients; Cerejeira & Mukaetova-Ladinska 2011; de la Varga-Martínez et al., 2023). In certain health situations and the case of some substances, delirium can indicate life-threatening complications. Older adults with delirium are at higher risk for functional decline and mortality (Wan & Chase, 2017). Delirium is usually expected to remit when the underlying etiology is treated or the substance or medication causing it is eliminated from the body. Although antipsychotic medications or benzodiazepines may be useful in the short-term treatment of delirium, they do not address the underlying causes and can also be associated with adverse side effects. Behavioral strategies effectively reduce the risk of delirium in some hospitalized populations (National Institute for Health and Care Excellence, 2019).

Etiology of Delirium

The *ICD-11* offers the following options to indicate the etiology of delirium. "Delirium due to disease classified elsewhere" should be used when it is known or presumed that the delirium is caused by a specific, identified medical condition, which should be diagnosed separately. Specific options for identifying the cause of "delirium due to psychoactive substances, including medications," are provided for 13 substance classes (e.g., alcohol, opioids, MDMA [ecstasy] or related drugs), as well as for multiple substances and unknown or unspecified substances. "Delirium due to multiple etiological factors" should be used when delirium is attributed to multiple medical conditions or to both one or more medical conditions and one or more substances. Categories are also provided for "delirium due to other specified causes" and "delirium due to unknown or unspecified causes."

Mild Neurocognitive Disorder

Mild neurocognitive disorder is characterized by mild impairment in one or more cognitive domains relative to expectations for age and general premorbid level of neurocognitive functioning, which represents a decline from the individual's previous level of functioning (Blazer, 2013). Mild difficulties in complex activities are often present (e.g., using transportation, meal preparation), but they are not severe enough to interfere significantly with the performance of activities of daily living or to cause substantial impairment in personal, family, social, educational, occupational, or other critical functional areas. The cognitive impairment in mild neurocognitive disorder is not attributable to normal aging, the typical syndrome of substance intoxication or substance withdrawal, or another mental disorder (e.g., schizophrenia, depressive or bipolar disorder, posttraumatic stress disorder, dissociative disorders). Behavioral and psychological symptoms (e.g., depressed mood, anxiety, sleep disturbance) that are insufficient for a separate mental disorder diagnosis are commonly present and are sometimes the primary complaint when the individual presents for care. A subjective report of impairment alone is not a sufficient basis for diagnosing mild neurocognitive disorder. Instead, cognitive impairment relative to a previous level of functioning should be corroborated by objective evidence from standardized neuropsychological/cognitive testing or, in its absence, another quantified clinical assessment (e.g., a neurobehavioral status examination; American Medical Association, 2022).

The risk for mild neurocognitive disorder increases with age, but it can occur at any point across the life span. The course of impairment depends on the specific etiology and available treatment options. Some forms may improve with treatment or resolution of the underlying condition, whereas patterns of impairment may be more stable or progressive. Mild neurocognitive disorder sometimes represents an early presentation of an underlying disease process that may later meet the diagnostic requirements for dementia.

Etiology of Mild Neurocognitive Disorder

The observed impairment in mild neurocognitive disorder may be attributable to an underlying acquired disease of the nervous system, a trauma, an infection, or other disease process affecting the brain, use of specific substances or medications, nutritional deficiency or exposure to toxins, or the etiology may be unknown (Saari, 2023). A wide range of medical conditions may potentially cause mild neurocognitive disorders, including all the exact causes observed in dementia. However, separate categories for different etiologies are not provided for mild neurocognitive disorder. When the etiological condition has been identified, the diagnosis corresponding to that disease, illness, or injury should be assigned in addition to mild neurocognitive disorder. For example, mild neurocognitive disorder diagnosed with the category Alzheimer disease from the chapter on diseases of the nervous system could be an appropriate diagnosis when the presence of Alzheimer disease has been established (e.g., via biomarkers), but the cognitive disturbance is subthreshold for dementia.

Amnestic Disorder

Amnestic disorder is characterized by prominent memory impairment, defined as reduced ability to acquire, learn, or retain new information relative to age and overall level of intellectual functioning, in the absence of significant impairment in other neurocognitive domains (e.g., executive functioning, attention, visuospatial abilities). This may include the inability to recall previously learned information. Recent memory is typically more impaired than remote memory, and the ability to immediately recognize a limited amount of information is usually relatively preserved. The memory impairment represents a marked decline from previous level of functioning. The onset of symptoms can be sudden, such as when due to stroke or trauma, or gradual, such as when caused by chronic exposure to certain psychoactive substances or nutritional deficiencies.

Normal aging is typically associated with some degree of memory change. Amnestic disorder should not be diagnosed if performance is consistent with expectations for the individual's age based on age-related norms for performance on a standardized assessment, or if the symptoms are better accounted for by delirium or other disturbance of consciousness or altered mental status, substance intoxication or withdrawal, or another mental disorder.

Symptoms may be stable or progress over time, depending on the underlying causal condition. Some symptoms may improve over time if the underlying etiology is treated. When memory impairment worsens progressively over time, amnestic disorder may represent an early presentation of dementia.

Etiology of Amnestic Disorder

The *ICD-11* offers the following options to indicate the etiology of amnestic disorder: "amnestic disorder due to disease classified elsewhere" should be used when it is known or presumed that the memory problems are caused by a specific, identified medical condition, which should be diagnosed separately. Particular options for identifying the cause of "amnestic disorder due to psychoactive substances, including medications," are provided for three substance classes known to be potential causes or contributors to amnestic disorder (i.e., alcohol; sedatives, hypnotics, or anxiolytics; volatile inhalants). A category for "amnestic disorder due to unknown or unspecified causes" is also provided.

Dementia

Dementia is characterized in the *ICD-11 CDDR* by impairment in two or more cognitive domains relative to expected performance based on the individual's age and general premorbid level of neurocognitive functioning, which represents a decline from the individual's previous level of functioning. Memory impairment is present in most forms of dementia, but neurocognitive impairment is not restricted to memory. Several cognitive domains are typically affected in dementia, such as executive functioning, attention, language, social cognition, judgment, psychomotor speed, or visuoperceptual or visuospatial functioning. Behavioral changes (e.g., changes in personality, disinhibition, agitator irritability) may also be present and, in some forms of dementia, may be the presenting symptom (Saari, 2023).

Different etiologies are associated with varying patterns of dementia symptoms (see the following discussion on the etiology of dementia). However, a common pattern in the development of dementia is a reduction over time of the individual's ability to remember, understand, and solve problems. Memory problems typically begin as short-term memory loss, expanding gradually to substantial problems with recall of all forms of recently learned information and eventually to long-term memory loss. In addition, impairment in the ability to attend and difficulty with organizing behavior to accomplish complex tasks and solve problems (executive functioning) often slowly emerge and become more significant over time. Associated impact on everyday functioning increases over time as cognitive impairments become increasingly pronounced.

Etiology of Dementia

The *ICD-11* provides detailed categories to identify the specific etiology of dementia, as shown in Exhibit 18.1. When dementia is due to a disease or condition classified elsewhere, the diagnosis for the etiological disease or condition should be assigned along with the dementia. Specific categories are also provided for dementia due to specific psychoactive substances known to be potential causes or contributors to dementia (i.e., alcohol, sedatives, hypnotics or anxiolytics, or volatile inhalants). When dementia is due to psychoactive substances or medication, the appropriate disorder due to substance

EXHIBIT 18.1

ICD-11 **Etiological Categories for Dementia**

Dementia due to diseases classified elsewhere
- Dementia due to Alzheimer disease
  - Dementia due to Alzheimer disease, mixed type, with cerebrovascular disease
  - Dementia due to Alzheimer disease, mixed type, with other nonvascular etiologies
- Dementia due to cerebrovascular disease
- Dementia due to Lewy body disease
- Frontotemporal dementia
- Dementia due to Parkinson disease
- Dementia due to Huntington disease
- Dementia due to exposure to heavy metals and other toxins
- Dementia due to human immunodeficiency virus
- Dementia due to multiple sclerosis
- Dementia due to prion disease
- Dementia due to normal pressure hydrocephalus
- Dementia due to injury to the head
- Dementia due to pellagra
- Dementia due to Down syndrome
- Dementia due to other specified diseases classified elsewhere

Dementia due to psychoactive substances including medications
- Dementia due to use of alcohol
- Dementia due to use of sedatives, hypnotics, or anxiolytics
- Dementia due to use of volatile inhalants
- Dementia due to other specified psychoactive substance

use diagnosis for the relevant substance (generally harmful pattern of psychoactive substance use or substance dependence) should also be assigned alongside dementia. Although the etiological categories for dementia provided in the *ICD-11* and shown in Exhibit 18.1 are numerous, they are not exhaustive. For this reason, a category is provided for dementia due to other specified causes. If the cause has not been identified, the category for dementia due to an unknown or unspecified cause should be used.

The onset and course of dementia symptoms vary considerably by etiology, and the symptom course may provide information about etiology. Most dementias are progressive, but some are reversible (e.g., when related to nutritional or metabolic abnormalities). Presentations may be stable or rapidly progressive. Sometimes dementia may have multiple etiologies, as in the "mixed type" etiological subcategories provided for dementia due to Alzheimer disease. The CDDR include information on the general characteristics and typical course of the etiological categories for dementia listed in Table 18.1.

The most prevalent forms of dementia, and therefore the types of dementia most likely to be seen in general psychological practice, are dementia due to Alzheimer disease, dementia due to cerebrovascular disease, dementia due to Lewy body disease, and frontotemporal dementia (Chan et al., 2013). Dementia is sometimes also seen in other common neurological disorders

TABLE 18.1. Typical Presenting Symptoms in Common Forms of Dementia

Etiology of dementia	Typical presenting symptoms
Dementia due to Alzheimer disease	Memory loss is sometimes accompanied by problems in attention, executive functions, processing speed, social cognition and judgment, visuoperceptual or visuospatial problems, and difficulties in behavior and/or mood.
Dementia due to cerebrovascular disease	Most common neurocognitive symptoms are in the areas of attention, executive function, and processing speed.
Dementia due to Lewy body disease	Initial presentation is commonly characterized by attention and executive function problems, which may be accompanied by visual hallucinations.
Frontotemporal dementia	Characterized by significant changes in personality and behavior, sometimes accompanied by apathy, decreased social cognition, stereotyped behaviors, language deficits, and movement disorders. Memory usually remains intact.
Dementia due to Parkinson disease	Problems with attention, executive functions, memory abilities, and visual functions. Changes in affect and behavior may also be present.
Dementia due to multiple sclerosis	Significant problems in attention, executive functions, memory, and processing speed, with changes in affect.
Dementia due to injury to the head	Initial deficits include disorientation and loss of consciousness; subsequent symptoms may include attention, executive function, memory, and speed of processing, along with changes in personality and social cognition.

such as Parkinson disease and multiple sclerosis, as well as in head injury. In each case, the patterns of deterioration and the domains affected are slightly different. Table 18.1 provides a summary of the prominent problems associated with each of these common types of dementia.

Dementia Severity

The severity of dementia for each dementia category is rated as mild, moderate, or severe according to the individual's degree of neurocognitive and functional impairment and their capacity for independence in activities of daily living. Dementia severity is a primary determinant of the level of support that an individual will require—and therefore, the treatment and residential options available to them. The CDDR indicate that persons with mild dementia may be able to live independently, but some supervision or support is often required. They are generally able to participate in community or social activities without help and may appear unimpaired to those who do not know them well. Persons with moderate dementia require support to function outside the home, and only simple household tasks are maintained. They have difficulties with basic activities of daily living, such as dressing and personal hygiene. Socializing is increasingly difficult as the individual may behave inappropriately. The difficulties are typically apparent to most individuals who have contact with the individual. In severe dementia, the person is usually unable to make

---

EXHIBIT 18.2

Specifiers for Behavioral or Psychological Disturbances in Dementia

Psychotic symptoms in dementia
Mood symptoms in dementia
Anxiety symptoms in dementia
Apathy in dementia
Agitation or aggression in dementia
Disinhibition in dementia
Wandering in dementia
Other specified behavioral or psychological disturbances in dementia
Behavioral or psychological disturbances in dementia, unspecified

---

judgments or solve problems. They may have difficulty understanding what is happening around them and are typically entirely dependent on others for primary personal care in bathing, toileting, and feeding. The *CDDR* provide additional information on the diagnostic requirements for mild, moderate, and severe dementia.

Behavioral or Psychological Disturbances in Dementia

The *ICD-11* provides specifiers for behavioral and psychological disturbances. These are shown in Exhibit 18.2 and may be used together with any dementia diagnosis. These disturbances are common in dementia—particularly moderate and severe dementia—and have specific implications for treatment and management. The appropriate specifier(s) should be used when the corresponding behavioral or psychological disturbance is severe enough to represent a focus of clinical intervention; multiple specifiers may be applied. Additional information about these specifiers is provided in the *CDDR*.

DIFFERENTIAL DIAGNOSIS

Normal aging is typically associated with some degree of cognitive change. Delirium is differentiated from age-related cognitive changes by the sudden onset of symptoms (e.g., within hours or days), significant confusion and/or global neurocognitive impairment, and transient and typically fluctuating symptom presentation. Other neurocognitive disorders diagnoses should not be assigned if performance is consistent with expectations for the individual's age based on age-related norms for performance on standardized assessments. When memory difficulties consistent with normal aging are present and clinically relevant, the category age-associated cognitive decline from the *ICD-11* chapter on symptoms, signs, or clinical findings, not elsewhere classified may be used to document a subjective or objective decline in cognitive neurocognitive functioning that is consistent with age-related norms.

Regarding differential diagnosis, care should be taken to distinguish delirium from substance intoxication and substance withdrawal when there is a history of use of psychoactive substances or medications. For delirium to be diagnosed, the duration or severity of the symptoms must be substantially in excess of the characteristic intoxication or withdrawal syndrome associated with the specified substance. In contrast to delirium, other neurocognitive disorders are more typically characterized by impairment in specific neurocognitive abilities, tend to be more gradual in onset, and are often progressive. Individuals with other neurocognitive disorders, particularly dementia, are at increased risk for delirium (Sachdev et al., 2014). A diagnosis of delirium and another neurocognitive disorders should be assigned together if the diagnostic requirements for each are met.

Unlike mild neurocognitive disorder, memory deficits in amnestic disorder and neurocognitive deficits in dementia are associated with significant impairment in functioning. This boundary is imprecise, however, so it is often a clinical judgment to determine when mild neurocognitive disorder crosses over into dementia based on the number and severity of symptoms and their effect on the patient's life. Amnestic disorder and dementia are distinguished in that specific and prominent memory impairment is the primary clinical feature of amnestic disorder. In contrast, dementia is characterized by significant impairment in two or more cognitive domains, which often includes memory.

Differentiating among different etiologies for neurocognitive disorders, especially among the different etiological categories for dementia, can be complex because they are all characterized by cognitive declines or alterations, as well as by behavioral changes. It is often difficult to distinguish the variability in presentation among different cases with the exactly the same etiology from variability due to different etiologies. To diagnose neurocognitive disorders, available data (e.g., records, medical tests, clinical and psychometric findings) are compared with the characteristic symptoms related to specific etiologies that have some symptomatic overlap with the individual's presentation. (See the section on assessment later in this chapter.)

Neurocognitive disorders should not be diagnosed if the symptoms are better accounted for by another mental disorder. This includes neurodevelopmental disorders, especially disorders of intellectual development. However, both disorders may be present, and adults with disorders of intellectual development are at greater and earlier risk of developing dementia (e.g., dementia due to Down syndrome). The symptoms of neurocognitive disorders, especially mild neurocognitive disorder, must be distinguished from other mental disorders, whether these are an intrinsic part of the diagnosis in question (e.g., problems with memory and concentration in depressive episodes; a range of cognitive deficits in schizophrenia) or an effect of having them (e.g., compromised test performance due to high levels of anxiety or paranoid delusions). The CDDR provide more detailed information about disorders that should be considered in the differential diagnosis. Cognitive changes due to other mental disorders typically improve with appropriate treatment of that disorder.

In reciprocal fashion, psychological symptoms are associated with many neurocognitive disorders. Some of the most common and significant psychological symptoms are found in frontotemporal dementia. The pathognomonic symptoms are unusual and unexpected changes in personality and behavior in comparison with longstanding characterological traits. The changes are difficult to understand, measure, and control. Some of these changes are misperceived initially as volitional, or they may be misunderstood as symptoms of mood disorders. Another important example of behavioral changes is found in dementia due to Parkinson disease, where there may be both perceptual changes (e.g., visual hallucinations) and changes in affect (e.g., flatness). The visual hallucinations are often perceived by patients as entertaining and non-threatening, unlike those usually found with schizophrenia or delirium. Another change in behavior that is often misinterpreted as mood changes is found in dementia due to multiple sclerosis. Depressive symptoms often appear, associated with a decrease in energy and stamina. The symptoms are not explained by an emotional reaction to the disease.

ASSESSMENT

Assessment in neurocognitive disorders typically focuses on neurocognitive and neurobehavioral functions, although other areas may be assessed as relevant (Armstrong & Morrow, 2019). Neurocognitive functions are organized into domains. Some domains are relatively simple to understand and measure, whereas others are complex and multidimensional. Essential neurocognitive functions include orientation (to time, place, person, and circumstance), attention (ability to focus and sustain attention), motor functions (such as lateralized, gross, and fine motor abilities), and sensory functions (primarily visual and auditory). Examples of more complex neurocognitive functions include linguistic skills, including receptive communication abilities (i.e., ability to understand verbal, written, and nonverbal information) and expressive communication abilities (i.e., ability to generate verbal, written, and/or nonverbal information). The most complex and challenging functions to conceptualize and assess are often referred to as higher cortical functions (referring to the cerebral cortex). These include but are not limited to learning (acquisition and storage of information); memory (the recall of such information); executive functions (including but not limited to planning, organizing, and executing purposeful behavior); and intellectual functions (which could be considered the amalgamation of the previously mentioned higher cortical functions). These domains form patterns of functioning that are characteristic of different diagnoses. In addition, measurement of psychopathology (e.g., affective states) and personality functioning, academic abilities, and social understanding and skills are often part of a comprehensive neuropsychological evaluation, which is the gold standard approach for assessing neurocognitive disorders.

A typical neuropsychological assessment involves reviewing available records (e.g., medical, educational, vocational), interviews of the patient and important informants (e.g., significant other, family members) and administering scientifically validated and appropriately normed, standardized neuropsychological and psychological tests. When the goal of the neuropsychological evaluation is to aid in diagnoses, the usual approach is to document the pattern of domain-specific performance, compare the results obtained with the characteristic pattern for different disorders and etiologies, and then use that information along with the results of other available information to arrive at a diagnostic hypothesis (American Psychological Association, 2020; Pérez-García, 2009). For example, in dementia due to Huntington disease, the motor symptoms often affect gross motor movements whereas motor symptoms in dementia due to Alzheimer disease tend to affect fine motor movements. Findings from clinical observation of different activities (e.g., walking vs. writing) and psychometric testing (e.g., simple tests of motor strength vs. finger tapping) are integrated in these situations. In other cases, such as frontotemporal dementia, the problematic behaviors are challenging to measure using standardized tests (Bang et al., 2015).

A complete neuropsychological testing battery would typically assess orientation, attention, motor functioning, sensory functioning, learning, memory, executive functions, intellectual abilities, academic achievement, and psychopathology (Roebuck-Spencer et al., 2017). The findings from the test instruments would be compared with appropriate samples for referencing. The variables used for referencing would include demographic status (e.g., age), neurological condition (e.g., poststroke), mental disorder diagnoses (e.g., patients with recurrent depressive disorder), socioeconomic status, and linguistic and cultural group (American Education Research Association, American Psychological Association, & National Council on Measurement in Education, 2014). The comparison of the testing results would often occur with several specific groups, such as in the case of an older adult who has experienced a stroke, is depressed, is from a lower economic group, and whose native language is Spanish. When relevant reference samples are not available, this places limits on the validity of the test interpretation. When that happens, available sources of objective documentation should be used (e.g., school and work history, daily functioning).

The most commonly used screening tests for cognitive dysfunction are the Mini-Mental Status Exam (MMSE; Folstein et al., 1983) and the Montreal Cognitive Assessment (MoCA; Nasreddine et al., 2005). These tests are in the public domain and have been translated into multiple languages. Although the MMSE is more frequently used, the MoCA has greater widespread acceptance by geriatric specialists (Siqueira et al., 2019). However, these tests have been criticized for their lack of usefulness in patients with low educational and economic levels (Lezak et al., 2012). For example, patients who do not have access to technology and digital media for economic reasons are less likely to be knowledgeable about social and political events and therefore will tend to perform less well on the questions in the General Information section of the MMSE. Similarly, items that require drawing or copying shapes, reciting sentences or a series of digits, and even computing arithmetical problems will be biased in favor of those with a sufficient level of formal schooling. Despite their challenges, these tests, especially the MoCA, are frequently considered the first step in assessing neurobehavioral functioning and may be the only psychometric measure used in many settings. Their widespread use is due to their acceptance, applicability, and availability in the public domain and various languages. The simplicity of these measures and the high frequency of their use makes the information they provide useful in communicating across a broad spectrum of health professionals as well as over time to document changes in basic neuropsychological functions.

If there is evidence of neurocognitive dysfunction based on screening tests or other sources of information, the next step would generally be a more detailed assessment of the essential domains of attention, language, and motor and sensory functioning. These domains are considered foundational to cognitive and behavioral functioning and are building blocks for subsequent, more complex evaluation if it is indicated (Lezak et al., 2012). Also, if any of these areas are compromised, it will affect the measurement of more complex functions. For example, if a patient has impaired communication abilities, it would be challenging to measure verbal memory. There are numerous measures of attention, including in the public domain. There are fewer public domain measures of language and motor and sensory functioning. Assessment of activities of daily living may also be incorporated at this phase. The Vineland Adaptive Behavior Scales–III (Sparrow et al., 2016) is the most frequently used test of adaptive functioning and is available in some languages other than English. However, the test is expensive and not yet adapted for global use. For additional information on standardized tests and nonstandardized approaches to assessing adaptive abilities, especially those involving the assessment of intellectual disabilities, see Reschly et al. (2002).

After these primary domains are measured, the evaluation of the most complex assessment domains is undertaken. This includes measuring learning, memory, executive functioning, and intellectual abilities (American Education Research Association, American Psychological Association, & National Council on Measurement in Education, 2014). For intellectual functioning, the most frequently used are the Wechsler intelligence scales (e.g., Wechsler, 2008, 2014), although other widely used tests such as Raven's Progressive Matrices (Raven et al., 1998) are applicable, global, and available in the public domain. Other areas, such as memory and executive function, are more challenging to measure and less well researched, although number scales are available in the public domain (see Morgan & Ricker, 2017). However, these domains are often the affected in neurocognitive disorders and tend to be involved earlier in the course of the disease. Assessment of additional areas, such as psychopathology and academic functioning, may be included depending on the scope and guiding questions of the evaluation. neurocognitive disorders have high rates of co-occurrence with other mental disorders, particularly depressive disorders. One of the most widely used measures in the area of psychopathology is the Minnesota Multiphasic Personality Inventory–3 (Ben-Porath & Tellegen, 2020); this measure is available in multiple languages but is proprietary. There are also tests of affective functioning that are in the public domain and available in multiple languages (e.g., Patient Health Questionnaire–9; Kroenke et al., 2001). Academic achievement and occupational functioning is measured as a means of understanding the individual's baseline as well as to help estimate eventual vocational training opportunities.

In recent years, there has been an increasing emphasis on understanding effort or performance validity in neuropsychological test performance. That is, sometimes patients may exaggerate or minimize their symptoms and functional problems for a variety of reasons. The assessment of effort or performance validity helps determine the validity of test performance across domains, and a range of strategies have been described for doing this (Schroeder & Martin, 2021).

It is important to emphasize that circumstances sometimes preclude using standardized, quantitative testing of the relevant domains due to the lack of available instruments and norms or the patient's inability or ability to take these tests. In these situations, the evaluator will need to use more flexible, ecologically based qualitative assessments (Luria, 1980). This approach emphasizes understanding the deficits, the person, and sociohistorical and cultural contexts. Assessment is based on hypothesis testing as the assessment progresses, designed to fit the patient's sociocultural and educational background (Glozman, 1999). The qualitative information generated in this manner provides rich diagnostic data relating to the relative impairment or preservation of various cognitive systems, allowing the assessor to formulate a picture of the pattern of individual cognitive deficits experienced by the patient (Melikyan et al., 2019). This approach aims to provide a more accurate assessment of the individual by reducing irrelevant constructs (e.g., tests of intellectual abilities that are in fact measuring linguistic limitations).

The most important part of the evaluation is integrating testing data with the available records, history, clinical findings, and behavior to address the referral question—in this case, the diagnosis of a neurocognitive disorder. Considerable training and expertise are needed to integrate a multidimensional, scientific analysis (both quantitative and qualitative) with a clinically focused, patient-centered, sociocultural perspective that emphasizes context and qualitative information. When this level of expertise is unavailable, the goal should be to acquire as much objective, although not necessarily quantitative, information as possible and to use that data as a basis for an objective interpretation of the symptoms and whether the diagnostic requirements for a specific neurocognitive disorder are met.

CULTURAL AND CONTEXTUAL CONSIDERATIONS

Most neuropsychological tests are North American- and European-centric because this is where the specialty of neuropsychology started and is most developed. This reduces the generalizability of the measurement of neurocognitive constructs but should not prevent addressing their objective assessment in other contexts. It is critical to be aware of the influence that cultural and linguistic factors may have on their results. The confounding of these variables with the construct being measured (e.g., memory) will contribute to false-positive diagnoses (Daughtery et al., 2016). When standardized tests are used to determine neurocognitive impairment, they should be appropriately normed for the linguistic and cultural population of which the individual being tested is a member (Glozman, 2012). Where linguistically and culturally appropriate norms are unavailable, assessment of neurocognitive disorders requires greater reliance on clinical judgment and on collateral and historical information from informants or records. A clinician not conscious of these issues is likely to confuse sequelae of the disorder with linguistic and cultural effects on test performance.

Test performance and diagnostic accuracy may be affected directly by cultural biases (e.g., references in test items to terminology or objects not familiar to a culture) as well as by limitations of translation and adaptation (Puente & Puente, 2009). In evaluating activities of daily living, the expectations of the individual's culture and social environment should be considered. Similarly, some degree of memory loss or neurocognitive impairment might be seen as expected in some family or social systems and may not be fully recognized when existing support systems in the family and community are able to adapt.

KEY POINTS

- Emerging evidence over the past 2 decades has supported the conceptualization of neurocognitive disorders as both psychological and neurological. The *ICD-11* approach to neurocognitive disorders, in which the cognitive syndrome is characterized separately from the underlying cause, is consistent with this approach.

- Delirium is characterized by a disturbance of attention, orientation, and awareness that develops quickly and typically presents as significant confusion or global neurocognitive impairment.

- Mild neurocognitive disorder is characterized by mild impairment in one or more neurocognitive domains but without impact on independent functioning in activities of daily living.

- Amnestic disorder is characterized by prominent memory impairment with other neurocognitive domains generally intact.

- Dementia is characterized by impairment in two or more neurocognitive domains with an associated impact on independent functioning in activities of daily living. Dementia is also described in terms of its severity and the presence of behavioral and psychological disturbances with direct implications for care (e.g., mood symptoms, agitation or aggression, wandering).

- A neurocognitive disorder diagnosis should be based on standardized testing when available. Tests should be appropriately developed and normed for the population to which the individual belongs. Assessment requires greater reliance on clinical judgment when appropriately normed and standardized tests are unavailable.

- Special attention must be paid to determining that the impairment is not attributable to the effects of aging alone, that it represents a marked decline from previous levels of functioning, and that test results are not biased by cultural or linguistic factors.

- The heterogeneity and complexity of neurocognitive disorders are best understood when neuropsychological assessment methodology is pursued. A pattern of neuropsychological domain deficits is placed in the context of the development of the disease, comorbid disorders, and the patient's history, gender, social, and cultural context.

REFERENCES

American Education Research Association, American Psychological Association, & National Council on Measurement in Education. (2014). *Standards for educational and psychological tests.* American Psychological Association.

American Medical Association. (2022). *Current procedural terminology.*

American Psychological Association. (2020). *APA guidelines for psychological assessment and evaluation.* https://www.apa.org/about/policy/guidelines-psychological-assessment-evaluation.pdf

Armstrong, C., & Morrow, L. (Eds.). (2019). *Handbook of medical neuropsychology.* Springer. https://doi.org/10.1007/978-3-030-14895-9

Artero, S., Ancelin, M. L., Portet, F., Dupuy, A., Berr, C., Dartigues, J. F., Tzourio, C., Rouaud, O., Poncet, M., Pasquier, F., Auriacombe, S., Touchon, J., & Ritchie, K. (2008). Risk profiles for mild cognitive impairment and progression to dementia are gender specific. *Journal of Neurology, Neurosurgery, and Psychiatry, 79*(9), 979–984. https://doi.org/10.1136/jnnp.2007.136903

Bamford, S.-M., & Walker, T. (2012). Women and dementia. *Maturitas, 73*(2), 121–126. https://doi.org/10.1016/j.maturitas.2012.06.013

Bang, J., Spina, S., & Miller, B. L. (2015). Frontotemporal dementia. *The Lancet, 386*(10004), 1672–1682. https://doi.org/10.1016/S0140-6736(15)00461-4

Ben-Porath, Y. S., & Tellegen, A. (2020). *The Minnesota Multiphasic Personality Inventory–3 (MMPI-3): Technical manual.* University of Minnesota Press.

Blazer, D. (2013). Neurocognitive disorders in *DSM-5. The American Journal of Psychiatry, 170*(6), 585–587. https://doi.org/10.1176/appi.ajp.2013.13020179

Cerejeira, J., & Mukaetova-Ladinska, E. B. (2011). A clinical update on delirium: From early recognition to effective management. *Nursing Research and Practice, 2011,* 875196. https://doi.org/10.1155/2011/875196

Chan, K. Y., Wang, W., Wu, J. J., Liu, L., Theodoratou, E., Car, J., Middleton, L., Russ, T. C., Deary, I. J., Campbell, H., Wang, W., Rudan, I., & the Global Health Epidemiology Reference Group. (2013). Epidemiology of Alzheimer's disease and other forms of dementia in China, 1990–2010: A systematic review and analysis. *The Lancet, 381*(9882), 2016–2023. https://doi.org/10.1016/S0140-6736(13)60221-4

Chêne, G., Beiser, A., Au, R., Preis, S. R., Wolf, P. A., Dufouil, C., & Seshadri, S. (2015). Gender and incidence of dementia in the Framingham Heart Study from mid-adult life. *Alzheimer's & Dementia, 11*(3), 310–320. https://doi.org/10.1016/j.jalz.2013.10.005

de la Varga-Martínez, O., Gutiérrez-Bustillo, R., Muñoz-Moreno, M. F., López-Herrero, R., Gómez-Sánchez, E., & Tamayo, E. (2023). Postoperative delirium: An independent risk factor for poorer quality of life with long-term cognitive and functional decline after cardiac surgery. *Journal of Clinical Anesthesia, 85,* 111030. https://doi.org/10.1016/j.jclinane.2022.111030

Folstein, M. F., Robins, L. N., & Helzer, J. E. (1983). The Mini-Mental State Examination. *Archives of General Psychiatry, 40*(7), 812. https://doi.org/10.1001/archpsyc.1983.01790060110016

Gaebel, W., Jessen, F., & Kanba, S. (2018). Neurocognitive disorders in *ICD-11*: The debate and its outcome. *World Psychiatry, 17*(2), 229–230. https://doi.org/10.1002/wps.20534

Gaebel, W., Reed, G. M., & Jakob, R. (2019). Neurocognitive disorders in *ICD-11*: A new proposal and its outcome. *World Psychiatry, 18*(2), 232–233. https://doi.org/10.1002/wps.20634

Glozman, J. (2012). *Developmental neuropsychology*. Taylor and Francis.

Glozman, J. M. (1999). Quantitative and qualitative integration of Lurian procedures. *Neuropsychology Review, 9*(1), 23–32. https://doi.org/10.1023/A:1025638903874

Kroenke, K., Spitzer, R. L., & Williams, J. B. (2001). The PHQ-9: Validity of a brief depression severity measure. *Journal of General Internal Medicine, 16*(9), 606–613.

Lezak, M., Howeison, L., Bigler, E., & Tranel, D. (2012). *Neuropsychological assessment* (5th ed.). Oxford University Press.

Luria, A. (1980). *Higher cortical functions in man* (2nd ed.). Basic Books. https://doi.org/10.1007/978-1-4615-8579-4

Melikyan, Z. A., Agranovich, A. V., & Puente, A. E. (2019). Fairness in psychological testing. In G. Goldstein, D. N. Allen, & J. DeLuca (Eds.), *Handbook for psychological assessment* (pp. 551–572). Elsevier Academic Press. https://doi.org/10.1016/B978-0-12-802203-0.00018-3

Morgan, J. E., & Ricker, J. H. (Eds.). (2017). *Textbook of clinical neuropsychology* (2nd ed.). Routledge. https://doi.org/10.4324/9781315271743

Nasreddine, Z. S., Phillips, N. A., Bédirian, V., Charbonneau, S., Whitehead, V., Collin, I., Cummings, J. L., & Chertkow, H. (2005). The Montreal Cognitive Assessment, MoCA: A brief screening tool for mild cognitive impairment [see correction at https://doi.org/10.1111/jgs.15925]. *Journal of the American Geriatrics Society, 53*(4), 695–699. https://doi.org/10.1111/j.1532-5415.2005.53221.x

National Institute for Health and Care Excellence. (2019). *Delirium: Prevention, diagnosis and management in hospital and long-term care* (2023 update). https://www.nice.org.uk/guidance/cg103/chapter/Recommendations#interventions-to-prevent-delirium-2

Niu, H., Álvarez-Álvarez, I., Guillén-Grima, F., & Aguinaga-Ontoso, I. (2017). Prevalencia e incidencia de la enfermedad de Alzheimer en Europa: Metaanálisis [Prevalence and incidence of Alzheimer's disease in Europe: A meta-analysis]. *Neurologia, 32*(8), 523–532. https://doi.org/10.1016/j.nrl.2016.02.016

Ospina, J. P., King, F., IV, Madva, E., & Celano, C. M. (2018). Epidemiology, mechanisms, diagnosis, and treatment of delirium: A narrative review. *Clinical Medicine and Therapeutics, 1*(1), 3. https://doi.org/10.24983/scitemed.cmt.2018.00085

Pérez-García, M. (2009). *Manual de neuropsicología clínica* [Manual of clinical neuropsychology]. Psicología Pirámide.

Peterson, R. C., Roberts, R. O., Knopman, D. S., Boeve, B. F., Geda, Y. E., Ivnik, R. J., Smith, G. E., & Jack, C. R. (2009). Mild cognitive impairment: Ten years later. *Neurological Review, 66*(12), 1447–1455. https://doi.org/10.1001/archneurol.2009.266

Puente, A. E., & McCaffrey, R. J., III, (Eds.). (1992). *Handbook of neuropsychological assessment: A biopsychosocial perspective*. Plenum Press. https://doi.org/10.1007/978-1-4899-0682-3

Puente, A. E., & Puente, A. N. (2009). The challenge of measuring abilities and competencies in Hispanics/Latinos. In E. L. Grigorenko (Ed.), *Multicultural psychoeducational assessment* (pp. 417–441). Springer.

Raven, J., Raven, J. C., & Court, J. H. (1998). *Manual for Raven's progressive matrices and vocabulary scale: Section 1: General overview*. Oxford Psychologists Press.

Reed, G. M., First, M. B., Kogan, C. S., Hyman, S. E., Gureje, O., Gaebel, W., Maj, M., Stein, D. J., Maercker, A., Tyrer, P., Claudino, A., Garralda, E., Salvador-Carulla, L., Ray, R., Saunders, J. B., Dua, T., Poznyak, V., Medina-Mora, M. E., Pike, K. M., . . .

Saxena, S. (2019). Innovations and changes in the *ICD-11* classification of mental, behavioural and neurodevelopmental disorders. *World Psychiatry, 18*(1), 3–19. https://doi.org/10.1002/wps.20611

Reschly, D. J., Myers, T. G., & Hartel, C. R. (Eds.). (2002). *Mental retardation: The role of adaptive behavior assessment*. National Academies Press. https://www.ncbi.nlm.nih.gov/books/NBK207541/

Roebuck-Spencer, T. M., Glen, T., Puente, A. E., Denney, R. L., Ruff, R. M., Hostetter, G., & Bianchini, K. J. (2017). Cognitive screening tests versus comprehensive neuropsychological test batteries: A National Academy of Neuropsychology education paper. *Archives of Clinical Neuropsychology, 32*(4), 491–498. https://doi.org/10.1093/arclin/acx021

Saari, T. T. (2023). Empirical and authoritative classification of neuropsychiatric syndromes in neurocognitive disorders. *The Journal of Neuropsychiatry and Clinical Neurosciences, 35*(1), 39–47. https://doi.org/10.1176/appi.neuropsych.21100249

Sachdev, P. S., Blacker, D., Blazer, D. G., Ganguli, M., Jeste, D. V., Paulsen, J. S., & Petersen, R. C. (2014). Classifying neurocognitive disorders: The *DSM-5* approach. *Nature Reviews Neurology, 10*(11), 634–642. https://doi.org/10.1038/nrneurol.2014.181

Schroeder, B. W., & Martin, P. K. (Eds.). (2021). *Validity assessment in clinical neuropsychological practice*. Guilford Press.

Siqueira, G. S. A., Hagemann, P. M. S., Coelho, D. S., Santos, F. H. D., & Bertolucci, P. H. F. (2019). Can MoCA and MMSE be interchangeable cognitive screening tools? A systematic review. *The Gerontologist, 59*(6), e743–e763. https://doi.org/10.1093/geront/gny126

Sparrow, S. S., Cicchetti, D. V., & Saulnier, C. A. (2016). *Vineland Adaptive Behavior Scales* (3rd ed.). Pearson.

Wan, M., & Chase, J. M. (2017). Delirium in older adults: Diagnosis, prevention, and treatment. *BC Medical Journal, 59*(3), 165–170.

Wechsler, D. (2008). *Wechsler Adult Intelligence Scale: Administration and scoring manual* (4th ed.). Pearson.

Wechsler, D. (2014). *WISC-V: Technical and interpretive manual*. Pearson.

World Health Organization. (2001). *The international classification of functioning, disability and health* (ICF). https://www.who.int/classifications/icf/en/

World Health Organization. (2022, September 20). *Dementia*. https://www.who.int/newsroom/fact-sheets/detail/dementia

World Health Organization. (2023). *ICD-11 for mortality and morbidity statistics* (Version: 01/2023). https://icd.who.int/browse11/l-m/en#/

World Health Organization. (2024). *Clinical descriptions and diagnostic requirements for ICD-11 mental, behavioural and neurodevelopmental disorders*. https://www.who.int/publications/i/item/9789240077263

II

IMPORTANT DIAGNOSES OUTSIDE MENTAL AND BEHAVIORAL DISORDERS

19

Sexual Dysfunctions and Sexual Pain Disorders

Brigitte Khoury, Elham Atallah, Iván Arango-de Montis, and Sharon J. Parish

OVERARCHING LOGIC

Across the world, sexual relationships play an important role in most people's lives (Bhugra & de Silva, 2007). Problems with sexual relationships and sexual functioning are common and affect the physical, psychological, and social well-being of both those who experience them and their partners (Brotto et al., 2016). The classification of sexual dysfunctions in the 10th revision of the *International Classification of Diseases* (*ICD-10*) was developed more than three decades ago, when sexual health and sexual medicine were still relatively new as distinct areas of research and practice. The World Association of Sexual Health was founded in 1978, the International Society for Sexual Medicine was founded in 1982, and *The Journal of Sexual Medicine* began publication in 2004. There have been both rapid growth and major advances in scientific knowledge and standards of practice related to sexual functioning since the publication of the *ICD-10*, making this an important area of focus in the development of the 11th revision of the *ICD* (*ICD-11*; Khoury et al., 2012; Parish et al., 2021; Reed et al., 2016; Sharan et al., 2019).

In the *ICD-11*, sexual dysfunctions are defined as "syndromes that comprise the various ways in which adult people may have difficulty experiencing personally satisfying, non-coercive sexual activities" (World Health Organization [WHO], 2023). The *ICD-11* classification of sexual dysfunctions represents

https://doi.org/10.1037/0000392-019
A Psychological Approach to Diagnosis: Using the ICD-11 as a Framework, G. M. Reed, P. L.-J. Ritchie, and A. Maercker (Editors)

an area of major innovation compared with the *ICD-10*; the term "paradigm shift" is, in this case, not an exaggeration. The *ICD-10* classification of sexual dysfunctions was based on a separation of mind and body, distinguishing "nonorganic" from "organic" conditions. The *ICD-10* chapter on mental and behavioral disorders included sexual dysfunctions that were considered to be "nonorganic" whereas most "organic" sexual dysfunctions were classified in the *ICD-10* chapter on diseases of the genitourinary system. However, such a view of sexual functioning has long been considered outdated by experts in the field. It is now universally acknowledged in the field of sexual health that the origin and maintenance of sexual dysfunctions frequently involves the interaction of physical and psychological factors (Carvalho & Nobre, 2011; Lewis et al., 2010; Parish et al., 2021; Perelman, 2009.)

On the basis of current evidence and best practices, the *ICD-11* contains a new, integrated classification of sexual dysfunctions as a part of a new chapter on conditions related to sexual health (Chou et al., 2015; Reed et al., 2016). This new chapter was considered necessary because sexual dysfunctions— and other conditions related to sexual health such as gender incongruence (Reed et el., 2016; Robles et al., 2022)—cannot be viewed as either disorders of the mind or disorders of the sexual organs (Jannini et al., 2010; Sachs, 2003). The *ICD-11* classification of sexual dysfunctions is based on the per- spective that sexual response is "a complex interaction of psychological, inter- personal, social, cultural and physiological processes and one or more of these factors may affect any stage of the sexual response" (WHO, 2023). This per- spective and the new integrated classification of sexual dysfunctions is a more accurate reflection of current research and practice (Reed et al., 2016).

The *ICD-11* organizes sexual dysfunctions into five main groups (see Exhibit 19.1):

1. Hypoactive sexual desire dysfunction
2. Sexual arousal dysfunctions
3. Orgasmic dysfunctions
4. Ejaculatory dysfunctions
5. Other specified sexual dysfunctions.

Where possible, *ICD-11* sexual dysfunction categories apply to both men and women, emphasizing commonalities in sexual response (e.g., hypoactive sexual desire dysfunction, orgasmic dysfunction) without ignoring estab- lished sex differences in their expression or subjective experience (Basson, 2000; Parish et al., 2021). Separate sexual dysfunctions categories for men and women are provided where sex differences are related to distinct clinical presentations (e.g., female sexual arousal dysfunction in women compared with male erectile dysfunction in men).

In addition, sexual pain disorders comprise two separate groupings in the *ICD-11*:

1. Sexual pain-penetration disorder
2. Other specified sexual pain disorders (see Exhibit 19.1)

EXHIBIT 19.1

ICD-11 Sexual Dysfunction and Sexual Pain Disorder Categories

Sexual dysfunctions
- Hypoactive sexual desire dysfunction
- Sexual arousal dysfunctions
  - Female sexual arousal dysfunction
  - Male erectile dysfunction
  - Other specified sexual arousal dysfunctions
  - Sexual arousal dysfunction, unspecified
- Orgasmic dysfunctions
  - Anorgasmia
    - Other specified orgasmic dysfunctions
    - Orgasmic dysfunction, unspecified
- Ejaculatory dysfunctions
  - Male early ejaculation
  - Male delayed ejaculation
  - Other specified ejaculatory dysfunctions
  - Ejaculatory dysfunction, unspecified
- Other specified sexual dysfunctions
- Sexual dysfunction, unspecified

Sexual pain disorders
- Sexual pain-penetration disorder
- Other specified sexual pain disorders
- Sexual pain disorder, unspecified

Although they are grouped separately in the *ICD-11*, sexual pain disorders can be conceptualized as a subgroup of sexual dysfunctions. *ICD-11* defines sexual pain disorders as

> marked and persistent or recurrent difficulties related to the experience of pain during sexual activity in adult people, which are not entirely attributable to an underlying medical condition, insufficient lubrication in women, age-related changes, or changes associated with menopause in women, and are associated with clinically significant distress. (WHO, 2023)

Sexual pain disorders also result in difficulty experiencing personally satisfying, noncoercive sexual activities; can represent a complex interaction of psychological, interpersonal, social, cultural, and physiological processes; and are associated with clinically significant distress. In this chapter, when we refer to "sexual dysfunctions," we intend to include sexual pain disorders unless we make an explicit distinction between the two groupings.

In the *ICD-10* classification of mental and behavioral disorders, there were two separate categories related to sexual pain: nonorganic dyspareunia and nonorganic vaginismus. However, the term "dyspareunia" has increasingly been used to refer to sexual pain that is caused by an underlying medical condition or other identified physical determinants (Basson, 2005; Binik, 2005). In dyspareunia, pain typically emerges not only as a response to penetration attempts during sexual intercourse but also in other situations such as insertion of tampons and gynecological exams. In addition, treatment approaches for dyspareunia differ from the those used for sexual pain disorders (Dias-Amaral & Marques-Pinto, 2018). For these reasons, the *ICD-11* category dyspareunia has been defined explicitly as caused by physical determinants and retained in the *ICD-11* chapter on diseases of the genitourinary system, along with other categories of pelvic and menstrual pain considered to have largely physical determinants.

In the *ICD-10*, nonorganic vaginismus referred to a "spasm of the muscles that surround the vagina, causing occlusion of the vaginal opening" (WHO, 1992, p. 152), making penile entry either impossible or painful. It is now recognized that fear or anxiety about vulvovaginal or pelvic pain is the central element of this condition (Binik, 2010). For this reason, sexual pain-penetration disorder has replaced nonorganic vaginismus in the *ICD-11*. In contrast to the treatments for pelvic pain conditions classified in diseases of the genitourinary system, treatment for sexual pain-penetration disorder generally focuses on reducing fear and anxiety rather than on muscle contractions or pain. Sexual pain-penetration disorder is the central diagnosis in the grouping of sexual pain disorders in the new chapter on conditions related to sexual health.

It is important to note that transgender people and those with nonbinary gender identities also have sexual dysfunctions and should have access to appropriate treatment. The discussion of male and female categories is not meant to be exclusionary in this sense but is partly based on sexual anatomy. This chapter refers to men and women to emphasize that these categories in the *ICD-11* are intended to apply to adults. Work on sexual dysfunctions with transgender people requires specialized knowledge and experience, particularly following gender-affirming medical procedures (Holmberg et al., 2019; Marinelli et al., 2023; Vedovo et al., 2020). This includes knowledge about the effects of hormone treatment and relevant surgical procedures on sexual functioning (Defreyne et al., 2020). Treatment approaches will be based on the person's anatomical, hormonal, and surgical status and desired forms of sexual functioning (Kerckhof et al., 2019), but also require open communication, a strong therapeutic relationship, and a fundamental respect for the individual's experiences and desires and the terminology they wish to use.

THE SEXUAL RESPONSE CYCLE

Recent evidence supports the idea that there are important differences in the sexual response cycle between men and women, which are also related to the organization of sexual dysfunction categories by gender in the *ICD-11*. For men, phases of sexual functioning are currently conceptualized as desire, excitement, orgasm, and resolution. The cycle starts with fantasies, followed by pleasure via penile tumescence and erection, then the sensation of ejaculation inevitability followed by ejaculation of semen, ending with muscle relaxation and physiological refraction for variable periods (Baldwin, 2001).

This model is quite similar to the one proposed by Masters and Johnson (1966) more than 50 years ago for both men and women.

More recent conceptualizations of the sexual response cycle in women describe a circular response cycle with overlapping phases rather than a linear process with physiological stages (Basson, 2001; Parish et al., 2021). For example, in some women, sexual arousal and desire occur simultaneously. Similarly, the orgasm of the woman does not necessarily signify a "peak event," but may occur multiple times and at any point of the cycle. It has also been found that, in contrast to male erections signifying arousal, the physiological reactions that women experience do not necessarily translate into subjective experiences of arousal (Meston, 2000). In fact, studies have shown that for women, using devices that measure vaginal lubrication and increases in vaginal vasocongestion have failed to be consistently accurate in predicting cognitive experiences of sexual arousal, which are more strongly related to emotions regarding the relationship and awareness of bodily changes (Basson, 2002).

A PSYCHOLOGICAL APPROACH TO SEXUAL DYSFUNCTIONS

The assessment and treatment of sexual dysfunctions have traditionally been a part of the scope of psychological practice, given appropriate training and experience. Approaches including cognitive behavior therapy, emotion-based therapy, couples communication techniques, and mindfulness are treatment mainstays for sexual problems (Peterson, 2017). The *ICD-11* classification of sexual dysfunctions strongly reflects a psychological approach in several ways.

First, the *ICD-11* places subjective experience at the center, making clear that there is no normative standard for sexual activity. The assessment of sexual dysfunctions may involve physical examinations or laboratory tests but should be based primarily on the reported, subjective experience of the individual. *Satisfactory* sexual functioning is defined as being satisfying to the individual; that is, the person is able to participate in sexual activity and in a sexual relationship as desired. A sexual dysfunction should not be diagnosed when the individual is satisfied with their pattern of sexual experience and activity, even if it is different from what might be satisfying to other people or from what is considered normative in a given culture or subculture. The individual's experience of their own sexual functioning is treated with attention and respect. Similarly, the adequacy of sexual functioning is not defined by the extent to which it conforms with the desires of others. This has historically been a problematic aspect in that women's sexual functioning has been viewed through the lens of male satisfaction (e.g., the concept of "frigidity"). Unrealistic expectations on the part of a partner, a discrepancy in sexual desire between partners, or inadequate sexual stimulation are all appropriate targets of treatment, but they are not valid bases for a diagnosis of sexual dysfunction.

Second, the *ICD-11* classification of sexual dysfunctions and sexual pain disorders includes a system of specifiers emphasizing important elements related to the developmental course and situational context of the dysfunction.

A *temporal specifier* indicates whether the dysfunction is *lifelong* (the person has always experienced the dysfunction from the time of initiation of relevant sexual activity) or *acquired* (the onset of the sexual dysfunction has followed a period of time during which the person did not experience it). A *situational specifier* indicates whether the dysfunction is *generalized* (the desired response is absent or diminished in all circumstances, including masturbation) or *situational* (the desired response is absent or diminished in some circumstances—e.g., with some partners or in response to some stimuli but not in others).

Third, a system of *etiological considerations specifiers* that indicate a wide range of potential contributing factors can be applied to all sexual dysfunctions and sexual pain disorders. These are not mutually exclusive, and as many may be applied as relevant to a particular case. Etiological considerations specifiers include the following (see WHO, 2023):

- "Associated with a medical condition, injury, or the effects of surgery or radiation treatment." This specifier is used when there is evidence that an underlying or comorbid medical condition, including hormonal, neurological, and vascular conditions; injuries; and consequences of surgical or radiation treatment is an important contributing factor to sexual dysfunctions or sexual pain disorders. Examples include diabetes mellitus, pituitary adenomas, multiple sclerosis, metabolic syndrome, hypothyroidism, hyperprolactinemia, female genital mutilation, radical prostatectomy, and injury to the spinal cord.

- "Associated with psychological or behavioral factors, including mental disorders." This specifier is used when the clinician judges that psychological and behavioral factors or symptoms are important contributing factors. Examples include low self-esteem, negative attitudes toward sexual activity, adverse past sexual experiences (including trauma), and behavioral patterns such as poor sleep hygiene and overwork. Mental disorders such as depressive disorders, anxiety and fear-related disorders, and disorders specifically associated with stress also frequently interfere with sexual functioning, as do subthreshold depressive, anxiety, or stress symptoms.

- "Associated with use of psychoactive substance or medication." This specifier is used when there is evidence that the direct physiological effects of a psychoactive substance or medication are an important contributing factor. Examples include selective serotonin reuptake inhibitors, histamine-2 receptor antagonists (e.g., cimetidine), alcohol, opioids, and amphetamines.

- "Associated with lack of knowledge or experience." This specifier is applied when the clinician's assessment indicates that the individual's lack of knowledge or experience of their own body, sexual functioning, and sexual response is an important contributing factor. This includes inaccurate information or myths about sexual functioning.

- "Associated with relationship factors." This specifier is available to the clinician to indicate that relationship factors are important contributing factors to the sexual dysfunction or sexual pain disorder. Examples include relationship conflict or lack of romantic attachment.

- "Associated with cultural factors." This specifier is used when the clinician's assessment indicates that cultural factors are important contributing factors to the sexual dysfunction or sexual pain disorder. Cultural factors may influence expectations or provoke inhibitions about the experience of sexual pleasure or other aspects of sexual activity. Other examples include strong culturally shared beliefs about sexual expression—for example, a belief that loss of semen can lead to weakness, disease, or death.

Together, these aspects of the *ICD-11* classification of sexual dysfunctions and sexual pain disorders support and promote a conceptualization of sexual disorders that is biopsychosocial, person-centered, relational, multidimensional, and richly contextual. This is a major innovation in the diagnosis of sexual dysfunctions that is fully consistent with a psychological approach.

PRESENTATIONS AND SYMPTOM PATTERNS

Several required features are common to all sexual dysfunctions. For an individual's experienced difficulty with sexual functioning to be diagnosable, it must (a) occur frequently; (b) have been present episodically or persistently for a period of at least several months, although it may fluctuate in severity or be absent on some occasions; and (c) be associated with clinically significant distress. These requirements separate sexual dysfunctions in the *ICD-11* from normal variation. Level and quality of sexual experience and functioning fluctuate over the life cycle and in response to life events or other stressors. Temporary or periodic fluctuations in sexual functioning in response to developmental changes or life events should not be diagnosed as a sexual dysfunction.

However, the *ICD-11* also indicates that in cases where there is an immediate acute cause of the sexual dysfunction (e.g., a radical prostatectomy or injury to the spinal cord in the case of erectile dysfunction; effects of breast cancer and its treatment in female sexual arousal dysfunction), the diagnosis can be assigned even though the duration requirement has not been met. This is intended to facilitate the initiation of treatment to support the individual in returning to sexual functioning they experience as satisfying. Similarly, there are no frequency or duration requirements for sexual pain disorders, so as not to impose any barrier to their rapid treatment.

The presenting features of the main sexual dysfunction and sexual pain disorder diagnoses are described in the following subsections.

Hypoactive Sexual Desire Dysfunction

Hypoactive sexual desire dysfunction is characterized by the absence or marked reduction in sexual desire. This may include reduced or absent spontaneous desire, such as sexual thoughts or fantasies; reduced or absent responsive desire to erotic cues and stimulation; or inability to sustain desire or interest in sexual activity once it has been initiated. As a result, the individual typically avoids initiating or participating in sexual activity or situations that might lead to such activity. Most individuals with hypoactive sexual desire dysfunction also report a subjective experience of diminished or absent enjoyment when they do participate in sexual activity.

Changes in the level of sexual desire are often related to relationship problems. In addition, sexual desire may be affected by a variety of medical conditions, including hormonal changes, endocrine disorders, and chronic illnesses. Use of certain medications (e.g., selective serotonin reuptake inhibitors, benzodiazepines, antipsychotics, hormones, anticonvulsants, and, in men, 5-alpha reductase inhibitors) or substances (e.g., opioids, long-term use of alcohol or amphetamines) can also affect sexual desire. Depressive episodes, anxiety and fear-related disorders, posttraumatic stress disorder, or subthreshold psychological and behavioral symptoms may also contribute to lack of sexual desire. Sexual desire may also be affected by a history of traumatic experiences, including sexual abuse. The contributions of these factors can be recorded using the etiological considerations specifiers for sexual dysfunction and sexual pain disorders.

Female Sexual Arousal Dysfunction

Female sexual arousal dysfunction is characterized by the absence or marked reduction in a sexual response to sexual stimulation. This may include an absence or marked reduction in genital response, including vulvovaginal lubrication, engorgement of the genitalia, and sensitivity of the genitalia; absence or marked reduction in nongenital sexual responses such as hardening of the nipples, flushing of the skin, increased heart rate, increased blood pressure, and increased respiration rate; or absence or marked reduction in subjective feelings of sexual arousal, excitement, or pleasure from any type of sexual stimulation. This absence or marked reduction in sexual response to sexual stimulation occurs even though the individual desires sexual activity and sexual stimulation is adequate. Like lack of sexual desire, lack of sexual arousal in response to stimulation in women can be a manifestation of relationship problems. It can also be affected by a range of medical conditions (e.g., diabetes mellitus, multiple sclerosis, metabolic syndrome, hypertension, and hyperlipidemia, injuries, radiation therapy, surgical treatments) as well as by psychological and behavioral symptoms and disorders. Furthermore, sexual arousal in women can be affected by substances or medications (e.g., antidepressants including selective serotonin reuptake inhibitors and serotonin and norepinephrine reuptake inhibitors, antihypertensives, antihistamines, antipsychotics). These factors can all be recorded using the etiological considerations specifiers.

Male Erectile Dysfunction

Male erectile dysfunction is characterized by inability or marked reduction in the ability to attain or sustain a penile erection of sufficient duration or rigidity to allow for sexual activity. The erectile difficulty occurs despite the desire for sexual activity and adequate sexual stimulation and has occurred episodically or persistently over a period of at least several months, although symptoms may fluctuate in severity or be absent on some occasions. Sexual activity that is experienced as unsatisfying because of difficulties with erectile functioning can lead to anxiety surrounding the inability to attain or sustain a penile erection that in subsequent sexual interactions may draw the man's attention away from erotic cues that normally serve to enhance arousal. In turn, this may contribute to the development and maintenance of erectile dysfunction.

Examples of medical conditions that can affect erectile functioning include those that affect the nervous and vascular systems, such as diabetes mellitus, cardiovascular disease, neurological disorders, and genitourinary diseases, as well as injuries and radiological or surgical treatments. In cases where there is an immediate acute cause of the male erectile dysfunction, such as radical prostatectomy or injury to the spinal cord, the diagnosis can be assigned to facilitate entry to treatment when this is important to the person, even though the duration requirement of several months has not been met. Depressive, anxiety, and other psychological and behavioral symptoms and disorders may interfere with erectile functioning, which can also be affected by a history of trauma, including sexual and psychological abuse. Use of certain medications (e.g., beta-blockers, antidepressants including selective serotonin reuptake inhibitors and serotonin and norepinephrine reuptake inhibitors) or substances (e.g., smoking, alcohol, amphetamines, opioids, cocaine) can also interfere with erectile functioning. Erectile dysfunction may also be related to relationship problems. These factors can be recorded using the etiological considerations specifiers.

Anorgasmia

Anorgasmia is characterized by the absence or marked infrequency of orgasm or markedly diminished intensity of orgasmic sensations. In women, this includes a marked delay in orgasm, which in men would typically be diagnosed as male delayed ejaculation. The pattern of absence, delay, or diminished frequency or intensity of orgasm occurs despite adequate sexual stimulation, including the desire for sexual activity and orgasm.

The experience of orgasm may be affected by a variety of medical conditions, including diabetes mellitus, multiple sclerosis, Parkinson disease, injuries (e.g., female genital mutilation, spinal cord pathology, brain injuries), and surgical treatments. Depressive, anxiety, and other psychological and behavioral symptoms may interfere with orgasmic functioning. Orgasmic functioning may also be affected by a history of trauma including sexual and psychological abuse. Use of certain medications (e.g., antidepressants including selective serotonin reuptake inhibitors and serotonin and norepinephrine reuptake inhibitors, anticonvulsants, antipsychotics) or substances (e.g., opioids) may affect orgasmic experience. These contributory factors should be documented using the etiological considerations specifiers.

Male Early Ejaculation

Male early ejaculation is characterized as ejaculation that occurs before or within a very short duration of the initiation of penetration (e.g., less than 1 minute) or other relevant sexual stimulation, with no or little perceived control over ejaculation. Ejaculatory latency can be influenced by multiple factors, including overall physical health; the frequency of sexual intercourse; the period of time elapsed since the previous ejaculation; the duration and content of foreplay; the sexual position; and the depth, force, and frequency of penile thrusting.

Unrealistic expectations on the part of the man or his partner regarding what should be his capacity to control his ejaculations or a discrepancy in sexual desire between partners is not a valid basis for a diagnosis of male early ejaculation. As a point of reference, for lifelong male early ejaculation involving vaginal penetration, an ejaculatory latency of less than 1 minute is commonly used as a diagnostic threshold in research, whereas for acquired male early ejaculation involving vaginal penetration, an ejaculatory latency of less than 3 minutes is commonly used.

Ejaculatory latency fluctuates over the life cycle, typically being shorter in younger men. Transient early ejaculation (e.g., following a period of sexual abstinence) is not uncommon. Ejaculatory latency may also be influenced by a variety of factors, including life events or other stressors. A temporary or periodic reduction of ejaculatory latency in response to developmental changes or life events should not be diagnosed as male early ejaculation.

Male Delayed Ejaculation

Male delayed ejaculation is characterized by the inability to achieve ejaculation or an excessive or increased latency to achieve ejaculation, despite adequate sexual stimulation and the desire to ejaculate. Men with delayed ejaculation may have little or no difficulty attaining or sustaining erections but often report low levels of subjective sexual arousal and pleasure, which may or may not meet the diagnostic requirements for hypoactive sexual desire dysfunction, and lower frequencies of coital activity. Sexual activity that is experienced as unsatisfying because of difficulties with ejaculatory functioning can lead to anxiety surrounding the inability to ejaculate that in subsequent sexual interactions may draw the man's attention away from erotic cues that normally serve to enhance arousal and later ejaculation. In turn, this may contribute to the development and maintenance of male delayed ejaculation.

Ejaculatory functioning may be affected by a variety of medical conditions, including diabetes mellitus, multiple sclerosis, and thyroid diseases, as well as injuries and surgical treatments (e.g., radical prostatectomy). Depressive, anxiety, and other psychological and behavioral symptoms can interfere with ejaculatory functioning, as can a history of trauma including sexual and psychological abuse. Use of certain medications (e.g., antidepressants including selective serotonin reuptake inhibitors and serotonin and norepinephrine reuptake inhibitors, antipsychotics, alpha-blockers) or substances (e.g., alcohol, amphetamines, methadone, opioids) can also interfere with ejaculatory functioning. Male delayed ejaculation may also be related to relationship problems. Contributing factors should be recorded using the etiological considerations specifiers.

Sexual Pain-Penetration Disorder

Sexual pain-penetration disorder is characterized by at least one of the following: marked difficulties with penetration during sexual intercourse, including due to involuntary tightening or tautness of the pelvic floor muscles during attempted penetration; marked vulvovaginal or pelvic pain during penetration; or fear or anxiety about vulvovaginal or pelvic pain in anticipation of, during, or as a result of penetration. The symptoms are recurrent during sexual interactions that potentially involve penetration, even though the individual experiences adequate sexual desire and stimulation. The symptoms are not explained by a mental disorder or medical condition that results in genital or penetrative pain, and they are not entirely attributable to insufficient vaginal lubrication or postmenopausal/age-related changes.

The experience of difficulties with penetration, vulvovaginal, or pelvic pain during intercourse, or fear or anxiety about engaging in sexual activity, can lead to anxiety that, in subsequent sexual interactions, is likely to draw the individual's attention away from erotic cues that normally serve to enhance arousal. In turn, this may contribute to the development and maintenance of sexual pain-penetration disorder. Avoidance of sexual activity as a result of sexual pain-penetration disorder is common, even if sexual desire is present. Over time, avoidance may generalize to a variety of stimuli associated with sex or sexual situations. The individual may experience difficulty with penetration or entry, including during attempted medical examinations or insertion of an object (such as a tampon), and may show signs of pelvic floor muscle involvement even at rest (i.e., in the absence of attempted penetration) exhibiting higher tone, more muscle spasm, more pain with medical examination, lower strength, and poorer muscle control. Treatment delays of months to years are common with sexual pain-penetration disorder. By the time individuals with the disorder come to clinical attention, both the individual and their partner may have given up on attempts at penetration during sex. The diagnosis should not be assigned based on isolated incidents but rather based on a pattern over time, involving repeated episodes of difficulty with penetration or associated pain, abandoned attempts, or avoidance of intercourse.

Examples of medical conditions that may underlie or contribute to sexual pain include provoked vestibulodynia, vulvodynia, pelvic floor muscle dysfunction, hypertonus, myalgia, postobstetric vulvar trauma, vulvovaginal atrophy, genitourinary syndrome of menopause, vaginal agenesis, pelvic inflammatory disease, endometriosis, interstitial cystitis, or female genital mutilation. If the symptoms are fully explained by the underlying medical condition and do not represent an independent focus of clinical attention, it is typically not necessary to assign an additional diagnosis of sexual pain-penetration disorder. Depressive, anxiety, and other psychological and behavioral symptoms may contribute to discomfort, anxiety, or pain related to penetration, which can also be related to a history of trauma including sexual and psychological abuse. Sexual pain-penetration disorder may also be related to relationship problems. The appropriate etiological specifiers should be used to document relevant contributing factors.

ASSESSMENT

In assessing sexual dysfunctions, it is important to take a detailed history of the problem, exploring the different factors that may have contributed to its onset and maintenance. The clinician should keep in mind that some initially precipitating or contributory factors (e.g., a depressive episode) may no longer be present even though the dysfunction has persisted after their remission. A medical examination is often important to understand the contribution made by medical conditions and their treatment.

Most of the information needed for identifying and managing sexual dysfunctions will be gathered by clinical interview. The clinician should particularly focus on the status of the relationship, including differences in partner desires, partner responses to sexual difficulties, and intimate partner violence (Brotto et al., 2016). When assessing sexual pain disorders, it is important to ask about arousal before the attempt, the possibility of vaginal entry, the timing and duration of the pain, relevant medical findings, and the partner's response to the individual's experience of pain.

Rather than comparing sexual functioning to what is considered normal by general society, it is important to compare an individual's desire, arousal, receptivity, and orgasm to their usual or previous experiences as well as to the sexual experience they would consider to be satisfactory or desirable. Past experiences of trauma, including sexual abuse, should be evaluated because these are often relevant factors. It is critical to achieve an understanding of how the individual's cultural background impacts their experience of sexual desire, sexual pleasure, sexual dysfunction, and related distress. An additional important enquiry in the assessment process is the partner's sexual response cycle because the presenting dysfunction may sometimes be secondary to the partner's sexual dysfunction.

There are a variety of standardized questionnaires that can be useful in the clinical assessment of sexual dysfunctions (Grover & Shouan, 2020). The Female Sexual Functioning Index (FSFI; Meston et al., 2019) is widely used for women and generally compatible with the *ICD-11*. The Female Sexual Distress Scale (Derogatis et al., 2002) could be used in conjunction with the FSFI, which does not assess distress related to sexual functioning. The Male Sexual Health Questionnaire (Rosen et al., 2004) is commonly used for men. All these scales are available in multiple languages and free of charge for clinical use or unfunded research projects (https://eprovide.mapi-trust.org/).

CO-OCCURRING DISORDERS

Sexual dysfunctions can co-occur with one another, and all diagnoses for which the diagnostic requirements are met and that represent a focus of clinical attention may be assigned. However, multiple diagnoses should not be assigned based entirely on overlapping features. For example, if a woman has difficulties with attaining or sustaining genital and nongenital responses but these are fully explained by diminished or absent sexual desire (i.e., hypoactive sexual desire dysfunction), an additional diagnosis of female sexual arousal dysfunction should not be assigned.

Sexual dysfunctions can be associated with a range of health issues that may be contributing factors in their development and maintenance, as described in the previous sections. These include diabetes mellitus, heart disease, hypertension, cancer, sexually transmitted infections, urinary tract conditions, and infertility (McCabe et al., 2016).

Individuals who experience sexual dysfunctions also have elevated rates of co-occurring mental health problems compared with those without sexual dysfunctions (Günzler & Berner, 2012; Heiman, 2002). In particular, the adverse effects of depressive episodes on sexual desire and sexual pleasure have been well documented (Angst, 1998; Baldwin, 2001). Moreover, some antidepressant medications interfere with sexual functioning (Kennedy et al., 2000). Other mental disorders including panic disorder, social anxiety disorder, and obsessive-compulsive disorder—as well as anxiety related to sexual performance—have also been shown to affect sexual functioning (Aksaray et al., 2001; Figueira et al., 2001; Kane et al., 2019; McCabe et al. 2016). The relationship of these psychological disorders to sexual dysfunctions is likely to be bidirectional, with relationship problems potentially exacerbating both (Catalan et al., 1990).

PREVALENCE

Approximately one third of both men and women report having sexual problems at some point during their lives (Brotto et al., 2016). The sexual dysfunctions most commonly reported by men are early ejaculation and male erectile dysfunction, whereas women are more likely to report hypoactive sexual desire dysfunction, followed by female sexual arousal dysfunction and sexual pain. A large proportion of women experience multiple sexual dysfunctions (McCabe et al., 2016).

CULTURAL CONSIDERATIONS

Sex is experienced subjectively, and that experience may be heavily influenced by one's cultural context and upbringing. Norms vary across cultures regarding individual sexual desire, arousal, sexual practices, duration of intercourse, and expectation of orgasm (Nicolosi et al., 2004). Care seeking and clinical distress related to sexual dysfunctions are influenced by sociocultural factors such as the expectations of the partner, sexual education, family and religious values, and messages from the media. Cultures differ regarding whether sexual activity is viewed as a means of experiencing pleasure or solely for procreation, particularly for women (Bhugra & de Silva, 2007). People from pleasure-oriented cultures are more likely to complain and seek care difficulties related to sexual arousal and pleasure because they are more likely to believe that they are entitled to these experiences.

In contrast, people from more strongly procreation-oriented societies may focus on difficulties with pain or male arousal and orgasm, which are perceived as signs of a physical problem (e.g., Dogan, 2009; Lo & Kok, 2014). For example, in a field study for *ICD-11*, Sharan et al. (2019) found in a sample of married Indian women with probable sexual problems that most had limited knowledge and felt unskilled in sex and reported being led by their husbands in sexual matters. Unlike lack of desire and sexual pain, they were unlikely to experience lack of arousal and absence of orgasm as problematic or distressing. Similarly, in some societies, sexual dysfunctions may be linked more strongly to satisfaction of the couple and related threats to the relationship, whereas in others they are more strongly related to feeling of shame and failure (e.g., for men in the expression of potency, masculinity, superiority, and power).

In societies that do not encourage conversation about sexuality, many sexual practices are likely to be unfamiliar to many individuals, and more so for women who are expected to limit and repress their sexual needs before marriage. Religious ideologies may depict sexual activity outside marriage as a sin and virginity as sacred (Khoury et al., 2012), strongly influencing the sexual norms of many belief-oriented societies. Indeed, sexual activity of women outside marriage could be punished through discrimination, destroyed reputations, and, in some traditional societies, death (Abu-Baker, 2005; Bhugra & de Silva, 2007). This leads to reactions that may mimic or help explain sexual dysfunctions or symptoms but that in some cases could be considered normal reactions rather than pathological. When women are taught to believe that being interested in sex is disgraceful, they may experience guilt and shame, both of which have been associated with low levels of sexual desire and arousal (Lau et al., 2005; Woo et al., 2012).

Finally, whereas moral and religious beliefs can shape attitudes about sex, media messages may also play an important role (Atallah et al., 2016). For example, media images suggesting that only slender females are sexually desirable or appealing can affect women's body image and perceptions of their desirability and right to enjoyment. Particularly in societies with limited access to accurate information about sex, learning about sex from pornographic videos can create unrealistic expectations about the nature of sexual interactions as well as size, performance, and duration (Khan et al., 2008).

KEY POINTS

- The *ICD-11* classification of sexual dysfunctions is an area of major innovation. It overcomes the traditional separation of mind and body that characterized *ICD-10* and instead provides a new, integrated classification of sexual dysfunctions as a part of a new chapter on conditions related to sexual health.

- The *ICD-11* classification of sexual dysfunctions is based on the perspective that sexual response is a complex interaction of psychological, interpersonal, social, cultural, and physiological processes. This biopsychosocial view of sexual dysfunctions is highly compatible with a psychological approach.

- The *ICD-11* organizes sexual dysfunctions into five main groups: hypoactive sexual desire dysfunction, sexual arousal dysfunctions, orgasmic dysfunctions, ejaculatory dysfunctions, and other specified sexual dysfunctions.

- Sexual pain disorders are characterized by marked and persistent or recurrent difficulties related to the experience of pain during sexual activity that is not entirely attributable to an underlying medical condition or other physical factors. Sexual pain-penetration disorder is the central diagnosis in the grouping of sexual pain disorders; fear or anxiety about vulvovaginal or pelvic pain in anticipation of, during, or as a result of penetration is one of its primary features.

- The *ICD-11* classification of sexual dysfunctions and sexual pain disorders includes a system of specifiers emphasizing important elements related to the developmental course and situational context of the dysfunction. A system of etiological considerations specifiers allows the clinician to document a wide range of potential contributing factors.

- Together, these aspects of the *ICD-11* classification of sexual dysfunctions and sexual pain disorders support and promote a conceptualization of sexual disorders that is biopsychosocial person-centered, relational, multidimensional, richly contextual, and psychological.

REFERENCES

Abu-Baker, K. (2005). The impact of social values on the psychology of gender among Arab couples: A view from psychotherapy. *The Israel Journal of Psychiatry and Related Sciences, 42*(2), 106–114.

Aksaray, G., Yelken, B., Kaptanoğlu, C., Oflu, S., & Özaltin, M. (2001). Sexuality in women with obsessive compulsive disorder. *Journal of Sex & Marital Therapy, 27*(3), 273–277. https://doi.org/10.1080/009262301750257128

Angst, J. (1998). Sexual problems in healthy and depressed persons. *International Clinical Psychopharmacology, 13*(Suppl. 6), S1–S4. https://doi.org/10.1097/00004850-199807006-00001

Atallah, S., Johnson-Agbakwu, C., Rosenbaum, T., Abdo, C., Byers, E. S., Graham, C., Nobre, P., Wylie, K., & Brotto, L. (2016). Ethical and sociocultural aspects of sexual function and dysfunction in both sexes. *The Journal of Sexual Medicine, 13*(4), 591–606. https://doi.org/10.1016/j.jsxm.2016.01.021

Baldwin, D. S. (2001). Depression and sexual dysfunction. *British Medical Bulletin, 57*(1), 81–99. https://doi.org/10.1093/bmb/57.1.81

Basson, R. (2000). The female sexual response: A different model. *Journal of Sex & Marital Therapy, 26*(1), 51–65. https://doi.org/10.1080/009262300278641

Basson, R. (2001). Human sex-response cycles. *Journal of Sex & Marital Therapy, 27*(1), 33–43. https://doi.org/10.1080/00926230152035831

Basson, R. (2002). Are our definitions of women's desire, arousal and sexual pain disorders too broad and our definition of orgasmic disorder too narrow? *Journal of Sex & Marital Therapy, 28*(4), 289–300. https://doi.org/10.1080/00926230290001411

Basson, R. (2005). Women's sexual dysfunction: Revised and expanded definitions. *Canadian Medical Association Journal, 172*(10), 1327–1333. https://doi.org/10.1503/cmaj.1020174

Bhugra, D., & de Silva, P. (2007). Sexual dysfunction across cultures. In D. Bhugra & K. Bhui (Eds.), *Textbook of cultural psychiatry* (pp. 364–378). Cambridge University Press. https://doi.org/10.1017/CBO9780511543609.029

Binik, Y. M. (2005). Should dyspareunia be retained as a sexual dysfunction in *DSM-V*? A painful classification decision. *Archives of Sexual Behavior, 34*(1), 11–21. https://doi.org/10.1007/s10508-005-0998-4

Binik, Y. M. (2010). The *DSM* diagnostic criteria for vaginismus. *Archives of Sexual Behavior, 39*(2), 278–291. https://doi.org/10.1007/s10508-009-9560-0

Brotto, L., Atallah, S., Johnson-Agbakwu, C., Rosenbaum, T., Abdo, C., Byers, E. S., Graham, C., Nobre, P., & Wylie, K. (2016). Psychological and interpersonal dimensions of sexual function and dysfunction. *The Journal of Sexual Medicine, 13*(4), 538–571. https://doi.org/10.1016/j.jsxm.2016.01.019

Carvalho, J., & Nobre, P. (2011). Biopsychosocial determinants of men's sexual desire: Testing an integrative model. *The Journal of Sexual Medicine, 8*(3), 754–763. https://doi.org/10.1111/j.1743-6109.2010.02156.x

Catalan, J., Hawton, K., & Day, A. (1990). Couples referred to a sexual dysfunction clinic: Psychological and physical morbidity. *The British Journal of Psychiatry, 156*(1), 61–67. https://doi.org/10.1192/bjp.156.1.61

Chou, D., Cottler, S., Khosla, R., Reed, G. M., & Say, L. (2015). Sexual health in the *International Classification of Diseases* (*ICD*): Implications for measurement and beyond. *Reproductive Health Matters, 23*(46), 185–192. https://doi.org/10.1016/j.rhm.2015.11.008

Defreyne, J., Elaut, E., Kreukels, B., Fisher, A. D., Castellini, G., Staphorsius, A., Den Heijer, M., Heylens, G., & T'Sjoen, G. (2020). Sexual desire changes in transgender individuals upon initiation of hormone treatment: Results from the Longitudinal European Network for the Investigation of Gender Incongruence. *The Journal of Sexual Medicine, 17*(4), 812–825. https://doi.org/10.1016/j.jsxm.2019.12.020

Derogatis, L. R., Rosen, R., Leiblum, S., Burnett, A., & Heiman, J. (2002). The Female Sexual Distress Scale (FSDS): Initial validation of a standardized scale for assessment of sexually related personal distress in women. *Journal of Sex & Marital Therapy, 28*(4), 317–330. https://doi.org/10.1080/00926230290001448

Dias-Amaral, A., & Marques-Pinto, A. (2018). Female genito-pelvic pain/penetration disorder: Review of the related factors and overall approach. *Revista Brasileira de Ginecologia e Obstetrícia, 40*(12), 787–793. https://doi.org/10.1055/s-0038-1675805

Dogan, S. (2009). Vaginismus and accompanying sexual dysfunctions in a Turkish clinical sample. *The Journal of Sexual Medicine, 6*(1), 184–192. https://doi.org/10.1111/j.1743-6109.2008.01048.x

Figueira, I., Possidente, E., Marques, C., & Hayes, K. (2001). Sexual dysfunction: A neglected complication of panic disorder and social phobia. *Archives of Sexual Behavior, 30*(4), 369–377. https://doi.org/10.1023/A:1010257214859

Grover, S., & Shouan, A. (2020). Assessment scales for sexual disorders: A review. *Journal of Psychosexual Health, 2*(2), 121–138. https://doi.org/10.1177/2631831820919581

Günzler, C., & Berner, M. M. (2012). Efficacy of psychosocial interventions in men and women with sexual dysfunctions—A systematic review of controlled clinical trials. *The Journal of Sexual Medicine, 9*(12), 3108–3125. https://doi.org/10.1111/j.1743-6109.2012.02965.x

Heiman, J. R. (2002). Sexual dysfunction: Overview of prevalence, etiological factors, and treatments. *Journal of Sex Research, 39*(1), 73–78. https://doi.org/10.1080/00224490209552124

Holmberg, M., Arver, S., & Dhejne, C. (2019). Supporting sexuality and improving sexual function in transgender persons. *Nature Reviews Urology, 16*(2), 121–139. https://doi.org/10.1038/s41585-018-0108-8

Jannini, E. A., McCabe, M. P., Salonia, A., Montorsi, F., & Sachs, B. D. (2010). Organic vs. psychogenic? The Manichean diagnosis in sexual medicine. *The Journal of Sexual Medicine, 7*(5), 1726–1733. https://doi.org/10.1111/j.1743-6109.2010.01824.x

Kane, L., Dawson, S. J., Shaughnessy, K., Reissing, E. D., Ouimet, A. J., & Ashbaugh, A. R. (2019). A review of experimental research on anxiety and sexual arousal: Implications for the treatment of sexual dysfunction using cognitive behavioral therapy. *Journal of Experimental Psychopathology, 10*(2). Advance online publication. https://doi.org/10.1177/2043808719847371

Kennedy, S. H., Jr., Eisfeld, B. S., Dickens, S. E., Bacchiochi, J. R., & Bagby, R. M. (2000). Antidepressant-induced sexual dysfunction during treatment with moclobemide, paroxetine, sertraline, and venlafaxine. *The Journal of Clinical Psychiatry, 61*(4), 276–281. https://doi.org/10.4088/JCP.v61n0406

Kerckhof, M. E., Kreukels, B. P. C., Nieder, T. O., Becker-Hébly, I., van de Grift, T. C., Staphorsius, A. S., Köhler, A., Heylens, G., & Elaut, E. (2019). Prevalence of sexual dysfunctions in transgender persons: Results from the ENIGI follow-up study [erratum at https://doi.org/10.1016/j.jsxm.2020.02.003]. *The Journal of Sexual Medicine, 16*(12), 2018–2029. https://doi.org/10.1016/j.jsxm.2019.09.003

Khan, S. I., Hudson-Rodd, N., Saggers, S., Bhuiyan, M. I., Bhuiya, A., Karim, S. A., & Rauyajin, O. (2008). Phallus, performance and power: Crisis of masculinity. *Sexual and Relationship Therapy, 23*(1), 37–49. https://doi.org/10.1080/14681990701790635

Khoury, B., Attallah, E., & Fayad, Y. (2012). Classification of sexual dysfunctions in the Arab world in relation to *ICD-11*. *Arab Journal of Psychiatry, 23*(Suppl.), 35–41.

Lau, J. T., Wang, Q., Cheng, Y., & Yang, X. (2005). Prevalence and risk factors of sexual dysfunction among younger married men in a rural area in China. *Urology, 66*(3), 616–622. https://doi.org/10.1016/j.urology.2005.04.010

Lewis, R. W., Fugl-Meyer, K. S., Corona, G., Hayes, R. D., Laumann, E. O., Moreira, E. D., Jr., Rellini, A. H., & Segraves, T. (2010). Definitions/epidemiology/risk factors for sexual dysfunction. *The Journal of Sexual Medicine, 7*(4 Pt 2), 1598–1607. https://doi.org/10.1111/j.1743-6109.2010.01778.x

Lo, S. S. T., & Kok, W. M. (2014). Sexual behavior and symptoms among reproductive age Chinese women in Hong Kong. *The Journal of Sexual Medicine, 11*(7), 1749–1756. https://doi.org/10.1111/jsm.12508

Marinelli, L., Cagnina, S., Bichiri, A., Magistri, D., Crespi, C., & Motta, G. (2023). Sexual function of transgender assigned female at birth seeking gender affirming care: A narrative review. *International Journal of Impotence Research*. Advance online publication. https://doi.org/10.1038/s41443-023-00711-7

Masters, W., & Johnson, V. (1966). *Human sexual response*. Little Brown.

McCabe, M. P., Sharlip, I. D., Lewis, R., Atalla, E., Balon, R., Fisher, A. D., Laumann, E., Lee, S. W., & Segraves, R. T. (2016). Incidence and prevalence of sexual dysfunction in women and men: A consensus statement from the Fourth International Consultation on Sexual Medicine 2015. *The Journal of Sexual Medicine, 13*(2), 144–152. https://doi.org/10.1016/j.jsxm.2015.12.034

Meston, C. M. (2000). The psychophysiological assessment of female sexual function. *Journal of Sex Education and Therapy, 25*(1), 6–16. https://doi.org/10.1080/01614576.2000.11074323

Meston, C. M., Freihart, B. K., Handy, A. B., Kilimnik, C. D., & Rosen, R. C. (2019). Scoring and interpretation of the FSFI: What can be learned from 20 years of use? *The Journal of Sexual Medicine*, *17*(1), 17–25. https://doi.org/10.1016/j.jsxm.2019.10.007

Nicolosi, A., Laumann, E. O., Glasser, D. B., Moreira, E. D., Jr., Paik, A., Gingell, C., & the Global Study of Sexual Attitudes and Behaviors Investigators' Group. (2004). Sexual behavior and sexual dysfunctions after age 40: The global study of sexual attitudes and behaviors. *Urology*, *64*(5), 991–997. https://doi.org/10.1016/j.urology.2004.06.055

Parish, S. J., Cottler-Casanova, S., Clayton, A. H., McCabe, M. P., Coleman, E., & Reed, G. M. (2021). The evolution of female sexual disorders/dysfunctions nomenclature and definitions: A review of *DSM*, *ICSM*, *ISSWSH*, and *ICD* classification systems. *Sexual Medicine Reviews*, *9*(1), 36–56. https://doi.org/10.1016/j.sxmr.2020.05.001

Perelman, M. A. (2009). The sexual tipping point: A mind/body model for sexual medicine. *The Journal of Sexual Medicine*, *6*(3), 629–632. https://doi.org/10.1111/j.1743-6109.2008.01177.x

Peterson, Z. D. (Ed.). (2017). *The Wiley handbook of sex therapy*. Wiley Blackwell.

Reed, G. M., Drescher, J., Krueger, R. B., Atalla, E., Cochran, S. D., First, M. B., Cohen-Kettenis, P. T., Arango-de Montis, I., Parish, S. J., Cottler, S., Briken, P., & Saxena, S. (2016). Disorders related to sexuality and gender identity in the *ICD-11*: Revising the *ICD-10* classification based on current scientific evidence, best clinical practices, and human rights considerations. *World Psychiatry*, *15*(3), 205–221. https://doi.org/10.1002/wps.20354

Robles, R., Keeley, J. W., Vega-Ramírez, H., Cruz-Islas, J., Rodríguez-Pérez, V., Sharan, P., Purnima, S., Rao, R., Rodrigues-Lobato, M. I., Soll, B., Askevis-Leherpeux, F., Roelandt, J.-L., Campbell, M., Grobler, G., Stein, D. J., Khoury, B., Khoury, J. E., Fresán, A., Medina-Mora, M. E., & Reed, G. M. (2022). Validity of categories related to gender identity in *ICD-11* and *DSM-5* among transgender individuals who seek gender-affirming medical procedures. *International Journal of Clinical and Health Psychology*, *22*(1), 100281. https://doi.org/10.1016/j.ijchp.2021.100281

Rosen, R. C., Catania, J., Pollack, L., Althof, S., O'Leary, M., & Seftel, A. D. (2004). Male Sexual Health Questionnaire (MSHQ): Scale development and psychometric validation. *Urology*, *64*(4), 777–782. https://doi.org/10.1016/j.urology.2004.04.056

Sachs, B. D. (2003). The false organic-psychogenic distinction and related problems in the classification of erectile dysfunction. *International Journal of Impotence Research*, *15*(1), 72–78. https://doi.org/10.1038/sj.ijir.3900952

Sharan, P., Purnima, S., Rao, R., Kedia, S., Khoury, B., & Reed, G. M. (2019). Field testing of *ICD-11* proposals for female sexual dysfunctions in India: Cognitive interviews with patients. *Archives of Medical Research*, *50*(8), 567–576. https://doi.org/10.1016/j.arcmed.2020.01.002

Vedovo, F., Di Blas, L., Perin, C., Pavan, N., Zatta, M., Bucci, S., Morelli, G., Cocci, A., Delle Rose, A., Caroassai Grisanti, S., Gentile, G., Colombo, F., Rolle, L., Timpano, M., Verze, P., Spirito, L., Schiralli, F., Bettocchi, C., Garaffa, G., . . . Trombetta, C. (2020). Operated male-to-female sexual function index: Validity of the first questionnaire developed to assess sexual function after male-to-female gender affirming surgery. *The Journal of Urology*, *204*(1), 115–120. https://doi.org/10.1097/JU.0000000000000791

Woo, J. S., Brotto, L. A., & Gorzalka, B. B. (2012). The relationship between sex guilt and sexual desire in a community sample of Chinese and Euro-Canadian women. *Journal of Sex Research*, *49*(2–3), 290–298. https://doi.org/10.1080/00224499.2010.551792

World Health Organization. (1992). *The ICD-10 classification of mental and behavioural disorders: Clinical descriptions and diagnostic guidelines*. https://www.who.int/publications/i/item/9241544228

World Health Organization. (2023). *ICD-11 for mortality and morbidity statistics* (Version: 01/2023). https://icd.who.int/browse11/l-m/en#/

20

Sleep–Wake Disorders

Gualberto Buela-Casal, Almudena Carneiro-Barrera, and
Katie Moraes de Almondes

OVERARCHING LOGIC

In the 11th revision of the *International Classification of Diseases* (*ICD-11*; World
Health Organization [WHO], 2023), sleep–wake disorders have been unified in
a new and separate chapter. This innovation corrects the inaccurate and frag-
mented distribution of these disorders in the 10th revision of the *ICD* (*ICD-10*),
in which sleep–wake disorders were distributed across several chapters. In the
ICD-10, so-called "nonorganic" sleep disorders were included in the chapter on
mental and behavioral disorders, whereas most of the "organic" sleep disorders
were included in the chapter on diseases of the nervous system. Other categories
included in the *ICD-11* chapter on sleep–wake disorders had previously been
classified in the *ICD-10* chapters on endocrine, nutritional, and metabolic
diseases; diseases of the respiratory system; certain conditions originating in the
perinatal period; and symptoms, signs, and abnormal clinical and laboratory
findings, not elsewhere classified.

The *ICD-11* resolves the outdated mind–body, nonorganic–organic split
inherent in the *ICD-10*. Many sleep–wake disorders comprise both physiological
and psychological/behavioral components; they are neither strictly mental disorders nor medical conditions. Forced compartmentalization of these disorders into
one or the other category resulted in misleading and inaccurate inferences
regarding the nature of these conditions, with potentially adverse effects on
treatment. The *ICD-11* reflects an integrated biopsychosocial conceptualization of

https://doi.org/10.1037/0000392-020
A Psychological Approach to Diagnosis: Using the ICD-11 as a Framework, G. M. Reed,
P. L.-J. Ritchie, and A. Maercker (Editors)

sleep–wake disorders that is in harmony with current evidence and best practices in the modern field of sleep medicine.

The unified *ICD-11* classification of sleep–wake disorders also corrects what are now understood to be misclassifications of some disorders. For example, parasomnias (e.g., sleepwalking, night terrors, and nightmares) have historically been classified as mental disorders, based on outdated and incorrect assumptions about their etiology. These conditions are now understood to be largely biologically determined, including a substantial genetic component (Baldini et al., 2021; Broughton, 2022; Schredl, 2021). Moreover, the *ICD-11* also allows for the specification of several important sleep-related conditions that were previously classified as "unspecified," including REM sleep behavior disorder and periodic limb movement disorder.

The *ICD-11* chapter on sleep–wake disorders seeks to enhance patient care and public health through a more visible and accurate system that will enhance clinician awareness and improve diagnostic accuracy and treatment. The conceptualization of sleep–wake disorders as a distinct area supports the awareness and consideration of health-related consequences and impact of these disorders in other conditions such as mental and substance use disorders, neurological, respiratory, metabolic and endocrine disorders, and pain syndromes. Emerging data suggest that clinical attention to these sleep disorders as independent conditions that significantly impact morbidity and mortality can improve health outcomes (Garbarino et al., 2016).

The *ICD-11* classification of sleep–wake disorders was intentionally designed to be fully consistent with the third edition of the *International Classification of Sleep Disorders* (*ICSD-3*; American Academy of Sleep Medicine [AASM], 2014). It was developed by an international expert working group appointed jointly by the WHO Department of Mental Health and Substance Use and the AASM and chaired by the editor of the *ICSD-3*. Unlike the areas covered in this book that are part of the *ICD-11* chapter on mental, behavioral and neurodevelopmental disorders, sleep–wake disorders are not included in the *ICD-11 Clinical Descriptions and Diagnostic Requirements* (*CDDR*). The main part of *ICD-11* contains descriptions of each disorder, which include a summary of the diagnostic requirements that would be sufficient for most clinical applications. For example, the *ICD-11* description of chronic insomnia is as follows:

> Chronic insomnia is a frequent and persistent difficulty initiating or maintaining sleep that occurs despite adequate opportunity and circumstances for sleep and that results in general sleep dissatisfaction and some form of daytime impairment. Daytime symptoms typically include fatigue, depressed mood or irritability, general malaise, and cognitive impairment. The sleep disturbance and associated daytime symptoms occur at least several times per week for at least 3 months. Some individuals with chronic insomnia may show a more episodic course, with recurrent episodes of sleep/wake difficulties lasting several weeks at a time over several years. Individuals who report sleep related symptoms in the absence of daytime impairment are not regarded as having an insomnia disorder. If the insomnia is due to another sleep–wake disorder, a mental disorder, another medical condition, or a substance or medication, chronic insomnia should only be diagnosed if the insomnia is an independent focus of clinical attention. (WHO, 2023)

Substantially more detailed guidance is provided in the *ICSD-3*, which will be particularly useful for specialists in sleep medicine.

A PSYCHOLOGICAL APPROACH TO SLEEP–WAKE DISORDERS

A psychological approach to sleep–wake disorders is an increasingly important element in the clinical assessment, diagnosis, and treatment of these disorders due to the bidirectional relationship between sleep disturbances and mental health conditions. Specific behavior patterns, stress, anxiety, and depression are important predisposing, priming, or triggering factors in the development and maintenance of sleep–wake disorders (Dzierzewski et al., 2021; Fang et al., 2019). In addition, sleep–wake disorders have important consequences for distress, mental health, and disability (Anderson & Bradley, 2013; Fang et al., 2019). Sleep disruption or sleep deprivation, which occurs in most sleep–wake disorders, usually leads to impaired daytime functioning and mood, reduced cognitive function, and behavioral disturbances (Medic et al., 2017), typically associated with daytime sleepiness. Psychology plays an essential role in understanding and addressing the psychological components of sleep–wake disorders, both as risk factors and as outcomes (Meltzer et al., 2009; Stepanski & Perlis, 2000). Accordingly, psychologists are increasingly being integrated in multidisciplinary sleep medicine teams, enhancing both research and clinical practice (Stepanski & Perlis, 2000).

This chapter includes information intended to be useful for the general clinical practice of psychologists and other mental health professionals on the following groupings within the sleep–wake disorders chapter: insomnia disorders; hypersomnolence disorders; circadian rhythm sleep–wake disorders; and parasomnia disorders. These groupings cover the areas that had been classified as nonorganic sleep disorders in *ICD-10* (WHO, 1992).

This chapter does not cover the groupings of sleep-related breathing disorders and sleep-related movement disorders. Sleep-related breathing disorders are characterized by abnormalities of respiration during sleep and include central sleep apneas, obstructive sleep apneas, and sleep-related hypoventilation and hypoxemia disorders. Sleep-related movement disorders are primarily characterized by relatively simple, usually stereotyped, movements that disturb sleep or its onset. Among the sleep-related movement disorders, restless legs syndrome is unique because it is partly a waking, sensorimotor experience that also typically involves periodic limb movements during sleep. Additional information on sleep-related breathing disorders and sleep-related movement disorders can be found in the *ICD-11* (WHO, 2023) and in the *ICSD-3* (AASM, 2014).

INSOMNIA DISORDERS

Presentations and Symptom Patterns

Insomnia disorders are characterized by persistent difficulty with sleep initiation, duration, maintenance, or quality that occurs despite adequate opportunity and circumstances for sleep. To be diagnosed as an insomnia disorder, the sleep problems must result in general sleep dissatisfaction and some form of daytime impairment, such as fatigue, depressed mood or irritability, general malaise, or cognitive impairment (e.g., deficits in executive functions, memory, and attention). For a diagnosis of an insomnia disorder, sleep onset latencies and periods of wakefulness during sleep must last for at least 30 minutes for middle- and older-aged adults or at least 20 minutes in children and young adults. Early morning awakening is operationalized as occurring at least 30 minutes earlier compared with the usual sleep pattern.

A diagnosis of chronic insomnia may be assigned if the sleep problems and associated daytime impairment have occurred at least several times per week for at least 3 months. Some individuals with chronic insomnia have a more episodic course, with episodes that last for several weeks at a time over a period of several years. A diagnosis of short-term insomnia may be assigned if the sleep difficulties and associated daytime impairment have lasted for less than 3 months. There is often an identifiable precipitant for short-term insomnia. Short-term insomnia may also occur sporadically, often coincident with daytime stressors. Insomnia and associated impairments in daytime functioning may be risk factors for cardiovascular disease, diabetes, depressive disorders, suicide, and cognitive decline (Buysse, 2013). Other outcomes include absenteeism at work, risk of accidents, and decreased productivity (Daley et al., 2009).

Differential Diagnosis

In making a diagnosis of chronic or short-term insomnia, it is important to consider the frequency, chronicity, and recurrence of the symptoms, as well as factors that appear to precipitate the episodes or contribute to their severity and maintenance. When insomnia is a part of the presentation of another sleep–wake disorder, a mental disorder (e.g., a mood disorder, an anxiety disorder), or a medical condition (e.g., pain, gastroesophageal reflux disease), it should be diagnosed only if the insomnia is an independent focus of clinical attention—for example, when the underlying condition has improved but insomnia persists. A similar rule should be applied to insomnia due to the effects of a substance or medication on the central nervous system (e.g., caffeine, methylphenidate). Environmental circumstances contributing to sleep disturbance should be identified (e.g., noise, light, relationship conflict). Insomnia disorders should be distinguished from insufficient sleep syndrome, which refers to voluntary restriction of sleep when individuals choose to forgo sleep in favor of other obligations or activities and typically does not require intervention other than providing the opportunity to sleep. Insomnia disorders should also be distinguished from delayed and advanced sleep–wake phase disorders, which refer to shifting of the major sleep period compared with the conventional or desired sleep time.

Developmental Course

The onset of insomnia disorders can be gradual or sudden (Buysse, 2013; Morin et al., 2009). When chronic or recurrent, individuals often report that the symptoms began in early life or young adulthood. Onset is often linked to major life events, daily stressors, or changes in sleep schedule. Short-term insomnia may remit with the resolution of the precipitating stressor, but not always. Most individuals with diagnosable insomnia will still have it a year later, and about half will still have it after 3 years (Buysse, 2013; Morin et al., 2009). If untreated, sleep disturbance, daytime impairment, and apprehension about insomnia may worsen over time.

Symptoms, as well as precipitating and maintaining factors, may change over the course of development, in part due to biological factors such as the delayed sleep–wake phase in circadian rhythm typical of adolescents and young adults (i.e., later sleep onset and later awakening), and the advanced sleep–wake phase (earlier sleep onset and earlier awakening) and increased number of awakenings observed among the older adults (Buysse, 2013; Morin et al., 2009). Other medical conditions and medications as precipitating or maintaining factors are more prominent among older adults. Younger people are more likely to complain of difficulty falling asleep, whereas older adults report more difficulty with maintaining sleep.

Assessment

The clinical assessment should include the onset and course of the insomnia, preexisting or comorbid medical conditions, pain, mobility impairment, menopause, complaints of cognitive decline, co-occurring mental disorders or symptoms, medication use, daytime functioning, sleep habits, sleep environment, and interventions for insomnia already attempted. The Athens Insomnia Scale (Soldatos et al., 2000) is a widely used eight-item scale available in multiple languages that can help to structure the assessment of occurrence, duration, and variability of insomnia as well as daytime sleepiness and functioning.

A medical examination may be important to understand the contribution made by underlying medical conditions and their treatment. Actigraphy is a noninvasive method for measuring motor activity and other sleep parameters that can be used in the individual's normal sleep environment and provide an objective assessment of the quantity and quality of sleep (Smith et al., 2018). In chronic and persistent cases, polysomnography (PSG), which must be performed in a sleep laboratory, can be useful in the differential diagnosis of conditions that may be associated with insomnia such as sleep apnea and periodic limb movement disorder. Individuals with persistent complaints of insomnia accompanied by daytime sleepiness may also warrant a multiple sleep latency test (MSLT), particularly if narcolepsy is suspected.

Prevalence

Insomnia disorders are by far the most prevalent sleep–wake disorders (Roth, 2007). Population-based estimates indicate that approximately one third of adults report insomnia symptoms at some point in their lives (30%–35% of the population), 10% to 15% experience associated daytime impairment, and 10% with symptoms that meet the diagnostic requirements for insomnia disorder.

Like most sleep–wake disorders, the prevalence of insomnia disorders increases with age. In children, insomnia associated with requirements of parental/caregiver presence at bedtime and/or during the night, along with insomnia due to limit-setting difficulties, are estimated to occur in 10% to 30% of children, depending on the exact definition used (Roth, 2007). Studies of adolescents indicate prevalence rates of 3% to 12% for chronic insomnia after puberty, depending in part on the definition used, with a higher frequency in girls than boys (Calhoun et al., 2014; Roth, 2007). Data on the prevalence of short-term insomnia among adolescents is limited, but some studies suggest a range of 15% to 20%.

HYPERSOMNOLENCE DISORDERS

Presentations and Symptom Patterns

Hypersomnolence disorders are characterized by excessive daytime sleepiness that is not due to disturbed or insufficient sleep or to another sleep–wake disorder (e.g., circadian rhythm disorder or a sleep-related breathing disorder). Excessive daytime sleepiness is defined as the inability to stay awake and alert during the major waking episodes of the day, resulting in periods of irrepressible need for sleep or unintended lapses into drowsiness or sleep. Excessive sleepiness may lead to irritability, lack of energy, problems with attention and concentration, reduced vigilance, reduced motivation, dysphoria, fatigue, restlessness, and lack of coordination. Type 1 and Type 2 narcolepsy, idiopathic hypersomnia, and Kleine–Levin syndrome are sometimes referred to as primary hypersomnia, with the remaining hypersomnia disorders sometimes referred to as secondary hypersomnia because they are due to another identified cause (e.g., a medical condition, a mental disorder, a substance, insufficient sleep).

Narcolepsy

Narcolepsy is characterized by daily periods of irrepressible need for sleep or daytime lapses into sleep occurring for at least several months, accompanied by abnormal manifestations of REM sleep. In Type 1 narcolepsy, there are abnormally low levels of hypocretin in the cerebrospinal fluid (CSF). Hypocretin is a hypothalamic neuropeptide thought to have an important role in the regulation of sleep and arousal states (Sutcliffe & de Lecea, 2000). The pathognomonic symptom of Type 1 narcolepsy is cataplexy, which is a sudden and uncontrollable loss of muscle tone arising during wakefulness that is typically triggered by a strong emotion, such as excitement or laughter. However, cataplexy may not manifest until years after the onset of daytime sleepiness. Hypnagogic hallucinations, sleep paralysis, and sleep fragmentation usually manifest later in the course of the disorder. A definitive diagnosis of Type 1 narcolepsy requires either (a) cataplexy and MSLT and/or PSG findings characteristic of narcolepsy, or (b) demonstrated CSF hypocretin deficiency. In Type 2 narcolepsy, neither cataplexy nor low levels of CSF hypocretin are present, but MSLT/PSG findings characteristic of narcolepsy are required for a diagnosis.

Idiopathic Hypersomnia

Idiopathic hypersomnia is characterized by daily periods of irrepressible need to sleep or daytime lapses into sleep over a period of at least 3 months, without cataplexy and with a confirmed finding of no more than one sleep-onset REM period (SOREMPs) on MSLT. The hypersomnolence is not better explained by another disorder (e.g., insufficient sleep syndrome, obstructive sleep apnea, circadian rhythm sleep–wake disorder, a substance or medication, or a medical condition). In addition, hypersomnolence should be noted in the MSLT demonstrating a mean of sleep latency of 8 minutes or less or by PSG or actigraphy showing a total sleep time ≥660 minutes over 24 hours. Prolonged difficulty waking up with repeated returns to sleep (sleep inertia) are present, and naps are generally long—often more than 60 minutes—and unrefreshing. For a diagnosis of idiopathic hypersomnia, hypersomnolence should persist for at least 3 months.

Kleine–Levin Syndrome

Kleine–Levin syndrome is characterized by recurrent episodes of severe sleepiness together with characteristic cognitive, psychological, and behavioral disturbances. During episodes, patients may sleep as long as 16 to 20 hours per day, waking up only to eat and void. When awake during episodes, most patients are exhausted, apathetic, confused, and slow in speaking and answering. Hyperphagia, hypersexuality, childish behavior, depression, anxiety, hallucinations, and delusions are often observed during the episodes. A typical episode lasts a median of 10 days (range 2.5–80 days), with rare episodes lasting several weeks to months. Following episodes, most individuals have amnesia for the episode. Amnesia, transient dysphoria, or elation with insomnia may signal the termination of an episode. Between episodes, individuals with Kleine–Levin syndrome have normal alertness, cognitive function, behavior, and mood.

In hypersomnia due to a medical condition, the daytime sleepiness, excessive nocturnal sleep, or excessive napping occurs as a direct physiological consequence of a significant underlying medical or neurological condition (e.g., head trauma; Parkinson disease; certain genetic conditions and metabolic, neurologic, or endocrine disorders). In hypersomnia due to a medication or substance, the hypersomnia is attributable to the sedating effects of a medication, alcohol, or other psychoactive substances, including withdrawal syndromes (e.g., from stimulants). In hypersomnia associated with a mental disorder, it is attributable to a co-occurring mental disorder such as a mood disorder or a dissociative disorder; this is most typical of depressive episodes. To assign any of these three diagnoses, the hypersomnia must be severe enough to be an independent focus of clinical intervention.

Insufficient sleep syndrome is characterized by difficulty in obtaining the amount of sleep required to maintain normal levels of alertness and wakefulness. The sleep restriction is voluntary given that the individual chooses to forgo sleep in favor of other obligations or activities. A detailed history of the sleep pattern reveals a substantial disparity between the amount of sleep needed and the amount actually obtained, leaving the individual chronically sleep deprived. Given the opportunity to sleep, the person's ability to initiate and maintain sleep is unimpaired. As a result, sleep time is often markedly extended on weekend nights or during holidays compared with weekdays. When adequate sleep is obtained, the symptoms of sleepiness remit.

Differential Diagnosis

Excessive daytime sleepiness may be an aspect of the presentation of other sleep–wake disorders, such as sleep apnea and circadian rhythm sleep–wake disorders, which should be included in the differential diagnosis. A mental health evaluation is important because daytime sleepiness can occur in mood disorders, dissociative disorders, and other mental disorders. Cataplexy, which is characteristic in narcolepsy, should be differentiated from hypotension, transient ischemic attacks, drop attacks, akinetic seizures, neuromuscular disorders, vestibular disorders, sleep paralysis, and catatonia. Normal variations in sleep duration should be considered because individuals who require more than average sleep may exhibit excessive sleepiness if the required amount of nighttime sleep is not obtained.

Developmental Course

Primary hypersomnolence disorders tend to have their onset sometime between middle childhood and early adulthood (Khan & Trotti, 2015), with a first peak occurring in adolescence, at about 15 years, and a second peak at about 35 years. In young children, sleepiness may be expressed as excessively long nocturnal sleep or discontinuous napping episodes, with hyperactive behavior or poor school performance (Khan & Trotti, 2015; Moreira & Pradella-Hallinan, 2017). The presence of inattention, fatigue, insomnia, and hallucinations that may occur in these disorders can lead to an inappropriate diagnosis of schizophrenia, ADHD, or depression. Normative data are not available for the MSLT in children younger than 6 years of age. In adulthood, impairment in work performance, obesity, and depression are common. Driving may be avoided for fear of a motor vehicle accident. The developmental course of secondary hypersomnolence disorders is based on the course of the underlying condition.

Assessment

The severity of daytime sleepiness can be assessed subjectively using severity scales such as the Epworth Sleepiness Scale (Johns, 1991). This eight-item scale assesses the subjective likelihood of falling asleep in different situations; it is freely available for clinical and unfunded research use and has been translated into multiple languages (see https://eprovide.mapi-trust.org/instruments/epworth-sleepiness-scale). Sleepiness can be assessed objectively using overnight PSG and the MSLT.

Prevalence

Compared with insomnia, narcolepsy is rare. Incidence of narcolepsy in the United States (the number of new cases per year) has been estimated at 7.7 persons per 100,000 population, including Types 1 and 2 narcolepsy, with incidence of narcolepsy without cataplexy several times more common than narcolepsy with cataplexy (Longstreth et al., 2007). The highest incidence was among individuals in their early 20s and late teens. Studies from other regions including Europe and Hong Kong have estimated a total prevalence of narcolepsy of between 20 and 50 persons per 100,000 population (Longstreth et al., 2007). The prevalence of idiopathic hypersomnia and insufficient sleep syndrome is unknown. Kleine–Levin syndrome is rare, with prevalence estimated at approximately one to two cases per million (Arnulf et al., 2005).

CIRCADIAN RHYTHM SLEEP–WAKE DISORDERS

Presentations and Symptom Patterns

Circadian rhythm sleep–wake disorders are persistent or recurrent disturbances of the sleep–wake cycle due to alterations of the circadian time-keeping system, its entrainment mechanisms, or a misalignment of the endogenous circadian rhythm and the external environment (social demands, work and school schedules, light–dark environment). The most common complaints are excessive sleepiness or insomnia, or both. Circadian rhythm sleep–wake disorders may be characterized by displacement of circadian rhythms (delayed sleep–wake phase disorder and advanced sleep–wake phase disorder), temporary desynchronization of endogenous rhythms and times of day (circadian rhythm sleep–wake disorder shift work type and jet lag type), reduced amplitude of circadian rhythms (irregular sleep–wake rhythm disorder), or synchronization failure in relationship to day length (non-24-hour sleep–wake rhythm disorder). To diagnose any circadian rhythm sleep–wake disorder, the symptoms must result in significant distress or significant mental, physical, social, occupational, or academic impairment. For all disorders in the grouping except jet lag type, the symptoms must have been present for several months (e.g., 3 months) to assign a diagnosis.

Delayed sleep–wake phase disorder is characterized by a persistent and stable delay in the major sleep period (to a later time), compared with conventional or desired sleep times. When individuals can establish their own sleep–wake schedules so that these occur on the delayed schedule, sleep quality and duration are normal. The complaint is a chronic or recurrent inability to fall asleep and difficulty awakening because of the delayed circadian rhythm.

Advanced sleep–wake phase disorder is characterized by persistent and stable advance in the major sleep period (to an earlier time), compared with conventional or desired sleep times. This results in evening sleepiness (before the desired bedtime) and awakening earlier than the desired or required times.

When individuals can establish their own sleep–wake schedules to occur on the advanced, sleep quality and duration are normal.

Irregular sleep–wake rhythm disorder is characterized by lack of a clearly defined circadian rhythm of sleep and awake periods. The chronic or recurring sleep–wake pattern is temporally disorganized so that sleep and wake episodes are variable throughout the 24-hour cycle. The clinical presentation includes symptoms of insomnia and excessive sleepiness, depending on the time of day and their particular sleep–wake pattern.

Non-24-hour sleep–wake rhythm disorder is characterized by symptoms of insomnia or excessive sleepiness that occur because the intrinsic circadian clock is not entrained to the 24-environmental cycle. The non-24-hour period is typically longer than 24 hours, although it can be shorter. Symptoms occur as the circadian-controlled sleep–wake propensity cycles in and out of phase with the environmental day–night cycle. Non-24-hour sleep–wake rhythm disorder is most commonly observed among individuals with complete blindness.

Circadian rhythm sleep–wake disorder, shift work type, is characterized by complaints of insomnia or excessive sleepiness that occurs in association with work shifts that overlap with all or a portion of conventional nighttime sleep periods. The disorder is also associated with a reduction in total sleep time.

Circadian rhythm sleep–wake disorder, jet lag type, is characterized by a temporary mismatch between the timing of the sleep and wake cycle generated by the endogenous circadian clock and that of the sleep and wake pattern required by travel across at least two time zones. Individuals complain of disturbed sleep, sleepiness and fatigue, somatic symptoms (e.g., gastrointestinal distress), or impaired daytime function. The severity and duration of symptoms is dependent on the number of time zones traveled, the ability to sleep while traveling, exposure to appropriate circadian times cues in the new environment, tolerance to circadian misalignment when awake during the biological night, and the direction of travel.

Differential Diagnosis

It is important to assess the pattern and normal variation of sleep throughout the individual's development so as not to confuse circadian rhythm sleep–wake disorders with irregular sleeping times that are not associated with distress or functional impairment. Insomnia disorders are important in the differential diagnosis. Some degree of delayed sleep–wake phase is normal for adolescents and young adults, and advanced sleep–wake phase is commonly observed among older adults without being associated with distress or functional impairment. Among children, advanced sleep–wake phase disorder can be confused with chronically insufficient sleep, and neurodevelopmental disorders should also be evaluated.

Developmental Course

Symptoms of delayed sleep–wake phase disorder generally begin in adolescence and early adulthood. Onset of circadian rhythm sleep–wake disorder, shift work type; advanced sleep–wake phase disorder; and irregular sleep–wake rhythm disorder is more common among adults, with increased incidence with increasing age. Recurrence of symptoms is common, although severity may decrease with age. Clinical expression may vary throughout life depending on social, educational, and professional obligations. These disorders often persist for years before a diagnosis is made.

Assessment

Assessment should include a careful history of sleep and sleep disorders to verify the misalignment of the major nocturnal sleep episode relative to the desired and socially established timing of sleep (Reid, 2019). A history of mental health and medical conditions is important as well as a developmental and social history, a sleep diary, and actigraphy of at least 1 week documenting the sleep timing complaint.

Prevalence

The prevalence of diagnosable delayed sleep–wake phase disorder is higher among adolescents and young adults, estimated at 7% to 16% (AASM, 2014). However, some degree of delayed sleep–wake phase is normal among this age group, so its occurrence alone does not necessarily indicate a disorder. It is estimated that approximately 10% of patients presenting to sleep clinics with recurrent complaints of insomnia have delayed sleep–wake phase disorder. There are few studies of advanced sleep–wake phase disorder, although available data suggest a prevalence of approximately 1% in adults between 40 and 64 years old. Again, it should be kept in mind that some degree of advanced sleep–wake phase is normal among this age group, although it is less likely to cause functional impairment. The prevalence of non-24-hour sleep–wake rhythm disorder is believed to be high among people with complete blindness but very low in individuals with sight (AASM, 2014). The prevalence of circadian rhythm sleep–wake disorder shift work type and jet lag type is not clear but would depend on the working and travel habits of the population. The prevalence of shift work disorder among rotating and night-shift workers has been estimated to be between 10% and 38%. Recent studies have estimated the prevalence of all sleep–wake disorders was 32.1% among night workers and 10.1% among day workers (AASM, 2014).

PARASOMNIA DISORDERS

Presentations and Symptom Patterns

Parasomnia disorders are characterized by abnormal behaviors, experiences, or physiological events that appear during the transition from wakefulness to sleep, while sleeping, or upon arousal from sleep. Problematic/unusual sleep-related complex movements, behaviors, emotions, perceptions, dreams, and/or autonomic nervous system activity are the core features of these disorders, affecting the patient, the bed partner, or both. On the basis of their characteristics and time of occurrence during the sleep cycle, parasomnias can be divided into three main subtypes: disorders of arousal from non-REM sleep, parasomnias related to REM sleep, and other parasomnias. A clinical diagnosis of these disorders requires symptoms to be of sufficient severity to cause significant distress or significant impairment in personal, family, social, educational, occupational, or other important areas of functioning or significant risk of injury to the individual or to others (e.g., thrashing or striking out in response to efforts to restrain the individual). Sleep disruption, anxiety, and fear of going to sleep can occur as consequences of parasomnia disorders and have an impact on the individual's functioning.

Disorders of Arousal From Non-REM Sleep

The *ICD-11* includes four disorders of arousal from non-REM sleep: confusional arousals, sleepwalking disorder, sleep terrors, and sleep-related eating disorder. These disorders are characterized by incomplete awakenings or arousals from deep non-REM sleep that generate episodes of mental confusion or confused behaviors while the patient is in bed (confusional arousals), complex behaviors out of bed or ambulation (sleepwalking disorder), intense terror with autonomic activation (sleep terrors), or involuntary excessive and dangerous eating or drinking (sleep-related eating disorder). Features of the episodes include absent or minimal responsiveness to others, limited cognitive functioning, and subsequent amnesia for the specific episode. Open eyes, talking, and shouting are commonly present.

Parasomnias Related to REM Sleep

Parasomnias related to REM sleep include REM sleep behavior disorder, recurrent isolated sleep paralysis, and nightmare disorder. REM sleep behavior disorder is characterized by repeated episodes of sleep-related vocalization or complex motor behaviors that typically represent enactment of dreams. Recurrent isolated sleep paralysis is characterized by recurrent inability to move the trunk and the limbs at sleep onset or upon awakening from sleep, with episodes typically lasting from a few seconds to a few minutes. In nightmare disorder, the individual experiences recurrent, vivid, and highly dysphoric dreams that generally occur during REM sleep and generally result in awakening with anxiety. Unlike confusional arousals or sleep terrors, individuals with nightmare disorder are rapidly oriented and alert upon awakening.

Other Parasomnias

Other parasomnias include hypnogogic exploding head syndrome, sleep-related hallucinations, parasomnia disorder due to a medical condition, and parasomnia disorder due to a medication or substance. Hypnogogic exploding head syndrome is characterized by episodic perception of a sudden, loud noise or sense of a violent explosion in the head that normally occurs during the wake-to-sleep transition, although it can also occur upon awakening. The episodes produce abrupt arousal and often a sense of fright. Sleep-related hallucinations arise at sleep onset or awakening from sleep. They are primarily visual but can also be auditory, tactile, or kinetic. Parasomnia disorder due to a medical condition and parasomnia disorder due to a medication or substance are characterized by abnormal sleep-related complex movements, behaviors, emotions, perceptions, dreams, or autonomic nervous system activity that is attributable to a neurological disorder or medical condition or to the effects of a medication or substance, respectively.

Differential Diagnosis

Disorders of arousal from non-REM sleep can be distinguished by their main occurrence in the first third or half of the sleep period, during which there is a predominance of non-REM sleep. In contrast, parasomnias related to REM sleep usually appear in the second half of the sleep period. Differential diagnoses of parasomnias should include other sleep-related disorders such as narcolepsy (where abnormal sensations or experiences usually occur during the day and are triggered by emotions) and sleep-related breathing disorders (in which autonomic nervous system activity occurs due to breathing cessations). The effects of alcohol or substance use, as well as nonpathological variants such as sleep talking, should also be considered when diagnosing parasomnias disorders.

Developmental Course

Disorders of arousal from non-REM sleep and parasomnias related to REM sleep most often appear at childhood, with no sex differences in onset or prevalence, and often resolve spontaneously by puberty (Bloomfield & Shatkin, 2009; Laberge et al., 2000; Mason & Pack, 2007). An exception is REM sleep behavior disorder, which usually appears in middle-aged men with a progressive and unremitting course (Iranzo et al., 2009) and has been associated with underlying neurological conditions, including Parkinson disease, multiple system atrophy, dementia with Lewy bodies, and stroke. The onset of other parasomnias such as hypnagogic exploding head syndrome and sleep-related hallucinations is most commonly during adulthood with a higher prevalence in women (Bjorvatn et al., 2010). Parasomnia disorders can be precipitated by sleep deprivation, distress or anxiety, environmental stimuli, or sleep-related breathing disorders.

Assessment

Assessment of parasomnia disorders is primarily by clinical interview, which should include an assessment of the impact of the symptoms on the individual's functioning in a broad range of areas, as well as the impact of the symptoms on others. PSG can support a more accurate differential diagnosis and is especially important for REM sleep behavior disorder (Malhotra & Avidan, 2012).

Prevalence

The prevalence of parasomnia disorders is highest among children and adults younger than 35 years old (AASM, 2014; Bjorvatn et al., 2010). Non-REM sleep arousal disorders are common in the general population (American Psychiatric Association, 2013). Episodes of sleepwalking and night terrors are frequent among children, with the prevalence of sleepwalking disorder and sleep terror disorder, marked by repeated episodes and significant distress, impairment, or injury, being much lower. Approximately 2% to 8% of the general population reports a current problem with nightmares, and this is higher among clinical populations. The prevalence of REM sleep behavior disorder is 0.38% to 0.5% in the general population. Estimates of the prevalence of sleep paralysis vary widely due to differences in the definition used, the age of the sampled population, and possibly cultural factors.

CO-OCCURRENCE OF SLEEP–WAKE DISORDERS AND MENTAL DISORDERS

There is evidence that the relationship between sleep–wake disorders and mental disorders is bidirectional and interactive (Van Dyk et al., 2016). Difficulty falling asleep or maintaining sleep, poor sleep quality, nightmares, and excessive daytime sleepiness are some of the major clinical symptoms of sleep disorders seen in people with major depression, generalized anxiety disorder, bipolar disorder, and posttraumatic stress disorder (PTSD). Available evidence suggests that approximately 90% of patients with a depressive disorder report sleep–wake symptoms, especially insomnia, 23% to 78% of patients with bipolar disorder report symptoms of hypersomnia during nonmanic phases of the disorder, and 60% to 70% of patients with generalized anxiety disorder and panic disorder report major problems with sleep (Papadimitriou & Linkowski, 2005). Trauma-related nightmares are among the most common symptoms reported by patients with PTSD. Sleep disturbance can have a negative impact on the course and treatment of mental disorders and increase the risk of relapse of depressive episodes, suicidal ideation, and development of mania in bipolar disorder or psychotic episodes in schizophrenia (Fang et al., 2019; Stewart et al., 2020). Disorders due to use of substances may also result from attempts to reduce sleep disturbance through the use of alcohol, medications (e.g., benzodiazepines), or other psychoactive substances.

GENDER-RELATED FEATURES

Chronic insomnia is more prevalent among women than men, with onset frequently associated with the birth of a child or menopause (Krishnan & Collop, 2006; Yoshioka et al., 2012). Despite the higher prevalence among older women, polysomnographic studies suggest that sleep continuity and slow-wave sleep are better preserved in older women than in older men. Short-term insomnia is also more prevalent in women and in older age groups. In contrast, the overall prevalence of hypersomnia disorders may be slightly higher in men. There are no known gender differences in circadian rhythm sleep–wake disorders. Gender differences related to parasomnias show that sleepwalking occurs more often in females during childhood and in males during adulthood. Eating during sleepwalking episodes is more common among women. Among children, sleep terrors are more common in boys than in girls; among adults, there is no difference in prevalence by gender (AASM, 2014). Adult women report nightmare disorder more often than men (AASM, 2014; Schredl, 2014).

KEY POINTS

- Due to the bidirectional relationship between sleep disturbances and mental health disorders, a psychological approach is an increasingly important element in assessment, diagnosis, and treatment. Changes in this grouping have been made to better reflect and support research and clinical practice to improve public health and patient health care.

- In the *ICD-11*, sleep–wake disorders have been incorporated into a single, integrated chapter. This innovation reflects the more accurate conceptualization of sleep disorders and is fully consistent with the *ICSD-3*.

- Sleep–wake disorders are characterized by difficulty initiating or maintaining sleep (insomnia disorders), excessive sleepiness (hypersomnolence disorders), respiratory disturbance during sleep (sleep-related breathing disorders), disorders of the sleep–wake schedule (circadian rhythm sleep–wake disorders), abnormal movements during sleep (sleep-related movement disorders), or problematic behavioral or physiological events that occur while falling asleep, during sleep, or upon arousal from sleep (parasomnia disorders).

- Sleep–wake disorder diagnoses are generally made based on information from clinical interviews involving self-reports of behavior and experience (such as attention and memory deficits or sleep disruptions), sometimes supported by standardized scales (e.g., the Athens Insomnia Scale, the Epworth Sleepiness Scale). Diagnostic physiological tests such as actigraphy, polysomnography, or multiple sleep latency tests are often useful and, in some cases, are required for accurate diagnosis.

- Difficulty falling asleep or maintaining sleep, poor sleep quality, nightmares, and excessive daytime sleepiness are some of the major clinical symptoms of sleep disorders seen in people with major depression, generalized anxiety disorder, bipolar disorder, and PTSD.

- In turn, sleep disturbance can have a negative impact on the course and treatment of mental disorders and increase the risk of relapse of depressive episodes, suicidal ideation, and development of mania in bipolar disorder or psychotic episodes in schizophrenia. Disorders due to use of substances may also result from attempts to self-medicate sleep disturbance.

REFERENCES

American Academy of Sleep Medicine. (2014). *International classification of sleep disorders* (3rd ed.).

American Psychiatric Association. (2013). *Diagnostic and statistical manual of mental disorders* (5th ed.).

Anderson, K. N., & Bradley, A. J. (2013). Sleep disturbance in mental health problems and neurodegenerative disease. *Nature and Science of Sleep, 5,* 61–75. https://doi.org/10.2147/NSS.S34842

Arnulf, I., Zeitzer, J. M., File, J., Farber, N., & Mignot, E. (2005). Kleine–Levin syndrome: A systematic review of 186 cases in the literature. *Brain: A Journal of Neurology, 128*(Pt. 12), 2763–2776. https://doi.org/10.1093/brain/awh620

Baldini, T., Loddo, G., Ferri, R., & Provini, F. (2021). Neurobiology of parasomnias. In L. M. DelRosso & R. Ferri, R. (Eds.), *Sleep neurology—A comprehensive guide to basic and clinical aspects* (pp. 121–145). Springer. https://doi.org/10.1007/978-3-030-54359-4_9

Bjorvatn, B., Grønli, J., & Pallesen, S. (2010). Prevalence of different parasomnias in the general population. *Sleep Medicine, 11*(10), 1031–1034. https://doi.org/10.1016/j.sleep.2010.07.011

Bloomfield, E. R., & Shatkin, J. P. (2009). Parasomnias and movement disorders in children and adolescents. *Child and Adolescent Psychiatric Clinics of North America, 18*(4), 947–965. https://doi.org/10.1016/j.chc.2009.04.010

Broughton, R. J. (2022). The parasomnias and sleep related movement disorders— A look back at six decades of scientific studies. *Clinical and Translational Neuroscience, 6*(1), Article 3. https://doi.org/10.3390/ctn6010003

Buysse, D. J. (2013). Insomnia. *JAMA, 309*(7), 706–716. https://doi.org/10.1001/jama.2013.193

Calhoun, S. L., Fernandez-Mendoza, J., Vgontzas, A. N., Liao, D., & Bixler, E. O. (2014). Prevalence of insomnia symptoms in a general population sample of young children and preadolescents: Gender effects. *Sleep Medicine, 15*(1), 91–95. https://doi.org/10.1016/j.sleep.2013.08.787

Daley, M., Morin, C. M., LeBlanc, M., Grégoire, J. P., & Savard, J. (2009). The economic burden of insomnia: Direct and indirect costs for individuals with insomnia syndrome, insomnia symptoms, and good sleepers. *Sleep, 32*(1), 55–64.

Dzierzewski, J. M., Sabet, S. M., Ghose, S. M., Perez, E., Soto, P., Ravyts, S. G., & Dautovich, N. D. (2021). Lifestyle factors and sleep health across the lifespan. *International Journal of Environmental Research and Public Health, 18*(12), 6626. https://doi.org/10.3390/ijerph18126626

Fang, H., Tu, S., Sheng, J., & Shao, A. (2019). Depression in sleep disturbance: A review on a bidirectional relationship, mechanisms and treatment. *Journal of Cellular and Molecular Medicine, 23*(4), 2324–2332. https://doi.org/10.1111/jcmm.14170

Garbarino, S., Lanteri, P., Durando, P., Magnavita, N., & Sannita, W. G. (2016). Co-morbidity, mortality, quality of life and the healthcare/welfare/social costs of disordered sleep: A rapid review. *International Journal of Environmental Research and Public Health, 13*(8), 831. https://doi.org/10.3390/ijerph13080831

Iranzo, A., Santamaria, J., & Tolosa, E. (2009). The clinical and pathophysiological relevance of REM sleep behavior disorder in neurodegenerative diseases. *Sleep Medicine Reviews, 13*(6), 385–401. https://doi.org/10.1016/j.smrv.2008.11.003

Johns, M. W. (1991). A new method for measuring daytime sleepiness: The Epworth Sleepiness Scale. *Sleep, 14*(6), 540–545. https://doi.org/10.1093/sleep/14.6.540

Khan, Z., & Trotti, L. M. (2015). Central disorders of hypersomnolence: Focus on the narcolepsies and idiopathic hypersomnia. *Chest, 148*(1), 262–273. https://doi.org/10.1378/chest.14-1304

Krishnan, V., & Collop, N. A. (2006). Gender differences in sleep disorders. *Current Opinion in Pulmonary Medicine, 12*(6), 383–389. https://doi.org/10.1097/01.mcp.0000245705.69440.6a

Laberge, L., Tremblay, R. E., Vitaro, F., & Montplaisir, J. (2000). Development of parasomnias from childhood to early adolescence. *Pediatrics, 106*(1, Pt. 1), 67–74. https://doi.org/10.1542/peds.106.1.67

Longstreth, W. T., Jr., Koepsell, T. D., Ton, T. G., Hendrickson, A. F., & van Belle, G. (2007). The epidemiology of narcolepsy. *Sleep, 30*(1), 13–26. https://doi.org/10.1093/sleep/30.1.13

Malhotra, R. K., & Avidan, A. Y. (2012). Parasomnias and their mimics. *Neurologic Clinics, 30*(4), 1067–1094. https://doi.org/10.1016/j.ncl.2012.08.016

Mason, T. B., II, & Pack, A. I. (2007). Pediatric parasomnias. *Sleep, 30*(2), 141–151. https://doi.org/10.1093/sleep/30.2.141

Medic, G., Wille, M., & Hemels, M. E. (2017). Short- and long-term health consequences of sleep disruption. *Nature and Science of Sleep, 9*, 151–161. https://doi.org/10.2147/NSS.S134864

Meltzer, L. J., Phillips, C., & Mindell, J. A. (2009). Clinical psychology training in sleep and sleep disorders. *Journal of Clinical Psychology, 65*(3), 305–318. https://doi.org/10.1002/jclp.20545

Moreira, G. A., & Pradella-Hallinan, M. (2017). Sleepiness in children: An update. *Sleep Medicine Clinics, 12*(3), 407–413. https://doi.org/10.1016/j.jsmc.2017.03.013

Morin, C. M., Bélanger, L., LeBlanc, M., Ivers, H., Savard, J., Espie, C. A., Mérette, C., Baillargeon, L., & Grégoire, J. P. (2009). The natural history of insomnia: A population-based 3-year longitudinal study. *Archives of Internal Medicine, 169*(5), 447–453. https://doi.org/10.1001/archinternmed.2008.610

Papadimitriou, G. N., & Linkowski, P. (2005). Sleep disturbance in anxiety disorders. *International Review of Psychiatry, 17*(4), 229–236. https://doi.org/10.1080/09540260500104524

Reid, K. J. (2019). Assessment of circadian rhythms. *Neurologic Clinics, 37*(3), 505–526. https://doi.org/10.1016/j.ncl.2019.05.001

Roth T. (2007). Insomnia: Definition, prevalence, etiology, and consequences. *Journal of Clinical Sleep Medicine, 3*(Suppl. 5), S7–S10.

Schredl, M. (2014). Explaining the gender difference in nightmare frequency. *The American Journal of Psychology, 127*(2), 205–213. https://doi.org/10.5406/amerjpsyc.127.2.0205

Schredl, M. (2021). Parasomnias. In B. A. Stuck, J. T. Maurer, A. A. Schlarb, M. Schredl, & H.-G. Weeß (Eds.), *Practice of sleep medicine: Sleep disorders in children and adults* (pp. 197–217). Springer. https://doi.org/10.1007/978-3-030-17412-5_7

Smith, M. T., McCrae, C. S., Cheung, J., Martin, J. L., Harrod, C. G., Heald, J. L., & Carden, K. A. (2018). Use of actigraphy for the evaluation of sleep disorders and circadian rhythm sleep–wake disorders: An American Academy of Sleep Medicine clinical practice guideline. *Journal of Clinical Sleep Medicine, 14*(7), 1231–1237. https://doi.org/10.5664/jcsm.7230

Soldatos, C. R., Dikeos, D. G., & Paparrigopoulos, T. J. (2000). Athens Insomnia Scale: Validation of an instrument based on *ICD-10* criteria. *Journal of Psychosomatic Research, 48*(6), 555–560. https://doi.org/10.1016/S0022-3999(00)00095-7

Stepanski, E. J., & Perlis, M. L. (2000). Behavioral sleep medicine: An emerging subspecialty in health psychology and sleep medicine. *Journal of Psychosomatic Research, 49*(5), 343–347. https://doi.org/10.1016/S0022-3999(00)00171-9

Stewart, E. M., Landry, S., Edwards, B. A., & Drummond, S. P. A. (2020). The bidirectional relationship between sleep and health. In K. Sweeny, M. L. Robbins, & L. M. Cohen (Eds.), *The Wiley encyclopedia of health psychology* (pp. 165–188). John Wiley & Sons. https://doi.org/10.1002/9781119057840.ch200

Sutcliffe, J. G., & de Lecea, L. (2000). The hypocretins: Excitatory neuromodulatory peptides for multiple homeostatic systems, including sleep and feeding. *Journal of Neuroscience Research, 62*(2), 161–168. https://doi.org/10.1002/1097-4547(20001015)62:2<161::AID-JNR1>3.0.CO;2-1

Van Dyk, T. R., Thompson, R. W., & Nelson, T. D. (2016). Daily bidirectional relation-ships between sleep and mental health symptoms in youth with emotional and behavioral problems. *Journal of Pediatric Psychology, 41*(9), 983–992. https://doi.org/10.1093/jpepsy/jsw040

World Health Organization. (1992). *The ICD-10 classification of mental and behavioural dis-orders: Clinical descriptions and diagnostic guidelines*. https://www.who.int/publications/i/item/9241544228

World Health Organization. (2023). *ICD-11 for mortality and morbidity statistics* (Version: 01/2023). https://icd.who.int/browse11/l-m/en#/

Yoshioka, E., Saijo, Y., Kita, T., Satoh, H., Kawaharada, M., Fukui, T., & Kishi, R. (2012). Gender differences in insomnia and the role of paid work and family responsibilities. *Social Psychiatry and Psychiatric Epidemiology, 47*(4), 651–662. https://doi.org/10.1007/s00127-011-0370-z

21

Relationship Problems and Maltreatment

Richard E. Heyman, Amy M. Smith Slep, and Claudia García-Moreno

OVERARCHING LOGIC

This chapter focuses on problems in intimate partner and caregiver–child relationships (i.e., relationship problems and maltreatment). A curious reader may
wonder why these problems are in the *International Classification of Diseases* (*ICD*)
or why they are included in this book focused on mental, behavioral, and neurodevelopmental disorders. To address these questions, this chapter (a) introduces
what health is and how it is affected by intimate and caregiving relationships;
(b) describes how and where the 11th revision of the *ICD* (*ICD-11*; World Health
Organization [WHO], 2023) covers relationship problems and maltreatment;
(c) provides a psychological orientation to these problems; (d) introduces their
assessment, clinical presentations, symptoms, and differential diagnoses; and
(e) discusses cultural and gender-related considerations. This chapter is intended
to supplement and extend the section on relationship problems and maltreatment included in the *Clinical Descriptions and Diagnostic Requirements for ICD-11
Mental, Behavioural and Neurodevelopmental Disorders* (*CDDR*; WHO, 2024).

The World Health Organization defines health as "a state of complete physical, mental and social well-being and not merely the absence of disease or
infirmity" (WHO, 2020, p. 1). Family relationships strongly influence individuals'
mental and physical health and well-being (e.g., Repetti et al., 2002; Robles
et al., 2014). Social well-being depends on the health of the pair-bonded units

https://doi.org/10.1037/0000392-021
A Psychological Approach to Diagnosis: Using the ICD-11 as a Framework, G. M. Reed,
P. L.-J. Ritchie, and A. Maercker (Editors)

individuals form, most notably those with parents (or other primary caregivers), intimate partners, and children (Flinn, 2011).

Given that health and disorder—for both individuals and couples/families—are on a continuum, classification systems such as the *ICD* that delineate disorder from health must grapple with (a) what constitutes healthy intimate and family relationships (and, conversely, what constitutes problems in these relationships) and (b) where to locate intimate and family relationships problems within the classification system. Decisions on both matters are challenging given that relationships are inherently *symbiotic* (i.e., a "close, prolonged association between two or more different organisms . . . that may, but does not necessarily, benefit each member"; American Heritage Dictionary, 2019), requiring consideration of both the health of each individual and the health of the relationship itself.

We define healthy intimate and family relationships as those that (a) safeguard members' physical integrity, (b) minimize their risk of preventable physical and mental disorders, and (c) promote their physical and mental well-being. Relationships that do not do so are of concern. Those that threaten physical integrity or increase risk for physical and mental disorders can be considered health problems in their own right (Foran et al., 2013). Next, we turn to the specifics of how the *ICD* classifies such problems.

CLASSIFICATION OF RELATIONSHIP PROBLEMS AND MALTREATMENT IN THE *ICD-11*

ICD-11 includes several ways of classifying problems and maltreatment in intimate and family relationships, depending on the context and the purpose of the assessment. One set of maltreatment codes, located in the chapter on external causes of morbidity or mortality, is used to indicate the cause of an individual's specific injury or death. It includes physical, sexual, and psychological maltreatment, and neglect. These categories refer to acts or omissions that have directly compromised physical integrity, caused or exacerbated mental problems, or degraded physical or mental well-being. These categories are used along with a classification of the associated physical injuries (e.g., fracture of nasal bones; burns of external body surface) or mental health consequences. The maltreatment codes in the chapter on external causes of morbidity or mortality can be further specified to indicate the perpetrator–victim relationship (e.g., spouse or partner, parent), the gender of the perpetrator, and the context of the maltreatment (e.g., altercation). These categories are used when the primary focus is on documenting the cause of death or injury or other presenting harm to physical or mental health.

Categories from the chapter on factors influencing health status or contact with health services are used when the focus is on recording one of three types of clinically important relationship phenomena. The first type of phenomenon covered in this chapter is a history of maltreatment that is being identified in its own right rather than in relation to a specific injury or other harm. Categories from the section on personal history of maltreatment are used to describe a current or past pattern of physical, sexual, or psychological abuse or neglect. The time in life when the maltreatment or neglect occurred can also be specified. A category for history of spouse or partner violence is also available. The second type is a pattern of clinically significant relationship conflict with an intimate partner, parent, or other caregiver. The categories from the section on problems associated with relationships—caregiver-child relationship problem and relationship distress with spouse or partner—are used to describe substantial and sustained dissatisfaction with intimate relationships associated with significant disturbance in functioning. Finally, the third type is a possible episode of maltreatment that is currently being evaluated. Categories from the section on examination or observation for suspected maltreatment—including physical, sexual, and psychological maltreatment as well as neglect or abandonment—are used when the focus is on a recent incident that is currently being assessed and/or adjudicated.

The *ICD-11 CDDR* provide consistent definitions of maltreatment and neglect across these different sets of codes (see WHO, 2023). All categories are applied to the victim of the maltreatment or neglect, not the perpetrator.

- Physical maltreatment or abuse is defined as "non-accidental acts of physical force that result, or have reasonable potential to result, in physical harm or that evoke significant fear." (Code PJ20 Physical maltreatment, Description section)

- Sexual maltreatment or abuse is defined in adults as "forced or coerced sexual acts or sexual acts with someone who is unable to consent" and in children as "sexual acts involving a child that are intended to provide sexual gratification to an adult." (Code PJ21 Sexual maltreatment, Description section)

- Psychological maltreatment or abuse is defined as "non-accidental verbal or symbolic acts that result in significant psychological harm." (Code PJ22 Psychological maltreatment, Description section)

- Neglect is defined as "egregious acts or omissions by a caregiver that deprive a child of needed age-appropriate care or an adult who is incapable of self-care and that result, or have reasonable potential to result, in physical or psychological harm." (Code QE82.3 Personal history of neglect, Description section)

As discussed in more detail later in the chapter, diagnostic requirements for each type of problem include a hallmark indicator (e.g., unhappiness with the relationship; physical, verbal/symbolic, or sexual acts) and signs of actual or potential harm.

A PSYCHOLOGICAL APPROACH TO RELATIONSHIP PROBLEMS AND MALTREATMENT

Intimate partner and caregiver–child bonds are among the most foundational to human health. All psychological theories—from attachment to behavioral to psychodynamic to neurobiological—recognize the biopsychosocial importance of these relationships. Thus, threats to these bonds, through acts or omissions, have vast impacts on physical, mental, and social well-being. Maltreatment involves actual or potential threats to an intimate partner's or child's physical or mental integrity. For physical and psychological forms, the acts are typically from a continuum of behaviors that partners or caregivers use to influence another's behavior. For example, nonaccidental physical force can range from a light spank on the child's bottom to the use of potentially lethal weapons; verbal or symbolic acts can range from a reprimand for a child's violating a rule to threats of serious bodily harm. For neglect, at issue is the failure to provide needed or expected care (e.g., food, shelter, safety). For sexual maltreatment between adults, the issue is whether the behavior involved is mutually consensual; for acts involving children, it is a caregiver introducing sexual behavior to a caregiver–child relationship.

Because these acts or omissions fall on a continuum from normative (e.g., physical contact, saying hostile things, failing to provide some needed care) to manifestly unhealthy (e.g., murder, caregiver–child sexual contact), establishing a line between potentially problematic behavior and maltreatment involves setting a standard that the act caused, or had a high potential to cause, injury or significant distress (i.e., a harm criterion). Thus, except in cases where the threat to bodily integrity is overt, unambiguous, and immediate (limited chiefly to sexual abuse and physical acts with injury), the standards for what constitutes maltreatment involve the violation of social expectations that intimate and caregiving relationships should not harm individuals' physical, mental, and social well-being.

Whereas maltreatment involves harm to an individual, problems associated with relationships involve threats to the relationship itself or the relationship's ability to function as needed. For most people, intimate partner or parental/caregiver bonds are the closest relationships they have; physical, mental, and social threats to these relationships present both acute and chronic challenges to health. However, because the threat to the relationship is via psychological processes—such as attributions, schema, and expectancies—the hallmark sign of relationship problems is at least one individual's negative perception of that relationship (e.g., feeling unhappy, desiring a severing of the relationship). Thus, relationship problem diagnoses are based on reporting or inferences of those within the relationship about its failure to provide a sense of physical, mental, or social well-being. Although maltreatment diagnoses sometimes similarly involve reporting or inferences of those involved, they frequently also involve a clinician, social service agent, or other outsider's inferences of the threat to an individual's well-being.

In summary, couples and families comprise individuals. Although they should promote health and growth, they can also pose important environmental risks to physical and psychological health. Professionals cannot appropriately diagnose those presenting for intimate partner or parent–child problems without also considering the individual physical and psychological problems that may be affecting their relationships; conversely, professionals cannot appropriately diagnose those presenting for individual problems without also considering whether intimate partner or parent–child problems may also be present and affecting health and problem presentations.

PRESENTATIONS AND SYMPTOM PATTERNS

Maltreatment

Symptoms related to recent maltreatment differ depending on whether the presenting problem is related to an act (abuse) or an omission (neglect). In the *ICD-11* CDDR, the essential features for physical and psychological maltreatment or neglect require impacts that meet or exceed the harm criterion. The diagnostic requirements for sexual maltreatment require only a qualifying act (that is, harm or potential for harm is presumed), due to the intensely personal violation involved and the distinct line drawn around any act of coercive, nonconsensual, or caregiver–child sexual contact (e.g., in the United Nations Convention on the Rights of the Child; United Nations, 1989). Past maltreatment can be a reason for seeking services, or it may exacerbate other physical or psychological problems.

Physical Maltreatment

As noted earlier, physical maltreatment refers to nonaccidental acts of physical force that result, or have reasonable potential to result, in physical harm or evoke significant fear. The behaviors most essential to screen for are pushing/shoving, scratching, slapping, throwing something that could hurt, punching, and biting (Heyman et al., 2021). The presence of any of these should be followed up with more detailed assessment, including assessing for more severe (but less common) behaviors such as burning or using weapons. Impacts comprise any physical injury (e.g., bruises, cuts, sprains, broken bones, loss of consciousness, pain that lasts at least four hours), reasonable potential for incurring a significant physical injury (e.g., a thrown hard object that barely misses the head, dangling a child over a balcony), or significant fear (e.g., fear of bodily harm accompanied by symptoms such as hypervigilance or sleep disturbance). Excluded are incidents in which the act was for physical protection of self (e.g., to ward off other's use of force) or others (e.g., prevent partner or child from attempting suicide).

Health care presentation for physical maltreatment is extremely variable, ranging from couple or parent–child interactional problems to some of the most prevalent individual adult or child psychological and behavioral problems. This is due to physical maltreatment's major effects on physical and psychological functioning, which often last for many years after the behavior occurred. For adult physical maltreatment, worldwide data from WHO indicate significantly elevated rates of psychological (including posttraumatic stress disorder [PTSD] and suicidal thoughts and attempts) and physical (e.g., overall poor health, pain, sleep problems) problems (Kessler et al., 2017; Potter et al., 2021). Likewise, childhood physical abuse increases the risk for PTSD (Kessler et al., 2017), depressive disorders, drug use, suicide attempts, risky sexual behavior, and sexually transmitted infections (Norman et al., 2012). This wide range of presenting problems in health care settings underscores the importance of screening for physical maltreatment to understand possible contributing factors.

Psychological Maltreatment

This refers to nonaccidental verbal or symbolic (e.g., harming a treasured object or pet) acts that result in significant psychological harm. Examples of qualifying acts are verbal hostility (e.g., berating, disparaging, degrading, humiliating), threats, harming people or things that the victim cares about, and controlling or isolating behaviors. Impacts comprise the following: significant fear; significant psychological harm or distress (e.g., causing or exacerbating psychological problems); somatic symptoms that interfere with normal functioning; and, in children, reasonable potential for disruption of physical, psychological, cognitive, or social development.

Of the various forms of maltreatment, psychological maltreatment requires the most inference from clinicians and other assessors about whether the behavior violates cultural norms enough to be considered an act of maltreatment. For example, in many cultures, adults have the right to come and go freely; in such societies, controlling such activity in adult partners could constitute a qualifying act. Caregivers of children, in contrast, are expected to oversee and set rules for the whereabouts of minors; similar controlling or isolating behaviors toward children would have to be far more restrictive to qualify as being an egregious violation of the children's rights (and thus a potential act).

Health care presentations for psychological maltreatment are similar to those discussed for physical maltreatment because the physical and psychological sequelae are comparable (e.g., Norman et al., 2012; Potter et al., 2021). Of note to mental health providers, the impact of for child psychological maltreatment on depression is markedly higher than the impact of physical maltreatment (Norman et al., 2012).

Sexual Maltreatment

In adults, sexual maltreatment refers to sexual acts that were forced, coerced, or with a partner who was unable to consent (e.g., asleep, incapacitated by drugs or alcohol). In children, sexual maltreatment refers to any sexual act involving a child that was intended to provide sexual gratification to an adult. This includes caregiver–child acts involving sexual contact and those involving noncontact exploitation (i.e., a caregiver getting a child to participate in acts for anyone's sexual gratification without direct sexual contact between child and caregiver, such as pornography, voyeurism, or prostitution).

Health care presentation can be for the acute physical or psychological sequelae of the maltreatment or for a wide array of child or adult problems. Sexual abuse is associated with significant increases in lifetime diagnoses of anxiety disorders, depressive disorders, eating disorders, PTSD, sleep–wake disorders, and suicide attempts (Chen et al., 2010). It is one of the strongest risk factors for PTSD (Kessler et al., 2017). Thus, although most individuals presenting for these problems will not be victims of sexual abuse, a disproportionate number will be.

Neglect

Neglect refers to egregious acts or omissions by a caregiver that deprive the child or dependent adult of needed age-appropriate care in health, nutrition, shelter, or safety (and, in children, education and emotional development). Examples include not supervising a 3-year-old (who then wanders into traffic) or failing to safeguard dangerous chemicals (resulting in serious burns). For acts or omissions to be potentially neglectful, they must not be merely inadvisable or deficient but must clearly fall below the lower bounds of caregiving norms for a community, demonstrating striking disregard for the dependent's well-being. This especially applies to lack of supervision (where norms vary widely) and exposure to physical hazards (where local expectations vary as to what exposure to environmental hazards or tools [e.g., weapons, sharp implements] is ordinary or exceptional). Furthermore, neglect should be distinguished from poverty; it should be considered only where reasonable resources are available to the caregiver but are not used. Neglect involves egregious oversights by a caregiver regarding health, nutrition, shelter, or safety (and, for children, education, and emotional development). Impacts on victims include causing or exacerbating any of the following: physical injury (or reasonable potential for injury), significant fear or psychological distress, or stress-related somatic symptoms. For child victims, the reasonable potential for significant disruption of physical, psychological, cognitive, or social development is also considered an impact.

Given the broad nature of caregiver acts/omissions involved in the various forms of child neglect (e.g., lack of supervision; exposure to physical hazards; failure to provide food, clothing, shelter, education, or medical care even when financially viable), health care presentations are varied. These can range from physicians noting children's failure to attain developmental milestones, to teachers or psychologists noting behavior problems, to community sentinels noting unusually advanced maturity and independence. Presentations such as diaper rash, chronic medical conditions, and repeated childhood injuries can also warrant further assessment for neglect. Furthermore, because childhood neglect increases the risk for depressive disorders, drug use, suicide attempts, and sexual problems (i.e., sexually transmitted infections and risky sexual behavior; Norman et al., 2012), current or historical child neglect may be a contributing factor to other clinical presentations.

Problems Associated With Relationships

The *ICD-11* includes separate diagnoses for intimate partner and caregiver-child relationship problems. These diagnoses are independent of maltreatment categories; relationships can be problematic with or without the presence of maltreatment (and vice versa). That is, most couples presenting for relationship distress will not meet criteria for partner maltreatment, and many individuals reporting maltreatment (especially during the early years of relationships) will not report relationship distress (e.g., Jose & O'Leary, 2009). The same is true for parent–child problems and maltreatment. Thus, although these diagnoses are related, they nevertheless can occur separately; conversely, relationship problem and maltreatment codes may be used together if the definitional requirements for each are met.

For adult relationships, relationship distress with spouse or partner involves substantial and sustained dissatisfaction with a spouse or intimate partner associated with significant disturbance in functioning (i.e., impact on behavior, cognition, affect, health, social interaction, or key life roles). This category is applicable to all intimate relationships, regardless of the sex, gender identification, or sexual orientation of the individuals in the relationship or other relationship characteristics (e.g., marriage, cohabitation, exclusivity).

Dissatisfaction is typically expressed via one or both partners' perceived pervasive unhappiness with the relationship (e.g., feeling dissatisfied more days than not for a month) or recurrent thoughts of ending the relationship. If only one partner is unhappy, it may still be appropriate to assign the diagnosis to both partners because the relationship comprises both parties. Disturbances in functioning can be across a range of domains: behavior (e.g., persistent and intense conflicts, pervasive withdrawal or neglect, lack of positive behaviors), cognition (e.g., widespread negative attributions of partner's intent); emotion (e.g., persistent and intense anger, contempt, sadness, or apathy), physical health (e.g., somatic symptoms), interpersonal interaction (e.g., social isolation, decreased involvement in social activities), or major life role activities (e.g., work, school, caregiving). The impacts related to or exacerbated by problems with an intimate partner may also be part of a constellation that meets the diagnostic requirements for one or more *ICD-11* mental disorders, in which case that diagnosis should also be assigned.

Caregiver-child relationship problem is described similarly: substantial and sustained dissatisfaction within a caregiver–child relationship associated with significant disturbance in functioning. This category is potentially applicable to all meaningful caregiver–child relationships, regardless of the biological relatedness of the caregiver and child or custodial caregiver status. The dissatisfaction can be on the part of either the caregiver or the child and should be prolonged (e.g., present on more days than not during the past month). Examples include an overarching sense of unhappiness with the relationship by either the caregiver or the child, a child's recurring thoughts of running away or fantasies of having another caregiver, or a caregiver's wish that the child were totally different or had not been born. Associated disturbance in functioning (in caregiver, child, or both) can be evidenced in myriad areas: behavior (e.g., persistent and intense conflicts; pervasive withdrawal or neglect; paucity of positive behaviors; caregiver's failure to socialize child through nonexistent or poorly enforced limits; caregiver's poor monitoring of child's activities or child's concealment of activities; caregiver's overinvolvement in child's activities; child's persistent rejection, denigration, and criticism of the parent without cause); cognition (e.g., caregiver's or child's pervasive negative attributions of other's intent);

emotion (e.g., persistent and intense anger, contempt, sadness, or apathy); or health (e.g., exacerbation of physical or psychological symptoms). As with intimate partner problems, the impacts of caregiver–child problems may also be part of a constellation that meets the diagnostic requirements for one or more *ICD-11* mental disorders, which should also be diagnosed.

DIFFERENTIAL DIAGNOSES

In the case of maltreatment, both a qualifying act and an impact must be present. An act that is impactful for one child might not be impactful for another: A father mocking a very resilient child who has many caring adults in her life might have little impact, whereas the same act toward a very vulnerable child with no other caring adults might be much more damaging. On the other hand, not all distress or even injury attributed to a caregiver or partner indicates maltreatment. Divorce often causes psychological distress among children but does not constitute maltreatment. Of course, caregiver–child or partner problems and conflicts that are not maltreatment may still meet the diagnostic requirements for a relationship problem diagnosis. Alternatively, intimate partner and caregiver–child relationships can be problematic without rising to the level of meeting the requirements for a relationship problem or maltreatment diagnosis.

Major mental health and medical problems can cause, be caused by, exacerbate, or be exacerbated by relationship problems or maltreatment; properly capturing both individual and relationship problem or maltreatment diagnoses allows for more appropriate intervention. For example, all forms of relationship problems and maltreatment are associated with a substantial risk for *ICD-11* mental and other medical disorders, including suicidal ideation and attempts (e.g., Norman et al., 2012; Potter et al. 2021). Maltreatment is associated with PTSD and complex PTSD (Kessler et al., 2017). Regarding health, relationship problems and maltreatment are one of the most common forms of chronic, unavoidable stress, with implications for immune functioning and a range of disease processes (Kiecolt-Glaser & Wilson, 2017; Repetti et al., 2002).

DEVELOPMENTAL COURSE OF PROBLEMS

Child maltreatment risk varies by the age of the child, with some studies showing risk for physical abuse higher among older children (e.g., Finkelhor et al., 2019) and others suggesting risk peaks when children reach age 6 (e.g., Slep et al., 2022). In high-income countries, the risk for partner maltreatment generally declines with age (O'Leary, 1999); WHO studies do not show such a decline in male-to-female partner maltreatment in low- and middle-income countries (WHO, 2021). (Of course, even if subpopulation-level risk decreases with age, the risk in a specific relationship may not decrease or could even escalate over time. In such relationships, it is the pattern of change over time that should be considered when evaluating likely future course.) Some developmental milestones also affect risk for partner maltreatment, such as the perinatal period, during which there is an elevated risk for interpersonal violence (Charles & Perreira, 2007) and a decrease in relationship satisfaction (e.g., Mitnick et al., 2009).

Although cross-sectional research previously implied that intimate partner relationship starts high, declines during child-raising years, and then recovers somewhat (e.g., S. A. Anderson et al., 1983), longitudinal research indicates that there are several trajectories, with two thirds showing stably high satisfaction and one third at risk to develop relationship distress with spouse or partner (e.g., J. R. Anderson et al., 2010). Finally, the developmental course of a caregiver-child relationship problem has not received research attention.

PREVALENCE

Extrapolating from WHO (2010) data, globally, approximately 15% of women (15 years of age or older) experience partner physical or sexual maltreatment meeting *ICD-11* criteria during their lifetimes. Worldwide estimates for men's victimization are not available. Finally, globally 38% of murders of women, and 6% of men, are by an intimate partner or former partner.

Global prevalences of *ICD-11* partner psychological maltreatment are not available; extrapolating from limited studies comparing *ICD-11* physical and psychological maltreatment, we estimate that more than one in three women, and one in four men, experience psychological maltreatment meeting *ICD-11* criteria during their lifetimes.

For childhood maltreatment, it is estimated that 23% of children are physically abused before they are 18 years old, 36% of children are emotionally abused, 18% of girls and 8% of boys are sexually abused, and 16% of children are neglected worldwide (WHO, 2014). Further, in high-income countries, neglect is by far the most prevalent form of maltreatment, and its prevalence may be considerably underestimated.

For partner and caregiver-child relationship problems, one representative national study in the United States found that an average of 32% of couples in the general population would likely meet the *ICD-11* diagnostic requirements for relationship problems (Beach & Whisman, 2013); no comparable studies for caregiver-child relationship problems have been conducted. Global prevalences are unknown.

ASSESSMENT

Given the prevalence of relationship problems and maltreatment and the aforementioned significant impacts on psychological and physical health, screening for these problems should be a regular component of psychological and physical health care. Positive screens should be followed up privately to assess whether the relationship problems or maltreatment meet diagnostic levels, to explore the connection between presenting symptoms and the presence or history of relationship problems or maltreatment, to provide emotional support, and to ensure safety (e.g., Liebschutz et al., 2008).

Screening and assessment tools for *ICD-11* relationship problems and maltreatment have been developed and tested. These include short screeners, full questionnaire assessments, and structured clinical interviews. For examples of each type of assessment, see Heyman et al., 2013 (partner maltreatment); Slep et al., 2013 (child maltreatment); Beach et al., 2013 (relationship distress with partner); and Wamboldt and Cordaro, 2013 (caregiver-child relationship problem).

Screening is vital because only a sliver of those with relationship problems or maltreatment will initiate a report to a health care professional about the problem, but will often report if explicitly asked (e.g., O'Leary et al., 1992). Given the high prevalence of lifetime experience of at least one of these problems, we recommend universal screening by those providing mental health, obstetrics/gynecology, and family practice services, among others.

Screening for intimate partner and parent–child relationship problems can be accomplished with a single item each asking about satisfaction with the relationship (e.g., "Please indicate the degree of happiness, all things considered, of your relationship"; Funk & Rogge, 2007). The various forms of maltreatment can be assessed efficiently (see Heyman et al., 2013; Slep et al., 2013). For example, male-to-female partner physical maltreatment can be optimally screened with four items (pushed or shoved, grabbed, punched or hit, bit) and female-to-male with six (pushed or shoved, punched or hit, bit, slapped, threw something that could hurt, scratched; Heyman et al., 2021) and child physical maltreatment with three (spanked, slapped, grabbed; Slep et al., 2013). Individuals screening positive can then be interviewed by a health care professional to ascertain whether the problem meets *ICD-11* diagnostic requirements (i.e., both acts and impacts) and how it relates to other presenting physical or mental health problems. Before screening for child maltreatment, providers should be aware of whether their jurisdiction mandates reporting and, if so, the applicable legal requirements and definitions. Although the screening items may not identify behaviors that warrant reporting, parents would need to be informed if there are reporting implications before being interviewed about acts and impacts.

Because impacts for relationship problems and maltreatment often involve significant degradation of physical health and of affective, behavioral, or cognitive psychological functioning, a comprehensive assessment for individuals presenting with physical or psychological problems would ideally include screening for relationship problems and maltreatment. In some contexts, clinicians have access to collateral information that goes beyond individual self-report (e.g., emergency department assessments, medical or dental x-rays, police reports, teacher reports); all sources available should be used in the evaluation. For example, a woman brought to the emergency department by the police following a documented intimate partner altercation may later deny to a mental health professional that acts of physical intimate partner maltreatment had occurred, even if they were documented by others contemporaneously. Given the contradictions and inconsistencies common to the inter- and intrareporter accounts of maltreatment, clinicians should weigh factors such as contemporaneousness, secondary gain from reporting or recantation, and trauma to infer which report appears most credible.

Given the considerably elevated risk posed by relationship problems and maltreatment, individuals presenting for suicidal ideation and depression, anxiety, and substance use disorders (Norman et al., 2012; Potter et al., 2021) and PTSD (Kessler et al., 2017) should be routinely screened for relationship problems and maltreatment. Furthermore, professional organizations have also recommended that health professionals screen all women of childbearing age for intimate partner maltreatment (Feltner et al., 2018).

Finally, as with all physical and mental health diagnoses, clinicians should assess whether the acts and impacts meet *ICD-11* diagnostic requirements and also factors such as severity, chronicity, and trajectory of the acts and impacts in creating treatment plans. Furthermore, assessments should be culturally sensitive, placing the family unit within the larger ecology of their community and subculture. For example, child physical maltreatment may be due to a parent's impulsive anger, their interpretation of religious mandates, or their desire to enforce rules intended to protect children from racist dangers. Treatment plans for each of these scenarios would have to be different to work with the family effectively.

CULTURAL CONSIDERATIONS AND GENDER ISSUES

Local social norms and values held by health care providers undoubtedly affect whether and how they approach relationship problems and maltreatment (e.g., Domínguez-Martínez et al., in press). Although people from various cultures worldwide may disagree on whether causing injury to an intimate partner or child is "wrong," *ICD-11*'s harm criterion provides a common standard from which to draw clear lines between abusive or neglectful acts on the one hand and nonabusive or nonneglectful acts on the other. The advantage of the *ICD-11* harm criterion is that it requires acts to be damaging (or have a reasonable potential to be damaging) for them to be considered maltreatment (and not just ill advised). The harm criterion is imperfect; when clear-cut harm is not present, it requires considerable inference from clinicians. However, field testing with standardized clinical vignettes indicated that mental health professionals across the globe appear to apply the *ICD-11* diagnostic requirements for relationship problems and maltreatment in relatively similar ways (Heyman et al., 2018).

Furthermore, cultural issues intersect with gender issues in the unequal status of women in many societies and the "normalization" of violence against them, particularly in the context of sexual or other intimate relationships. This contributes to partner maltreatment prevalence variability by regions worldwide and across income levels (WHO, 2021). Globally, the following gender-related factors are related to higher local levels of male-to-female partner violence: norms related to male authority over female behavior; norms justifying "wife beating"; the extent to which law and practice disadvantage women, compared with men, in access to land, property, and economic resources; and gender-related discrimination within families (Heise & Kotsadam, 2015).

Gender is also an important factor in child maltreatment. The prevalence of self-reported sexual abuse is higher for females, whereas physical abuse prevalence is higher for males (Moody et al., 2018). Prevalences of self-reported emotional abuse and neglect differed by gender in some regions and not in others (Moody et al., 2018). There is not a large enough body of research to make conclusions about caregiver gender as a risk factor (Stith et al., 2009).

Although creating a threshold between what is socially sanctioned and what is problematic is an inherently culture-based decision, there are similar difficulties in creating international standards in other areas with strong cultural influences, such as the rights of women and children. Yet countries around the world have agreed on the United Nations' Convention on the Rights of the Child (United Nations, 1989) and the Convention on the Elimination of all Forms of Discrimination Against Women (United Nations, 1979) that establish these types of standards. The more elaborated guidance in the *ICD-11* CDDR provides mental health professionals worldwide with an improved standard to use in coding abusive and neglectful acts and omissions. We hope that the *ICD-11* CDDR for relationship problems and maltreatment will contribute to the assessment of these powerful factors in health and mental health and to relevant data collection and statistics, policy development, and health care practices that support the WHO's 1946 objective of "the attainment by all peoples of the highest possible level of health" (as cited in WHO, 2020, p. 2).

KEY POINTS

- Relationship problem codes involve a threat to the well-being of an intimate relationship or caregiver–child relationship. Maltreatment categories comprise problems that threaten the health or well-being of an individual (maltreatment—comprising physical, sexual, and psychological maltreatment and neglect).

- Maltreatment codes in the section on external causes of morbidity or mortality are used to indicate (a) the cause of an individual's specific injury or death and (b) whether the individual is the perpetrator or victim. Maltreatment codes are also in the section on factors influencing health status or contact with health services to record a history of maltreatment; codes in this section are also available for spouse/partner and caregiver–child problems. Finally, *ICD-11* has codes to document the examination or observation for suspected maltreatment.

- The *ICD-11 CDDR*'s line between problematic behavior and maltreatment (the "harm criterion") requires that acts or omissions cause, or have a high potential to cause, substantial harm to health.

- Relationship problems and maltreatment are common, affecting close to half of individuals during their lifetimes.

- Relationship problems and maltreatment can cause, be caused by, exacerbate, or be exacerbated by, mental, behavioral, and neurodevelopmental disorders. Thus, appropriate treatment of both individual and relational depends on careful assessment of both types of problems.

- Because of the prevalence of and risk inherent in relationship problems and maltreatment, screening for these problems should be a regular component of psychological and physical health care. Positive screens should be followed up privately to assess whether the relationship problems and/or maltreatment meet diagnostic levels, to explore the connection between presenting symptoms and the presence or history of relationship problems and/or maltreatment, to provide emotional support, and to ensure safety.

- Relationship problems and maltreatment are best understood through a developmentally and culturally informed assessment aimed at understanding how the behaviors within the family unit fit within the larger ecology of their community and subculture. Furthermore, such assessments need to consider the intersection of gender and culture in partners, caregivers, and children in the behavioral, cognitive, and affective factors that influence (a) risk for perpetration and victimization and (b) the meaning attached to these problems.

REFERENCES

American Heritage Dictionary. (2019). *American Heritage dictionary of the English language* (5th ed.). Houghton Mifflin Harcourt Publishing Company.

Anderson, J. R., Van Ryzin, M. J., & Doherty, W. J. (2010). Developmental trajectories of marital happiness in continuously married individuals: A group-based modeling approach. *Journal of Family Psychology, 24*(5), 587–596. https://doi.org/10.1037/a0020928

Anderson, S. A., Russell, C. S., & Schumm, W. R. (1983). Perceived marital quality and family life cycle categories. *Journal of Marriage and the Family, 45*(1), 127–139. https://doi.org/10.2307/351301

Beach, S. R. H., & Whisman, M. A. (2013). Relationship distress: Impact on mental illness, physical health, children, and family economics. In H. M. Foran, S. R. H. Beach, A. M. S. Slep, R. E. Heyman, & M. Z. Wamboldt (Eds.), *Family problems and family violence: Reliable assessment and the* ICD-11 (pp. 91–100). Springer.

Beach, S. R. H., Whisman, M. A., Snyder, D. K., & Heyman, R. E. (2013). Practical tools for assessing marital or intimate partner relational problems in clinical practice and public health settings. In H. M. Foran, S. R. H. Beach, A. M. S. Slep, R. E. Heyman, & M. Z. Wamboldt (Eds.), *Family problems and family violence: Reliable assessment and the* ICD-11 (pp. 101–109). Springer.

Charles, P., & Perreira, K. M. (2007). Intimate partner violence during pregnancy and 1-year post-partum. *Journal of Family Violence, 22*(7), 609–619. https://doi.org/10.1007/s10896-007-9112-0

Chen, L. P., Murad, M. H., Paras, M. L., Colbenson, K. M., Sattler, A. L., Goranson, E. N., Elamin, M. B., Seime, R. J., Shinozaki, G., Prokop, L. J., & Zirakzadeh, A. (2010). Sexual abuse and lifetime diagnosis of psychiatric disorders: Systematic review and meta-analysis. *Mayo Clinic Proceedings, 85*(7), 618–629. https://doi.org/10.4065/mcp.2009.0583

Domínguez-Martínez, T., Arango de Montis, I., Robles García, R., García, J. A., Medina Mora, M. E., Burns, S. C., Kogan, C. S., Heyman, R. E., Foran, H. M., Slep, A. M. S., Keeley, J. W., & Reed, G. M. (in press). Clinicians' diagnostic accuracy of intimate partner relational problems and maltreatment: An international *ICD-11* field study. *Psychology of Violence*.

Feltner, C., Wallace, I., Berkman, N., Kistler, C. E., Middleton, J. C., Barclay, C., Higginbotham, L., Green, J. T., & Jonas, D. E. (2018). Screening for intimate partner violence, elder abuse, and abuse of vulnerable adults: Evidence report and systematic review for the US Preventive Services Task Force. *Journal of the American Medical Association*, *320*(16), 1688–1701. https://doi.org/10.1001/jama.2018.13212

Finkelhor, D., Turner, H., Wormuth, B. K., Vanderminden, J., & Hamby, S. (2019). Corporal punishment: Current rates from a national survey. *Journal of Child and Family Studies*, *28*(7), 1991–1997. https://doi.org/10.1007/s10826-019-01426-4

Flinn, M. (2011). Evolutionary anthropology of the human family. In T. Shackelford & C. Salmon (Eds.), *The Oxford handbook of evolutionary family psychology* (pp. 12–32). Oxford University Press. https://doi.org/10.1093/oxfordhb/9780195396690.013.0002

Foran, H. M., Beach, S. R. H., Slep, A. M. S., Heyman, R. E., & Wamboldt, M. Z. (Eds.). (2013). *Family problems and family violence: Reliable assessment and the* ICD-11. Springer.

Funk, J. L., & Rogge, R. D. (2007). Testing the ruler with item response theory: Increasing precision of measurement for relationship satisfaction with the Couples Satisfaction Index. *Journal of Family Psychology*, *21*(4), 572–583. https://doi.org/10.1037/0893-3200.21.4.572

Heise, L. L., & Kotsadam, A. (2015). Cross-national and multilevel correlates of partner violence: An analysis of data from population-based surveys. *The Lancet Global Health*, *3*(6), e332–e340. https://doi.org/10.1016/S2214-109X(15)00013-3

Heyman, R. E., Baucom, K. J. W., Xu, S., Slep, A. M. S., Snarr, J. D., Foran, H. M., Lorber, M. F., Wojda, A. K., & Linkh, D. J. (2021). High sensitivity and specificity screening for clinically significant intimate partner violence. *Journal of Family Psychology*, *35*(1), 80–91. https://doi.org/10.1037/fam0000781

Heyman, R. E., Kogan, C. S., Foran, H. M., Burns, S. C., Smith Slep, A.M., Wojda, A. K., Keeley, J. W., Rebello, T. J., & Reed, G. M. (2018). A case-controlled field study evaluating *ICD-11* proposals for relational problems and intimate partner violence. *International Journal of Clinical and Health Psychology*, *18*(2), 113–123. https://doi.org/10.1016/j.ijchp.2018.03.001

Heyman, R. E., Slep, A. M. S., Snarr, J. D., & Foran, H. M. (2013). Practical tools for assessing partner maltreatment in clinical practice and public health settings. In H. M. Foran, S. R. H. Beach, A. M. S. Slep, R. E. Heyman, & M. Z. Wamboldt (Eds.), *Family problems and family violence: Reliable assessment and the* ICD-11 (pp. 43–70). Springer.

Jose, A., & O'Leary, K. D. (2009). Prevalence of partner aggression in representative and clinic samples. In K. D. O'Leary & E. M. Woodin (Eds.), *Psychological and physical aggression in couples: Causes and interventions* (pp. 15–35). American Psychological Association. https://doi.org/10.1037/11880-001

Kessler, R. C., Aguilar-Gaxiola, S., Alonso, J., Benjet, C., Bromet, E. J., Cardoso, G., Degenhardt, L., de Girolamo, G., Dinolova, R. V., Ferry, F., Florescu, S., Gureje, O., Haro, J. M., Huang, Y., Karam, E. G., Kawakami, N., Lee, S., Lepine, J., Levinson, D., . . . Koenen, K. C. (2017). Trauma and PTSD in the WHO World Mental Health Surveys. *European Journal of Psychotraumatology*, *8*(Suppl. 5), Article 1353383. https://doi.org/10.1080/20008198.2017.1353383

Kiecolt-Glaser, J. K., & Wilson, S. J. (2017). Lovesick: How couples' relationships influence health. *Annual Review of Clinical Psychology*, *13*(1), 421–443. https://doi.org/10.1146/annurev-clinpsy-032816-045111

Liebschutz, J., Battaglia, T., Finley, E., & Averbuch, T. (2008). Disclosing intimate partner violence to health care clinicians—What a difference the setting makes: A qualitative study. *BMC Public Health*, *8*(1), 229–237. https://doi.org/10.1186/1471-2458-8-229

Mitnick, D. M., Heyman, R. E., & Smith Slep, A. M. (2009). Changes in relationship satisfaction across the transition to parenthood: A meta-analysis. *Journal of Family Psychology, 23*(6), 848–852. https://doi.org/10.1037/a0017004

Moody, G., Cannings-John, R., Hood, K., Kemp, A., & Robling, M. (2018). Establishing the international prevalence of self-reported child maltreatment: A systematic review by maltreatment type and gender. *BMC Public Health, 18*(1), 1164. https://doi.org/10.1186/s12889-018-6044-y

Norman, R. E., Byambaa, M., De, R., Butchart, A., Scott, J., & Vos, T. (2012). The long-term health consequences of child physical abuse, emotional abuse, and neglect: A systematic review and meta-analysis. *PLoS Medicine, 9*(11), Article e1001349. https://doi.org/10.1371/journal.pmed.1001349

O'Leary, K. D. (1999). Developmental and affective issues in assessing and treating partner aggression. *Clinical Psychology: Science and Practice, 6*(4), 400–414. https://doi.org/10.1093/clipsy.6.4.400

O'Leary, K. D., Vivian, D., & Malone, J. (1992). Assessment of physical aggression against women in marriage: The need for multimodal assessment. *Behavioral Assessment, 14*, 5–14.

Potter, L. C., Morris, R., Hegarty, K., García-Moreno, C., & Feder, G. (2021). Categories and health impacts of intimate partner violence in the World Health Organization multi-country study on women's health and domestic violence. *International Journal of Epidemiology, 50*(2), 652–662. https://doi.org/10.1093/ije/dyaa220

Repetti, R. L., Taylor, S. E., & Seeman, T. E. (2002). Risky families: Family social environments and the mental and physical health of offspring. *Psychological Bulletin, 128*(2), 330–366. https://doi.org/10.1037/0033-2909.128.2.330

Robles, T. F., Slatcher, R. B., Trombello, J. M., & McGinn, M. M. (2014). Marital quality and health: A meta-analytic review. *Psychological Bulletin, 140*(1), 140–187. https://doi.org/10.1037/a0031859

Slep, A. M. S., Heyman, R. E., Snarr, J. D., & Foran, H. M. (2013). Practical tools for assessing child maltreatment in clinical practice and public health settings. In H. M. Foran, S. R. H. Beach, A. M. S. Slep, R. E. Heyman, & M. Z. Wamboldt (Eds.), *Family problems and family violence: Reliable assessment and the* ICD-11 (pp. 159–183). Springer.

Slep, A. M. S., Rhoades, K. A., Lorber, M. F., & Heyman, R. E. (2022). Glimpsing the iceberg: Parent-child physical aggression and abuse. *Child Maltreatment*. Advance online publication. https://doi.org/10.1177/10775595221112921

Stith, S. M., Liu, T., Davies, L. C., Boykin, E. L., Alder, M. C., Harris, J. M., Som, A., McPherson, M., & Dees, J. E. M. E. G. (2009). Risk factors in child maltreatment: A meta-analytic review of the literature. *Aggression and Violent Behavior, 14*(1), 13–29. https://doi.org/10.1016/j.avb.2006.03.006

United Nations. (1979). *Convention on the elimination of all forms of discrimination against women*. https://www.un.org/womenwatch/daw/cedaw/cedaw.htm

United Nations. (1989). Convention on the rights of the child (Treaty no. 27531), *United Nations Treaty Series, 1577*, 3–178. https://treaties.un.org/doc/Treaties/1990/09/19900902%2003-14%20AM/Ch_IV_11p.pdf

Wamboldt, M. Z., & Cordaro, A. R. (2013). Practical tools for assessing marital or intimate partner relational problems in clinical practice and public health settings. In H. M. Foran, S. R. H. Beach, A. M. S. Slep, R. E. Heyman, & M. Z. Wamboldt (Eds.), *Family problems and family violence: Reliable assessment and the* ICD-11 (pp. 216–228). Springer.

World Health Organization. (2010). *Global and regional estimates of violence against women: Prevalence and health effects of intimate partner violence and non-partner sexual violence.* https://www.who.int/publications/i/item/9789241564625

World Health Organization. (2014). *Global status report on violence prevention 2014.* https://www.who.int/publications/i/item/9789241564793

World Health Organization. (2020). *Basic documents* (49th ed., amended effective May 31, 2019). https://apps.who.int/gb/bd/

World Health Organization. (2021). *Violence against women prevalence estimates, 2018.* https://www.who.int/publications/i/item/9789240022256

World Health Organization. (2023). *ICD-11 for mortality and morbidity statistics* (Version: 01/2023). https://icd.who.int/browse11/l-m/en#/

World Health Organization. (2024). *Clinical descriptions and diagnostic requirements for ICD-11 mental, behavioural and neurodevelopmental disorder*s. https://www.who.int/publications/i/item/9789240077263

INDEX

ABOUT THE EDITORS

Geoffrey M. Reed, PhD, is a professor of medical psychology and the director of the World Health Organization Collaborating Center for Capacity Building and Training in Global Mental Health, department of psychiatry, Columbia University Vagelos College of Physicians and Surgeons. He is also a consultant to the department of mental health and substance use, World Health Organization (WHO) and works closely with the National Institute of Psychiatry Ramón de la Fuente Muñiz, Mexico, where he was a founder of the Center for Global Mental Health Research. He is a level 3 member (highest level) of the National System of Researchers, National Council of Science and Technology, Mexico.

Professor Reed was based at WHO in Geneva between 2008 and 2016, where he was the senior project officer for the development of the classification of mental, behavioral, and neurodevelopmental disorders for the 11th revision of WHO's *International Classification of Diseases (ICD-11)*. A foundation of the revision process was a rigorous program of international field studies involving thousands of clinicians around the world and producing hundreds of research articles in leading scientific journals. The *ICD-11* was approved by the World Health Assembly in 2019 and came into effect around the world in 2022. Professor Reed was cochair of the 2021 American Psychological Association Presidential Task Force on Psychology and Health Equity. His numerous awards include the Robert L. Spitzer, MD Memorial Award for Outstanding Contributions to Nosology and Diagnosis, Department of Psychiatry, Columbia University Medical Center and the 2021 American Psychological Association Award for Outstanding Lifetime Contributions to Psychology.

Pierre L.-J. Ritchie, PhD, is a professor emeritus in the school of psychology at the University of Ottawa. He was previously responsible for clinical training in the school's PhD program in clinical psychology and also served as director of the Center for Psychological Research and Services. He served as the main representative for psychology to the World Health Organization from 1997 to 2016. In this role, he was closely involved in the inception and implementation of the plan for the revision of the classification of mental, behavioral, and neurodevelopmental disorders for the 11th revision of WHO's *International Classification of Diseases (ICD-11)*.

Professor Ritchie has extensive leadership experience in the governance and management of national and international organizations as well as in health policy. He served as CEO of the Canadian Psychological Association and as executive director of the Canadian Register of Health Service Psychologists as well as a member of the Council of Representatives of the American Psychological Association. He was the longest serving secretary-general of the International Union of Psychological Science (1996–2012). At the International Council for Science, he was a member of the Committee on Scientific Planning and Review where he contributed to the creation of its Science Plan and was instrumental in the establishment of the multidisciplinary Urban Health and Well-being Programme for which he was a member and chair of its Science Committee.

Andreas Maercker, PhD, MD, is a professor of psychopathology and clinical intervention at the University of Zurich, Switzerland, and codirector of the department's outpatient clinical services. He received his academic training in psychology and medicine in East Germany and, after the fall of the Berlin Wall, in reunified Germany. Professor Maercker is particularly well known in the field of national and international studies in traumatic stress research. He was president of the German-speaking Society for Traumatic Stress Studies and subsequently held leading positions in the European and International Societies for Traumatic Stress Studies. He has chaired various committees and sections on research ethics and clinical psychology in the German and Swiss Psychological Associations and the European Association of Clinical Psychology and Psychological Treatment, which he cofounded in 2017. His ongoing research interests include e-mental health interventions and cultural clinical psychology.

From 2011 to 2019, Professor Maercker chaired the WHO Working Group responsible for developing proposals for the revision of trauma- and stress-related disorders in the *ICD-11*. He is a lead member of the international committee responsible for translation of the *ICD-11* into German. He has been awarded the Swiss Prize for Anthropological and Humanistic Psychology and the Wolter de Loos Award for Distinguished Contribution to Psychotraumatology in Europe from the European Society for Traumatic Stress Studies.

Tahilia J. Rebello, PhD, is an assistant professor of clinical medical psychology and research, the program manager of the WHO Collaborating Center for Capacity

Building and Training in Global Mental Health, Department of Psychiatry, Columbia University Vagelos College of Physicians and Surgeons. She also served as a consultant to WHO's Department of Mental Health and Substance Use from 2013 to 2018.

For over a decade, Dr. Rebello managed the implementation of the systematic program of more than 20 multilingual internet-based field studies that tested and strengthened the reliability, clinical utility, and global applicability of the *ICD-11* classification of mental, behavioral, and neurodevelopmental disorders. Dr. Rebello also managed the expansion and engagement of WHO's Global Clinical Practice Network, now consisting of more than 18,000 mental health and primary care health professionals from 164 countries, which contributed to the *ICD-11* directly by participating in these studies. Dr. Rebello's other responsibilities included contributing to the development of the data collection infrastructure, protocols, and trainings, and managing their implementation for the clinic-based reliability and utility field studies, which were successfully conducted in 14 countries representing all global regions. She played a leadership role in the design and development of a comprehensive online training program for global clinicians aimed at facilitating the integration of *ICD-11* into clinical practice across the world (https://gmhacademy.dialogedu. com/icd11).